Atopic dermatitis

Atopic dermatitis or eczema is an increasingly common skin disease, but its distribution, frequency and underlying causes have not yet been systematically reviewed in depth: this is the very first book to look at the epidemiology of atopic dermatitis, its prevalence and possible causes. Uniquely, this volume draws on international experts from a wide range of disciplines, including dermatologists, epidemiologists, paediatricians and immunologists. Atopic dermatitis has much in common with other allergic diseases and this comprehensive account will shed new light on the causes and mechanisms that underlie the allergic response.

Whilst atopic eczema is primarily a disease of childhood, and therefore a common problem in paediatric practice, its prevalence in adulthood continues to pose a challenge to dermatologists and primary care physicians. This wide-ranging new publication will be an invaluable resource for all involved in the study or treatment of atopic dermatitis.

Hywel Williams trained in dermatology at King's College Hospital and St. John's Dermatology Centre (London) and then also in epidemiology at the London School of Hygiene and Tropical Medicine. He was appointed Foundation Professor in Dermato-Epidemiology at the University of Nottingham in 1998. He has had a lifelong passion for researching the distribution, causes and treatment of atopic dermatitis, perhaps because he is an eczema sufferer himself. He has published over 100 peer-reviewed articles and one textbook. Professor Williams also has a keen interest in promoting evidence-based dermatology and he is the Co-ordinating Editor of the Cochrane Skin Group.

Atopic dermatitis

The epidemiology, causes and prevention of atopic eczema

Edited by

Hywel C. Williams

Foundation Professor of Dermato-Epidemiology
University of Nottingham, Queen's Medical Centre,
Nottingham

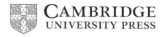

PUBLISHED BY THE PRESS SYNDICATE OF THE UNIVERSITY OF CAMBRIDGE
The Pitt Building, Trumpington Street, Cambridge, United Kingdom

CAMBRIDGE UNIVERSITY PRESS
The Edinburgh Building, Cambridge CB2 2RU, UK   http://www.cup.cam.ac.uk
40 West 20th Street, New York, NY 10011–4211, USA   http://www.cup.org
10 Stamford Road, Oakleigh, Melbourne 3166, Australia
Ruiz de Alarcon 13, 28014 Madrid, Spain

First published 2000

Printed in the United Kingdom at the University Press, Cambridge

Typeface Utopia 8½/12. System QuarkXPress® [SE]

A catalogue record for this book is available from the British Library

Library of Congress Cataloguing in Publication data

The epidemiology of atopic dermatitis / edited by Hywel C. Williams.
    p.   cm.
ISBN 0 521 57075 1
1. Atopic dermatitis – Epidemiology.   I. Williams, Hywel C.
RL243.E65   2000
614.5′9521–dc21   99–31355   CIP

0 521 57075 1 hardback

To Molly and Siân,
for their patience, understanding
and support

Contents

Contributors

Clive Archer
Department of Dermatology, University of Bristol, Bristol Royal Infirmary (UBHT), Bristol, BS2 8HW, UK

Carol Burrell-Morris
Department of Dermatology, University of West Indies, PO Box 504, Mandville, Jamaica, West Indies

Pieter-Jan Coenraads
Centre for Eczema and Occupational Dermatoses, Academisch, Ziekenhuis, Groningen, Hanzeplein 1, Postbus 30.001, 9700RB, Groningen, The Netherlands

Tim J. David
Professor of Child Health and Paediatrics, University of Manchester, Booth Hall Children's Hospital, Blackley, Manchester, M9 7AA, UK

Michael J. Day
Department of Pathology and Microbiology, University of Bristol, Langford, Bristol, BS18 7DU, UK

Thomas L. Diepgen
Biostatistics and Epidemiology Section of the Dermatology Department, University of Erlangen, Friedrich-Alexander University, Erlangen-Neurenberg, Germany
current address: Department of Dermatology, Heidelberg, Germany

Carol I. Ewing
Consultant Paediatrician, University of Manchester, Booth Hall Children's Hospital, Blackley, Manchester, M9 7AA, UK

Keith Godfrey
MRC Environmental Epidemiology Unit, University of Southampton, Southampton General Hospital, Southampton, SO16 6YD, UK

Robert M. Herd
Department of Dermatology, Western Infirmary, 56 Dumbarton Road, Glasgow, G11 6NT, UK

Harriett Kolmer
Asthma and Allergic Disease Center, University of Virginia Medical School, Box 225, Charlottesville, VA 22908, USA

Finn Schultz Larsen
Dermatology Clinic, Dronningensgade 72, DK-7000, Fredericia, Denmark

Adrian Mar
Department of Medicine (Dermatology), St Vincent's Hospital, Melbourne, Fitzroy, Victoria 3065, Australia

Robin Marks
Department of Medicine (Dermatology), St Vincent's Hospital, Melbourne, Fitzroy, Victoria 3065, Australia

Nicholas McNally
Department of Public Health, Kensington & Chelsea and Westminster Health Authority, 50 Eastbourne Terrace, London, W2 6LX, UK

Anne Braae Olesen
Department of Dermatology, University of Åarhus, Marseillesborg Hospital, DK-8000, Åarhus C, Denmark

Leena Patel
Senior Lecturer in Child Health, University of Manchester, Booth Hall Children's Hospital, Blackley, Manchester, M9 7AA, UK

David Phillips
Director, Asia-Pacific Institute of Ageing Studies, Faculty of Social Sciences, Lingnan College, Tuenmun, Hong Kong

Thomas A.E. Platts-Mills
Asthma and Allergic Disease Center, University of Virginia Medical School, Box 225, Charlottesville, VA 22908, USA

Johannes Ring
Director of the Department of Dermatology and Allergy, Biedersteiner Str. 29, Munich, Germany

Torsten Schäfer
Department of Dermatology and Allergy, Munich Technical University, Biedersteiner Str. 29, Munich, Germany

Susan E. Shaw
Department of Clinical Veterinary Science, University of Bristol, Langford, Bristol, BS18 7DU, UK

R.H.J. Stanton
Head of Service, Department of Nutrition and Dietetics, Booth Hall Children's Hospital, Blackley, Manchester, M9 7AA, UK

David P. Strachan
Professor in Epidemiology, Department of Public Health Sciences, St George's Hospital Medical School, Cranmer Terrace, London, SW17 0RE, UK

Kristian Thestrup-Pedersen
Department of Dermatology, University of Åarhus, Marseillesborg Hospital, DK-8000, Åarhus C, Denmark

Hywel C. Williams
Department of Dermatology, Queen's Medical Centre, University Hospital, Nottingham, NG7 2UH, UK

Brunello Wüthrich
Allergy Unit, Department of Dermatology, University Hospital, Zurich, Switzerland

Foreword

Due to its clinical importance atopic dermatitis is the subject of several dermatological books reflecting our present knowledge. In the opinion of the Editor of this book, Professor Hywel C. Williams, it is necessary, however, to emphasize the epidemiological aspects which constitute the starting point of our understanding of this multi-aetiological and still problematic skin disease. Thus, a framework has been provided in this work within which the basic genetic and environmental factors, in addition to clinical features and natural history, are discussed by well known experts.

Immunological and allergic mechanisms are not the only cornerstone of this condition – another being the impaired, characteristically dry skin. In this volume immunoregulatory dysfunction and inhalent allergens, as well as dietary factors, are reviewed and the possible protective effect of early infections is suggested. Of other causative factors the maternal influences and environmental pollution are also emphasized.

A certain shift in our concept of the disease has occurred. We have to shed more light on the global aspects of atopic dermatitis including migrant populations and geographical epidemiology. We must also consider more thoroughly the socioeconomic perspectives, occupational relationships and disease prevention.

In order to attempt to clarify the problems, we have to redefine some earlier conclusions such as the clearing rate of atopic dermatitis, and consequently be aware that not only children but many adults are still affected by the disease.

The final chapter is devoted to the perspectives of future research. I agree with the Editor who hopes that more discoveries will appear in the epidemiology of this condition where the interest, compared with other disciplines, has so far been relatively low.

This will, as an ultimate goal, hopefully provide better help for our atopic dermatitis patients.

Georg Rajka
Oslo, October 1999

Preface

Why a book devoted to the epidemiology of atopic dermatitis?

The title of this book may seem a little esoteric at first glance. But stop for a moment and consider the importance of atopic dermatitis and the need for its epidemiology to be studied.

Atopic dermatitis now affects around 5 to 20% of children worldwide and, like asthma, its prevalence has probably increased two- to threefold over the last 30 years. Recent studies suggest that it is not just a problem confined to northern temperate areas, and that rapidly developing cities throughout the world are witnessing an epidemic of cases. As well as the personal cost to sufferers and their families in terms of itching leading to sleep loss, disfigured skin and secondary infections, recent economic studies have suggested that the financial costs of atopic dermatitis to families and the State are comparable to those of asthma. Unlike asthma, atopic dermatitis is rarely life threatening, yet it is the product of the moderate morbidity multiplied by the high prevalence of this chronic disease which results in an enormous burden of disease in public health terms worldwide.

The last 30 years has witnessed a boom of research into the cellular and molecular mechanism of atopic dermatitis and there have been some interesting breakthroughs. But how has this helped a practitioner like me to help my patients?

Apart from a few drug treatments, which at best partly modify the disease symptoms, the answer is 'not very much'. We still do not know the genetic basis for atopic dermatitis and we do not know what makes it appear for the first time and whether genetic predisposition is a prerequisite for disease expression. We do not know for certain which factors cause flare-ups of established cases, and we do not know why some children clear and others do not. We do not know why only some children go on to develop asthma, or whether the long-term natural history of atopic dermatitis can be modified by any intervention.

Only epidemiology offers the methodological framework to answer these questions, yet it is only during the last five years or so that research into the epidemiology of atopic dermatitis has started in earnest. Thanks to such studies, we now know a lot more about the prevalence, morbidity and cost of atopic dermatitis so that funding bodies are now more likely to take notice of requests for research support. There have been some significant advances in methodological issues such as disease definition, and it will not be long before several genes which play a part in disease predisposition will be discovered. Migrant studies, geographical studies, links with social class and family size all indicate that the environment may be crucial for disease expression. This is good news for atopic dermatitis sufferers because if we discover specific environmental risk factors, such as hard water, which can be directly manipulated, this brings us one step nearer to our dream of disease prevention. Prevention is so much more logical than treating sick individuals, who present to us after a long chain of pathological events, with potentially toxic drugs which at best only ameliorate symptoms.

This book summarizes what is currently known about the epidemiology of atopic dermatitis and is intended for dermatologists, paediatricians, epidemiologists, public health physicians, immunologists, allergy specialists, medical geographers, sociologists, geneticists, primary care practitioners, patients and their representatives, and anyone with an interest in finding out more about the causes and distribution of this common yet enigmatic disease. A multidisciplinary approach is necessary to understand the problem of atopic dermatitis, and this is reflected in the wide range of backgrounds represented by the chapter contributors. The book takes the reader on a journey through the hierarchy of epidemiological studies, starting with descriptive studies of disease definition and disease burden, progressing to analytical studies which point to possible causes. The book goes on to deal with intervention studies and then draws on some useful lessons from related fields of research such as asthma and allergic diseases in small animals. The book concludes with a summary of where we are in terms of current research and what needs to be done in the future to address the current gaps in knowledge.

It is time that atopic dermatitis lost its image as the poor third cousin of allergic disease epidemiology. That time is now.

Hywel Williams

Acknowledgments

I would like to thank the following people and organizations for their help with this book: Dr John English, Dr Roger Allen and Dr Carolyn Charman (Nottingham) for their help with proof reading the chapters and for making helpful comments; the British Skin Foundation and the Wellcome Trust for funding many of the Editor's research projects which have contributed to this book; and the Economic and Social Research Council Data Archive and the National Child Development Study User Support Group for making data available for Chapters 3, 5, 10 and 17.

PART I

The nature of the problem

What is atopic dermatitis and how should it be defined in epidemiological studies?

Hywel C. Williams

Developing reliable diagnostic criteria may be as tedious as filling in muddy holes with concrete but both provide the foundation on which all else depends (Professor R.E. Kendell, 1975)

What is atopic dermatitis?

A distinct 'entity' or a continuum?

A particular problem hindering understanding of disease classification in dermatology today is 'binary thought disorder'. Binary thought disorder is a state whereby individuals are unable to appreciate that most biological phenomena do not fit neatly into all-or-nothing 'either/or' categories. Ever since Pickering shook the medical world by daring to suggest that essential hypertension, a major cause of death, was a graded characteristic which shaded insensibly into normality (Oldham et al., 1960), many physicians still have difficulties in viewing diseases as a quantitative or multidimensional process. Yet in a population setting, even with diseases like hepatitis, which might at first appear to conform well to a dichotomous disease definition, one sees a gradation of sickness ranging from those who are apparently healthy (many of whom will have subclinical infection), those who have mild gastrointestinal symptoms (some of whom are not infected), some who are moderately ill and some who are moribund or dead. Similarly, in atopic dermatitis (AD) one sees some children with normal skin (but with high IgE and positive skin prick tests to allergens), children with mucosal atopy and dry skin only, some with one episode of itching and erythema in just one

flexure, and others with classical persistent flexural disease. Perhaps the most appropriate question therefore is not to ask 'has he/she got atopic dermatitis, yes/no?' but rather 'how *much* atopic dermatitis does he/she have?' (Barker & Rose, 1979).

It is still not clear whether 'degree of atopic dermatitis' (if it can truly be expressed on a quantitative scale) is normally distributed in populations, or whether a bimodal distribution exists, the trough of which indicates a point of rarity or cut-off between 'disease' and 'normality'. Particular care has to be given to small population studies which claim disease bi- or trimodality, as artefactual peaks and troughs can easily be produced by chance or by manipulating the way in which individual features are scored. Two population-based studies in Germany (Figure 1.1) using an AD 'score' (Diepgen & Fartasch, 1992) suggest that 'degree of AD' could well be part of an underlying Gaussian distribution (Diepgen, T., personal written communication, 1998). It is possible that genetic factors, such as IgE hyper-responsiveness, and environmental triggers, such as high concentrations of house dust mite, shift the whole distribution of individuals to the right (Figure 1.2a), thereby increasing the proportion of individuals within the threshold whereby AD becomes manifest. The corollary of such a theory is that *any* individual could develop the clinical syndrome of 'AD' under the right circumstances, and that there is no ceiling to the prevalence of AD that could be theoretically achieved under appropriate adverse conditions.

Another viewpoint is that there exists in any one

(*a*)

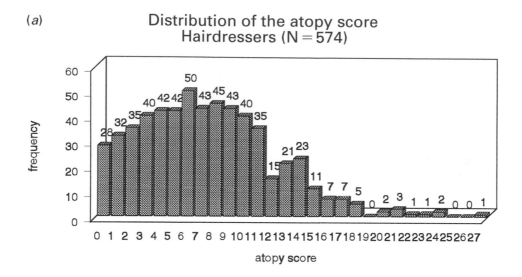

(*b*)

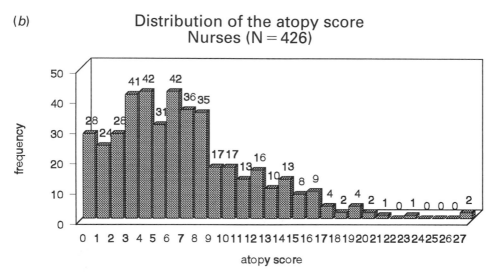

Fig. 1.1. Distribution of score of atopic skin diathesis amongst an unselected population of 574 hairdressers in Germany (Diepgen, T., written communication, 1998). A similar distribution is seen for 426 junior nurses

population a finite proportion of people who are genetically predisposed to AD, with additional perinatal or environmental factors determining the proportion of such people who will express disease at any one given time (Figure 1.2b). This concept could be one possible explanation of why the prevalence of AD has appeared to remain stable at around 20% in Japanese cities over the last 20 years (Sugiura et al., 1997), whereas it has increased two- to threefold at levels below 20% in Northern Europe (Williams, 1992). In other words, Japan has already witnessed its maximum prevalence in AD due to exposures correlated with rapid industrial and social development ahead of Western cultures, so that a 'state of saturation' has now been reached whereby nearly all predisposed subjects express disease. Such a notion would appear to fit well with the idea that a genetic

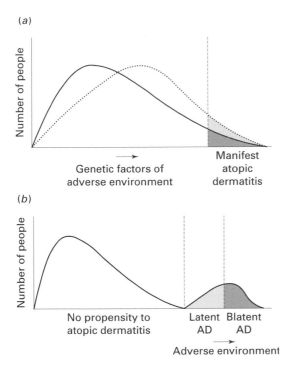

(a)

Number of people

Genetic factors of
adverse environment

Manifest
atopic
dermatitis

(b)

Number of people

No propensity to
atopic dermatitis

Latent   Blatent
AD   AD

Adverse environment

Fig. 1.2. (a) and (b) Is 'degree of atopic dermatitis' a continuum
that is normally distributed in populations, with factors that
enhance predisposition (genes) or precipitancy (allergenic
environment) shifting the whole distribution to the right
(Figure 2a)? Or are AD scores distributed bimodally, with only
a fixed proportion of the population capable of expressing a
manifest disease (Figure 2b)?

about individuals. Thus, whilst a log odds score of
AD of 3.27 might mean something to a researcher
trying to predict the degree to which a hairdressing
apprentice is likely to develop irritant hand dermatitis (Fartasch & Diepgen, 1994), such a score would
have little meaning to the thousands of doctors in
primary care who wish to describe the disease
pattern in their population. Comparing mean AD
scores between populations may be an interesting
academic exercise, but its biological significance
may be obscure. Another danger of quantitative
scales is that they are open to statistical abuse on the
erroneous assumption that such scales behave like
other continuous variables such as height and
weight. It is a natural reflex for workers to attempt
mathematical manipulations when faced with a
scale of numbers. Whereas it is true that a person
who weighs 100 kg is twice as heavy as a person
weighing 50 kg, it may not be assumed that a person
with an AD score of 6 has twice the amount of AD as
someone with a score of 3. In addition, the weights
applied to individual disease features derived from
regression models are highly dependent upon the
population who were selected to derive the criteria
(Wells, Feinstein & Walter, 1990), and ten different
studies could produce ten different sets of criteria,
each with different weighting, leading to international disputes on which weighting was 'correct'
(Kendell, 1975).

Dichotomous or categorical disease definitions,
on the other hand, require a line to be drawn
between disease and nondisease. Even the word
'diagnosis', which is derived from the Greek words
$\delta\iota\acute{\alpha}$ (the number two), and $\gamma\iota\gamma\nu\acute{\omega}\sigma\kappa\epsilon\iota\nu$ (to per-
ceive), implies a dichotomous outcome. Such
dichotomous definitions are far more widely used
and easily understood in public health settings, and
are therefore logical choices for promoting international communication. Their main drawback is that
the imposition of boundaries between those who are
sick and those who are apparently healthy, *almost
always results in the misclassification of some subjects*. Unless the disease in question has an abrupt
natural cut-off between normal and abnormal, the
imposition of an arbitrary dividing line will always

factor such as atopy or IgE responsiveness is that
necessary predisposing influence but, as is discussed later, IgE responsiveness is neither necessary
nor sufficient to diagnose AD. Until the genetic basis
for AD and its subtypes becomes clearer, it would be
wise not to make any assumptions on where normality ends and AD begins.

Measuring the total amount of disease in a population on a quantitative scale may sound attractive
in that it provides us with information on all of the
individuals in that population, but it also presents
some serious difficulties for epidemiologists. There
is a need to return to our main purpose of disease
definition, i.e. to assist in the comparison of groups
of people and to increase our predictive abilities

be subject to a trade off between sensitivity (proportion of true positives correctly identified by the test criteria) and specificity (proportion of genuine 'noncases' correctly identified) (Sackett et al., 1991). Thus, very sensitive symptoms such as 'itchy skin' might include all subjects with AD, but it would also be highly nonspecific, including subjects with other pruritic skin diseases such as lichen planus or tinea pedis (Williams et al., 1994a). By contrast, very specific signs such as infra-auricular fissure (Tada et al., 1994), might exclude all other skin diseases in a population survey, but it would also exclude most cases of AD as the sign is encountered so infrequently in a population setting where mild cases predominate (Williams et al., 1994a).

Exclusion of those who have extremely mild or asymptomatic disease may be desirable in public health surveys, but it must be realized that drawing the line between disease and nondisease has to be an arbitrary process. Various techniques such as receiver–operator curves (Freiman et al., 1978) may be used to assist in deciding the optimal cut-off between sensitivity and specificity for continuous data, but these techniques need to be evaluated in the clinical context of the question being addressed, and not as a means of abrogating responsibility for decision making. As is seen later in this chapter, sometimes very specific criteria are needed at the expense of sensitivity, and using a cut-off derived from a receiver–operator curve may be inappropriate for this purpose. Despite its limitations, it is felt that a binary definition for AD would be far more readily understood and used by clinicians and epidemiologists throughout the world (Kendell, 1975).

More than one disease?

Some have suggested that more than one type of atopic dermatitis exists (Imayama et al., 1992; Wüthrich & Schudel, 1983). There are clinicians who, having observed individuals in a hospital setting, have favoured a division of AD into those with 'pure' AD limited to childhood and those with more chronic disease associated with respiratory atopy (Roth, 1987). Great care has to be taken in making inferences about such disease associations from hospital studies since disease co-occurrence and disease severity are positively associated with hospital referral. This selection bias can result in all sorts of misleading inferences (Gerber et al., 1982). Others have suggested an intrinsic and extrinsic form of AD based on the presence or absence of reactivity to allergens (Wüthrich & Schudel, 1983). Such a division may be practical when advising individual patients, but its validity is limited by our incomplete knowledge of which allergens to test for, which type of test one should use (e.g. skin prick test, aeroallergen patch test, oral challenge, or combinations of these), the relevance of such skin test results to clinical disease (David, 1991), and because allergen reactivity can fluctuate over time. In adults, further confusion may arise from irritant or allergic contact dermatitis mimicking or exacerbating AD.

Some workers have taken things much further by suggesting that there may be at least four different subtypes of AD based on different combinations of skin prick and aeroallergen testing (Imayama et al., 1992). Inevitably, the number of apparent subcategories of disease will increase according to the number of tests and cross-tabulations performed. For example, even in normal individuals, the probability of getting an abnormal serum biochemistry blood test result at the 5% significance level is 0.64 when 20 tests are performed. Data-driven post hoc subdivisions for AD are therefore only useful if they are subsequently shown to increase our predictive ability such as prognosis or responsiveness to treatment. No such studies have been performed to date.

An important consideration in relation to the subgroup issue in AD is the extent to which failure in recognizing subgroups can obscure important epidemiological disease associations. One indirect response to such a question might be that if misclassification was gross, important epidemiological disease associations would have been obscured. This has certainly not been the case to date for studies which have considered the clinical syndrome of AD (Williams, 1997a). Whilst it is true that perfect classification might have increased the magnitude of such associations, the fact that so many relatively weak associations have been consistently shown for AD as it is currently classified, argues against major misclassification, at least in studies of children. The key question for researchers investigating AD in populations is not 'how can I be sure that all individual cases in my study have a homogeneous disease?' but 'is what is defined as atopic dermatitis in this study measuring a concept that is *useful* for health care workers?'

Is atopic dermatitis atopic?

The concept of 'atopy' has troubled many scientists since Coca and Cooke introduced the term in 1923 as meaning 'strange disease' (Coca & Cooke, 1923). Strange disease it certainly is, for whilst many physicians are content with the notion that 'atopy' represents a familial hypersensitivity of skin and mucous membranes against environmental substances associated with increased IgE production, the quest for consistent clinical, immunological or genetic markers that encompass all individuals fitting the above clinical picture has been fruitless. Some define atopy as the development of IgE antibody in response to antigen exposure (Turner, 1987), although individuals who make large amounts of IgE are not all atopic, e.g. those infected with parasites and, conversely, 20 to 50% of individuals with typical clinical AD exhibit normal values of total or specific IgE (Dotterud et al., 1995; Edenharter et al., 1998). It is also unclear whether the immediate hypersensitivity reactions encountered are relevant to the atopic dermatitis as concurrent mucosal allergy is often also present. Some have defined definite atopy on the basis of more than one positive skin prick test to common allergens, although such a definition could include 50% of the population (Barbee et al., 1987), most of whom will not have clinical disease. In addition, such 'atopy' may be inherited independently from the propensity to specific allergic disease (Sibbald, 1986). Ring has recognized the shortcomings of the traditional use of the term 'atopy' and has proposed that it should be redefined as a 'familial hypersensitivity of skin and mucous membranes against environmental substances,

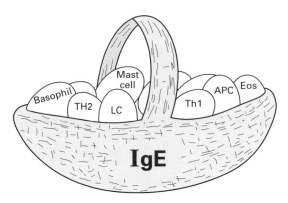

Fig. 1.3. We should not put all our atopic dermatitis eggs in the IgE basket

associated with increased IgE production and/or altered nonspecific reactivity' (Ring, 1991).

Recent research suggests that a type IV delayed-type hypersensitivity response involving different subsets of sensitized T-helper lymphocytes may be an important mechanism of allergic response in atopic dermatitis (Leung & Geha, 1986; Bos et al., 1992). Altered nonspecific skin reactivity such as increased α and decreased β adrenergic responsiveness and abnormalities in vasoactive mediators may also be key abnormalities underlying AD (Hanifin, 1992a). Another school of thought proposes that the crucial underlying problem of AD is that there is a primary defect in the barrier function of the epidermis, leading to a constellation of changes such as inflammation, itch and enhanced allergen–irritant penetration (Ogawa & Yoshiike, 1993).

Thus, although AD is strongly *associated* with increased total or specific IgE responsiveness, the role of classical immediate hypersensitivity in AD as a *necessary* phenomenon may have been overemphasized (Figure 1.3). As further research at a cellular level highlights the interaction between mast cell, eosinophil, Langerhans cell and T-lymphocyte in AD (Hanifin, 1992a), perhaps it would be wiser not constraining ourselves into the Gell and Coombs classification of hypersensitivity phenomena (Coombs & Gell, 1963) or a discussion of whether AD is atopic or not, but rather to ask ourselves to what degree is AD atopic?

In immunological terms, therefore, some might feel that the word 'atopy' when used in the term 'atopic dermatitis' is inappropriate or does not have a precise meaning. Although raised total and specific IgE levels and skin prick tests are frequently abnormal in atopic dermatitis subjects, their precise role in the pathogenesis of atopic dermatitis is still far from clear. The main argument for retaining the word 'atopic' in atopic dermatitis is to assist in separating our clinical concept of AD, a chronic pruritic disorder of early onset with inflammatory skin changes favouring flexural sites in individuals with a propensity to develop concomitant inhalant allergy, from other forms of dermatitis such as seborrhoeic, discoid, asteatotic, irritant and allergic contact dermatitis.

Dermatitis or eczema?

A detailed argument of the pros and cons of each term is beyond the scope of this chapter and may be found elsewhere (Ackerman, 1982). It is a sad reflection on modern dermatology that so much useful scientific energy has been wasted on arguing whether the term eczema or dermatitis should be used. Such debates have generated more heat than light on our understanding of the condition. Internationally, perhaps the term atopic dermatitis is more widely used than atopic eczema. The author accepts that the terms atopic eczema and atopic dermatitis are synonymous, and that in some countries such as the UK, others might prefer to use terms such as atopic eczema in order to avoid connotations of an occupationally acquired dermatosis.

Regressive and progressive nosology of disease

Based on the above discussion, some would argue that 'atopic dermatitis' is neither 'atopic' nor 'dermatitis'. Although the term 'atopic dermatitis' may have a scientific and objective ring to it, in practice it may not increase our predictive ability much more than the phrase 'itchy red rash in the skin folds'. Attaching a name to a condition can sometimes create a spurious impression of understanding so

that we cease to investigate the nature of the disease further (Kendell, 1975). Hardin coined the word panchreston (meaning 'explain-all', by analogy with panacea, or 'cure-all') to draw attention to the ways in which jargon is used to provide comforting but meaningless explanations for things we do not really understand (Hardin, 1956). Pearce has suggested that many fashionable 'new' diseases, such as posttraumatic syndrome, posttraumatic stress disorder, chronic fatigue syndrome and repetitive strain injury, are simply labels which hinder appropriate treatment and further research (Pearce, 1994). Such regressive nosology was highlighted by Abrams (1994), who pointed out that the term 'prostatism' has been used for many years to imply a prostatic cause for urinary symptoms when, in reality, almost no evidence exists for such a cause. Nosology is not simply a matter of semantics, as many men with 'prostatism' without bladder outflow obstruction are still being subjected unnecessarily to prostatectomy. Other terms such as 'benign prostatic hyperplasia' carry a spurious diagnostic authority, which may be translated into treatment without a proper diagnosis. Both Abrams and Pearce suggest that we would be better advised to adhere to established phenomena, and to be unashamed at honest diagnoses such as 'facial pain of unknown aetiology' or 'lower urinary tract symptoms' – terms which at least prompt further description, consideration and research. The situation is summed up nicely by Pearce who points out that 'diagnoses are not diseases, but are ever changing representations of disease to permit convenient communication and to allow brief descriptive insights into their nature'.

Progressive nosology, on the other hand, defines disease on the basis of a hierarchy of external evidence ranging from clinical descriptions to aetiological agents. As Scadding (1963) points out, myxoedema was originally defined as a clinical syndrome, but came to be defined as a disorder of function – a disorder of deficiency or utilization of thyroxine. This new definition will include some patients such as those with hypopituitarism who were not embraced by the original syndrome, and will exclude others with localized myxoedema in the absence of hypothyroidism, who were included in the original description. This is an example of progressive nosology, and similar examples are to be found in dermatology, such as the division of 'pemphigus', which formally referred to several diseases in which blistering was a feature (Pye, 1986) into pemphigoid, pemphigus and linear IgA disease on the basis of immunological discoveries. Changes of this sort are not a problem providing they are explicit, and that they confer benefits to patients (Kendell, 1975). By analogy, what we recognize as a clinical syndrome of atopic dermatitis today may in time be shown to be caused by three or four different agents. This does not imply that the original older criteria were 'wrong' at the time, provided they measured something useful or that they were instrumental in stimulating further research into the aetiology of that syndrome.

The need for a disease definition

Trying to define one of the most common skin diseases is not easy. Quite apart from the formidable difficulties of trying to define a disease which is variable in morphology, distribution and periodicity, and which lacks a laboratory reference standard, attempts to propose diagnostic criteria may be viewed as an imposition by other experienced physicians who are perfectly happy with the way in which they diagnose atopic dermatitis in individuals. Therein lies the crux of the matter. Diagnosis by physicians based on many years of clinical pattern recognition is entirely appropriate when dealing with individual patients. Problems begin, however, when *groups* of patients have to be described and compared. Whether this be the comparison of different prevalence rates from around the world, or comparison of therapeutic regimens, it is essential to know that different workers all refer to the same entity. Disease definition is essentially an aid to communication. Without it, all scientific communication would be impossible and our professional journals would be limited to case reports, anecdotes and statements of opinion.

There is always the possibility that the methodology for developing disease definitions becomes an end in itself. Disease definitions have meaning only in context to the biological question which is being asked. Different types of studies may require different types of definition. Disease definition is an evolutionary process which should be modified in the light of new knowledge.

Ways of defining atopic dermatitis

Various strategies can be employed in empidemiological studies for defining a disease dichotomy. For ordinal data (e.g. atopic dermatitis score) a statistical approach may be suitable. For example, any subject displaying a value above or below two standard deviations of a range of values of AD scores obtained from a representative population may be considered as abnormal. The biological meaning of such definitions may be obscure, however, and definitions based on two or more standard deviations from the mean also presupposes that the prevalence of all disease is 2.5% in each tail.

Prognostic definitions utilize elements of the condition which are associated with impaired outcome, such as sleep loss. Such an approach is useful for excluding asymptomatic or trivial disease, but the precise effects of disease on functional ability in many skin diseases is unknown.

Operational definitions are based on defining features for which action (in the form of cost effective treatment) is preferred to inaction. These are highly dependent on available resources and competing needs. This approach may be useful for implementing public health policies such as treatment of infestations in individual countries, but would be of little use in prevalence or aetiological studies.

On balance, a clinical approach of summarizing a constellation of symptoms and signs seems to be the most relevant to studying the epidemiology of AD today.

What is a good disease definition?

Before describing the various definitions for AD which have been used in epidemiological studies, it

Table 1.1. A good epidemiological definition for atopic dermatitis

1. Valid (sensitive and specific)
2. Repeatable (between and within observer)
3. Acceptable to the population
4. Rapid and easy to perform by field workers
5. Coherent with prevailing clinical concepts
6. A reflection of some degree of morbidity
7. Comprehensive in its applications
8. Comparable with other studies

Table 1.2. Synonyms for atopic dermatitis

- 'Eczema'
- Atopic eczema
- Infantile eczema
- Eczéma constitutionnel
- Flexural eczema
- Prurigo Besnier
- Allergic eczema
- Childhood eczema
- Lichen Vidal
- Endogenous eczema
- Spätexudatives Ekzematoid
- Neurodermatitis (constitutionalis)

is wise to consider what constitutes a good disease definition. These are summarized in Table 1.1 and are discussed in detail elsewhere (Williams, 1997b).

Diagnostic criteria for use in epidemiological studies

The dark ages

Although disease definition is perhaps the most fundamental step in any form of medical research, at least 12 synonyms for atopic dermatitis (AD) were in widespread use in Northern Europe (Table 1.2) up until the late 1970s (Sulzberger, 1983). Even dermatology texts use reflexive statements to define atopic dermatitis such as 'atopic dermatitis is the characteristic clinical type of dermatitis usually associated with atopy' (Champion & Parish, 1986), or 'eczema is a disease which shows eczematous features'. Such problems can be viewed in terms of nominalistic versus essentialist classification of disease (Burton, 1981). Nominalistic disease definitions imply that diseases have no real existence outside the individual patient. Even infectious agents such as the tubercle bacillus, which can be 'captured' and kept in a culture bottle like some demon, can produce a very wide range of clinical manifestations ranging from commensal existence to acute miliary tuberculosis. Similarly, atopic dermatitis does not conform to an essentialistic disease model (i.e. the disease is an entity in itself which 'attacks' patients), but rather a syndrome of related clinical features arising in response to a number of endogenous and exoge-

nous factors. The classification of a disease such as atopic dermatitis is thus the classification of patients, all of whom are different. 'Dis-ease' implies a complex interaction between external agents and host which will depend on a range of factors such as genetic predisposition, previous exposure to sensitizing agents and irritants, age, nutrition, hygiene, emotional and social well being and access to medical services.

Such a nominalistic approach can be taken to the extreme, however, for if we maintain that every patient is unique, then there could be as many diseases as there are patients. Whilst tailoring treatment to suit a unique constellation of problems in a particular individual might have some advantages in a clinical setting, as might have been the case in the 'dark ages', it is of little use in an epidemiological context where *groups* of patients need to be compared. Although some degree of nominalism is to be encouraged in order to reflect host factors, it is important that any patients defined by such an approach should behave similarly, so that we are able to communicate our findings on the morbidity and causes of the condition described by such a disease label.

The Hanifin, Lobitz and Rajka diagnostic criteria

The unsatisfactory situation of the dark ages came to an end with the suggestion by Rajka, Lobitz and

Table 1.3. The Hanifin and Rajka diagnostic criteria for atopic dermatitis

---

Must have three or more basic features
- Pruritus
- Typical morphology and distribution:
  Flexural lichenification or linearity in adults. Facial and extensor involvement in infants and children
- Chronic or chronically relapsing dermatitis
- Personal or family history of atopy (asthma, allergic rhinitis, atopic dermatitis)

Plus three or more minor features
Xerosis
Ichthyosis/palmar hyperlinearity/keratosis pilaris
Immediate (type I) skin test reactivity
Elevated serum IgE
Early age of onset
Tendency towards cutaneous infections
Tendency towards nonspecific hand or foot dermatitis
Nipple eczema
Cheilitis
Recurrent conjunctivitis
Dennie–Morgan infraorbital fold
Keratoconus
Anterior subcapsular cataracts
Orbital darkening
Facial pallor/facial erythema
Pityriasis alba
Anterior neck folds
Itch when sweating
Intolerance to wool and lipid solvents
Perifollicular accentuation
Food intolerance
Course influenced by environmental/emotional factors
White, dermographism/delayed blanch

Hanifin of a set of major and minor diagnostic criteria for atopic dermatitis (Rajka, 1975; Hanifin & Lobitz, 1977; Hanifin & Rajka, 1980) based on 24 clinical symptoms and signs (Table 1.3). In order to qualify as a case, subjects are required to have at least three out of four major features, or four out of five in a recent modification (Hanifin, 1992b), and at least three of the minor features listed in Table 1.3. These criteria undoubtedly represented a major step forward in ensuring some degree of uniformity of atopic dermatitis subjects in subsequent hospital studies and as a framework for further developments.

However, as Schultz Larsen and others have found out (Schultz Larsen & Hanifin, 1992; Seymour et al., 1987; Svensson, Edman & Möller, 1985; Visscher, Hanifin & Bowman, 1989; Diepgen & Fartasch, 1991) these criteria are unworkable in population-based studies. Many of the criteria, e.g. 'pityriasis alba', are not precisely defined (Hanifin, 1983), some (e.g. keratoconus) are very infrequent (Kennedy, Bourne & Dyer, 1986; Gelmetti, 1992), and some, such as white dermographism, are nonspecific (Svensson et al., 1985). They were derived in an empirical fashion in relation to clinical experience with predominantly white hospital-based cases of AD, and division into major and minor criteria was also empirical. More importantly, the criteria were not formally validated against the physician's diagnosis or tested for repeatability. In addition, the criteria contain invasive tests which are rarely used in routine clinical practice, and which might not be suitable for large studies involving children (Seymour et al., 1987).

Although the list of major criteria can usually be memorized, the list of over 30 minor criteria is difficult to assimilate into working practice, and introduces a large potential source of between- and within-observer variation. It has been shown that the human mind can process only about seven items of information simultaneously (Miller, 1956), and accuracy of diagnosis is usually diminished when physicians are presented with superfluous data (de Dombal et al., 1972). In addition, clinicians seldom incorporate arborizing strategies such as algorithms for diagnosis in clinical practice (Barrows et al., 1982). Although the Hanifin and Rajka criteria have been deployed in some population-based studies (Neame, Berth-Jones & Graham-Brown, 1993; Bakke, Gulsvik & Eide, 1990), the author suspects that what often happens in such cases is that physicians first decide whether or not a subject has AD using a pattern recognition approach (Sackett et al., 1991; Neufield et al., 1981), then seek confirmatory features from a wide choice of criteria in order to justify their initial clinical impression. Whilst the

Hanifin and Rajka diagnostic criteria may continue to be useful in some hospital studies because of their probable high sensitivity, their complexity and unknown validity makes them unsuitable for use in population-based studies or as a diagnostic aid to doctors in primary care.

The modern age

A number of groups have examined the usefulness of Hanifin and Rajka's diagnostic criteria (Mevorah et al., 1988; Diepgen, Fartasch & Hornstein, 1989; Kang & Tian, 1987; Kanwar, Dhar & Kaur, 1991; Kim, Chung & Park, 1993; Sehgal & Jain, 1993; Rudzki et al., 1994), but instead of addressing the crucial issues such as validation against the physician's diagnosis or deciding which should be designated major and minor criteria, these groups have tended to focus on small differences in the application of the 30 minor criteria mentioned in Hanifin and Rajka's original abstract. A recent editorial in *The Lancet* fuelled this preoccupation with minor criteria for AD (Rothe & Grant-Kels, 1996). These minor features may vary considerably following slight adjustments in their definition and interpretation. Features such as infra-orbital folds, periorbital pigmentation and hyperlinear palms are probably highly dependent on the age, sex and ethnicity of the population under study, which may explain the large discrepancies between these studies (Mevorah et al., 1988; Williams et al., 1996a). The atopic dermatitis cases used in these studies have all been hospital-based, which might explain the high frequency of odd signs such as anterior neck folds, Hertoghe's sign, hyperlinear palms, etc. – which are probably more frequently seen in a severe or chronic subset of AD cases. In none of the studies has the observers' recording of the presence or absence of these signs been blinded to the exposure status of the patient, and repeatability (between- and within-observer) of signs seems to have been overlooked.

A notable exception to these studies is the work of Diepgen et al. who derived a scoring system of useful diagnostic features of AD based on χ^2 values (Diepgen, Fartasch & Hornstein, 1989). They compared established hospital-ascertained AD cases ($n = 428$) with normal young adults from the community who did not have AD ($n = 628$), with respect to a number of Hanifin and Rajka's diagnostic criteria. They used clinical evidence of recurrent flexural itching or lichenified dermatitis as a gold standard for cases. This implied that it was impossible to assess the usefulness of history or visible flexural involvement as a feature of AD since, by definition, this criterion had 100% specificity and 100% sensitivity. On the basis of their χ^2 results, Diepgen et al. showed that some features, such as personal or family history of atopy, which are considered as 'major' features in Hanifin and Rajka's original criteria, are not as useful as some previously designated 'minor' features such as xerosis. They also showed that raised total serum IgE (>150 units/ml) and a positive radioallergosorbent test (RAST) for inhalant allergens were neither particularly sensitive nor specific for AD, the corresponding χ^2 values being less than most of the anamnestic and clinical features. Using their scoring system, they demonstrated good separation between cases and controls, although the scoring system was tested on the same data set from which the criteria were derived, as opposed to an independent sample. It should also be noted that their scoring system refers to discrimination of hospital-based AD cases from community controls who do not have AD, and when tested against a sample of 329 adults with skin disease recruited from hospital outpatients, specificity dropped from 97% to 84% (Diepgen, Sauerbrei & Fartasch, 1994). More importantly, repeatability of individual features has not been taken into account. Their study is nevertheless by far the largest and most systematic analysis of diagnostic criteria of AD to date, and their scoring system in particular may prove to be useful in estimating the risk of unmasking AD in nonaffected individuals, as might be considered in preemployment examinations. The author agrees with their conclusion that the diagnosis of AD should be based on traditional anamnestic and clinical features.

Schultz Larsen & Hanifin (1992) have proposed a questionnaire method for estimating AD, which includes many features which other workers have considered to be important in the diagnosis of AD. It is written using clear language, although the diagnostic label of 'eczema' (which might have many determinants) is mentioned throughout. Instead of using a binary disease definition (i.e. atopic dermatitis, yes/no), Schultz Larsen and Hanifin have chosen the categories of 'definite AD', 'possible AD' and 'no AD' as the main outcome measures based on a points system, the derivation of which is unclear. Such an approach is an attractive simplification of numerical estimations of the probability of AD in what may well be a disease continuum, but it is not clear how researchers comparing prevalences should deal with the 'possible AD' category, which could form the bulk of cases in community surveys. Defining opposite ends of the AD continuum is easy, but most prevalence or morbidity surveys will require a binary definition which offers a reasonable compromise between specificity of diagnosis and exclusion of asymptomatic disease.

Buser et al. have explored the validity of another questionnaire based on anamnestic criteria derived from the Hanifin and Rajka list against dermatologist's diagnosis in a sample of German schoolchildren (Buser et al., 1993). Although the questions have not yet been tested on an independent population or for repeatability, encouraging results were shown for a combination of three major and one minor feature. The authors chose to exclude ten children with equivocal diganosis from the main analysis, which perhaps defeats the purpose of the exercise.

The UK refinement of Hanifin and Rajka's criteria

In view of the absence of a definition for atopic dermatitis with known validity and repeatability, a UK working party set about the task of developing a minimum list of reliable discriminators for AD in 1990, using the Hanifin and Rajka list of clinical features as the building blocks. In addition to validity,

Table 1.4. The UK refinement of the Hanifin and Rajka diagnostic criteria for atopic dermatitis

---

In order to qualify as a case of atopic dermatitis with the UK diagnostic criteria, the child must have:

An itchy skin condition in the last 12 months

Plus three or more of:
1. Onset below the age of two*
2. History of flexural involvement
3. History of a generally dry skin
4. Personal history of other atopic disease†
5. Visible flexural dermatitis as per photographic protocol

---

*Not used in children under four years of age.
†In children aged under four years, history of atopic disease in a first-degree relative may be included.

repeatability and simplicity, a further requirement of the definition was that it should correspond well to our clinical concept of disease, be applicable to different ages and ethnic groups and be acceptable to subjects under study (Williams, 1997b). The detailed development of these criteria is to be found in six key papers published in the *British Journal of Dermatology* (Williams et al., 1994a, 1994b, 1994c, 1995a, 1996b; Popescu et al., 1998). Briefly, the study involved a national case-control study to examine the validity of specific symptoms and signs in relation to experienced physicians' diagnosis of AD. These physicians were consistent in their diagnosis of AD, and repeatability of signs was investigated in a separate study. Regression techniques and clinical consensus were used to derive a minimum list of reliable discriminators, which were then tested in independent validation studies. In order to capture the intermittent nature of AD and to minimize possible seasonal fluctuations in AD activity, the diagnostic criteria are recommended to be used as a 12-month period prevalence measure. The UK refinement of Hanifin and Rajka's criteria is shown in Table 1.4. Five out of the six UK diagnostic criteria are included as major features in a later refinement of the Hanifin and Rajka criteria (Hanifin, 1992b) which is a tribute to their original proposal. The exact wording of the questions is to be found in a manual that has been developed by the author for field studies (Williams, 1997c). This manual also contains a set of training photographs and a set of quality control photographs which can be checked centrally.

Performance

The UK criteria have performed well in subsequent independent hospital and community validation studies (Williams et al., 1994c, 1996b; Popescu et al., 1998). In a validation study of children attending hospital dermatology outpatients, the criteria were shown to have a sensitivity and specificity of 85% and 96%, respectively, when compared with a dermatologist's diagnosis (Williams et al., 1994c). When used as a one-year period prevalence measure in a community survey of London children aged 3–11 years of mixed ethnic groups where the prevalence of AD was approximately 10%, sensitivity and specificity were 80% and 97%, respectively (Williams et al., 1996b). Positive and negative predictive values in this survey were 80% and 97%, respectively. In an identical community validation study of 1114 Romanian schoolchildren (Popescu et al., 1998) the sensitivity and specificity of the criteria were 74% and 99%, respectively, when tested against the dermatologist's diagnosis. Acceptable repeatability has been demonstrated for the six features contained within the UK criteria (Williams et al., 1994b). The criteria appear to be equally applicable to children of different ethnic and socioeconomic groups. They have worked well in children down to the age of one year, but further evaluation in infants and adults needs to be done. The criteria are easy to ascertain (taking under two minutes per person, including examination for flexural dermatitis), and they have proven to be highly acceptable to children and adults because of their relatively simple and noninvasive nature. They correspond well to our clinical concept of atopic dermatitis in that they contain all of the key elements that previous researchers have emphasized. Several groups studying allergic diseases have used the UK criteria without any major problems. Further validation studies of these criteria in developing countries are currently underway.

The concept of using different versions of the same criteria

The idea that several versions of the UK refinement of Hanifin and Rajka's diagnostic criteria may be used at any one time to define atopic dermatitis may seem odd at first, considering that one of the driving forces to develop diagnostic criteria is to obtain one overall standardized definition so that groups of people can be compared. However, it should be pointed out that different studies have different requirements of their definitions, especially in terms of the relative importance of sensitivity and specificity. Suggestions for the most appropriate format of features for diagnosing atopic dermatitis in various study scenarios are given below and are discussed in more detail elsewhere (Williams, 1997c).

Simple prevalence survey to assess the burden of disease

Itch, plus three or more of the features shown in Table 1.4, is used as a one-year period prevalence measure to overcome potential problems with seasonal fluctuations. It will be noted that since the presence of an itchy skin condition is the sole necessary criterion, then only subjects responding affirmatively to this question need to be examined further for evidence of visible flexural dermatitis. Such a strategy might save considerable expense and time, although some researchers may also wish to examine a sample of those without a history of an itchy rash to assess the proportion of false negatives. If examining individuals is out of the question, then the questions-only version (itch plus two or more of the remaining four features in Table 1.4) should be used, or a single compound question that has been widely used in the International Study of Asthma and Allergies in Childhood (Williams et al., 1999). A similar criteria format can be used for comparative prevalence surveys.

Mixed asthma–hay fever–atopic dermatitis surveys

One of the six criteria for diagnosing AD is a personal history of hay fever or asthma. It is possible that the inclusion of asthma–hay fever within the definition of AD may be undesirable in some surveys which wish to keep the elements of the three allergic diseases entirely separate. If the inclusion of asthma–hay fever as part of the diagnosis of AD is unacceptable to an investigator, it is recommended that AD should be defined in terms of single unambiguous items, such as history of flexural itchy rash or visible flexural dermatitis.

Case-control studies

Since only a fraction of cases are sampled in most case-control studies, more specific, less sensitive criteria formats, such as itch plus four or more features, might be more suitable to minimize the inclusion of false positive cases. Similarly, very specific definitions of AD should be used in economic assessments of AD cases, as the inclusion of costs for noncases would be very misleading.

Cohort studies

Measurement of disease incidence poses difficulties as AD is usually an intermittent disease. The criteria proposed to date all refer to prevalent cases since they all contain elements of past disease or chronicity. In a cohort study, it might be appropriate to use the one-year period prevalences as a measure of disease incidence if they are recorded annually. Alternatively, an incident case of AD could be defined as any person who develops an itchy skin condition for the first time which is also compatible with AD (i.e. visible flexural dermatitis with modifications for young infants as outlined in the protocol). It is also possible to use the criteria to measure lifetime prevalence of AD by using 'has your child *ever* had an itchy skin condition?' for question 1 of the questionnaire shown in Table 1.4.

Hospital-based studies of AD subjects

There is no reason why the preferred criteria format of itchy skin plus three or more features could not be used in hospital studies which seek to recruit a representative population of AD cases. This would permit the selection of cases who are not necessarily active at the time of recruitment, and this might reduce the tendency to record epiphenomena associated with disease activity and severity.

Clinical trials

These would probably require subjects to have active disease on entry into a trial. Because cases referred to hospital are usually quite severe, it is likely that all hospital-ascertained cases of AD will have active dermatitis, and the normal criteria format of itch plus three or more features could be used.

Definite atopy

Some laboratory-based studies or clinical trials might require a stricter definition of the use of the word 'atopy' when defining subjects with atopic dermatitis. In such a context atopy, as defined by a positive skin prick test reaction (or raised allergen specific IgE) to one or more common environmental allergens, could be included as an additional necessary criterion for all cases.

As a diagnostic aid in the primary care setting

Although the UK refinements of Hanifin and Rajka's criteria were primarily designed for use in population surveys, they may be useful to family practitioners who wish to describe groups of subjects for audit studies. They may also be useful as a diagnostic aid to those less familiar with AD, but care must be taken in not interpreting failure to fulfil the diagnostic criteria as proof of excluding AD, as opposed to the correct interpretation that AD is not *probable* within a certain degree of confidence at that moment. The use of likelihood ratios may help in this respect and these are discussed further in the manual (Williams, 1997c).

Thus, for one disease, there may be a range of definitions with slightly different validity indices, each of which may be better suited to specific study designs or requirements. They all define the *same* disease, but with differing precision and practical suitablility for different study designs and constraints.

It is important for the researcher to appreciate one further point which might influence the way in which the data are recorded and coded. It would be naïve to expect that the preferred format of itch plus three or more features could not be replaced by better criteria in the light of future discoveries on disease aetiology. Whatever new disease definitions emerge, the separate elements which make up the UK diagnostic criteria (e.g. history of flexural itchy rash) are still likely to be useful in describing the AD phenotype in future studies, especially for investigating secular trends and international comparative prevalence estimates. For this reason, in addition to composite measures such as atopic dermatitis 'yes/no', it is strongly recommended that the subjects' responses to individual criteria are retained separately on file.

Problem areas with the UK refinement of Hanifin and Rajka's criteria

Misclassification

As with most diagnostic tests, some degree of misclassification is inevitable. The gains and losses conferred by different sensitivities and specificities will depend very much on the nature of the study to which the criteria are applied. It is anticipated that one of the most common epidemiological uses for the proposed diagnostic criteria will be to compare prevalence rates between countries or in the same population at different points in time. Even though

Table 1.5. The relationship between true prevalence of AD, positive predictive value, prevalence of AD by UK criteria and systematic error using the validity indices (sensitivity 74% and specificity 99%) derived from a validation study in Bucharest

True prevalence of atopic dermatitis (%)	Positive predictive value (%)	Prevalence of AD by UK criteria (%)	Systematic error
1	34	1.8	1.8
2	58	2.6	1.3
3	67	3.3	1.1
4	73	4.0	1.0
5	79	4.7	0.9
6	81	5.4	0.9
7	84	6.2	0.9
8	86	6.9	0.9
9	87	7.7	0.9
10	88	8.4	0.8
11	89	9.1	0.8
12	90	9.9	0.8
13	91	10.6	0.8
14	91	11.4	0.8
15	92	12	0.8
16	92	12.7	0.8
17	93	13.5	0.8
18	94	14.2	0.8
19	94	15.0	0.8
20	94	15.7	0.8

the sensitivity and specificity of the UK criteria for AD appear quite high, the underlying prevalence of AD has a critical influence on the positive predictive value (proportion of all those who fulfil the criteria and who are genuine cases) as shown in Table 1.5.

The effects of misclassification error in comparative prevalence studies can be examined directly by calculating the error for prevalence differences likely to be encountered in such studies. Take, for example, two populations of 1000 people in two different countries A and B. Suppose that the one-year period prevalence of AD in country A is 20% (200/1000) and in country B it is 10% (100/1000). Thus, the relative risk of AD is twice as high in country A when compared with country B (95% confidence intervals 1.6 to 2.5, χ^2 for difference between the two proportions 38.4, $p<0.001$). If it is assumed that the sensitivity and specificity of our criteria for AD are 80% and 97%, respectively, when applied to these countries, then the prevalence of AD in country A will become 18.4% compared with 10.7% in country B. This represents a slightly lower relative risk of 1.72 (95% confidence interval of 1.38 to 2.15) of AD in country A when compared with country B, and a fall in the χ^2 value from 38.4 to 23.2 (still highly statistically significant). This reduction in the risk estimate towards unity is to be expected with such nondifferential misclassification, but this example illustrates how the new criteria are unlikely to obscure the true prevalence differences of the magnitude specified in these two populations. If the true prevalence of AD in countries A and B is 10% and 5%, respectively, then the estimated prevalence with the new criteria will be 10.7% and 6.8% in countries A and B, respectively. This difference is still highly significant ($p = 0.003$), but the χ^2 value has fallen from 17.3 to 9.1.

Difficulties are likely to be encountered when very low disease prevalences occur. Although low prevalences for AD are unlikely in temperate climates, they could occur in tropical developing countries. Thus, a true prevalence difference of 5% and 2.5% in two countries may be obscured when the diagnostic criteria are applied. In addition, since the positive predictive values in these scenarios is more dependent on specificity, more specific alternative criteria formats, such as itch plus four or more features, could be used in populations with low disease prevalence.

Conversely, if significant differences are shown in a study where the new criteria are applied, then nondifferential misclassification is unlikely to have been a serious problem. Thus, in our community study of 695 schoolchildren in West Lambeth (Williams et al., 1995b), it was found that the prevalence of atopic dermatitis based on examination by a dermatologist was almost twice as high (16.3%) in Black children as in White children (8.7%, $p = 0.03$). When the UK criteria for atopic dermatitis were used, almost identical findings were observed, suggesting that nondifferential misclassification introduced by our criteria did not obscure important ethnic group variations in the prevalence of AD, even in a study as small as this.

For prevalence surveys which simply wish to assess accurately the total burden of disease caused by AD, it may be imperative to establish the right count of cases. The degree to which the total number of true cases differs from the total number ascertained by the criteria can be expressed by a ratio called the 'systematic error', which refers to the ratio of the total number of cases positive to the survey and the reference tests. In a hypothetical prevalence survey of a community of 1000 children where, say, 100 children (10%) have had AD in the last year then, using the newly proposed criteria, 107 children will be described as having AD, representing a very similar prevalence rate (10.7%) and a very low systematic error of 1.07 when applied to these absolute counts. Although on an individual basis, a physician might take great exception to one child with keratosis pilaris being classified as atopic dermatitis in such a study, in epidemiological terms such misclassification is less serious when comparing populations. The relationship between systematic error, predictive values and prevalence of atopic dermatitis is shown in Table 1.5, assuming a sensitivity of 80% and specificity of 97% for the criteria. It can be seen that the systematic error is lowest when the prevalence of AD is around 10 to 12%, which fortunately also happens to be the most likely value of AD prevalence in most modern studies. True prevalence is underestimated by the criteria when the true prevalence is over 15%, and overestimated under this value. Systematic error is unacceptable when the true prevalence of AD is very low ($<4\%$).

Even in a clinical situation where, for example, the diagnostic criteria are used by family practitioners as a diagnostic guide, the effects of misclassification of cases do not seem too serious. As our validation study showed (Williams et al., 1996b), nearly all of the false negative cases were inactive or asymptomatic cases of AD, and the consequences of a family practitioner not treating these cases with emollients or very mild topical corticosteroids is unlikely to cause problems. Most of the false positive cases were mild forms of AD who were considered inactive by the validator. Even the nonAD false positive cases were composed mainly of other mild inflammatory dermatoses such as keratosis pilaris, frictional lichenoid dermatosis and pityriasis alba, all of which have been considered as being possible variants of AD, and all of which are treated using a similar therapeutic approach to mild AD. Thus at an operational level, the consequences of misclassification produced by the criteria in a clinical setting seem quite minor.

Asymptomatic disease

It is possible to derive diagnostic criteria in a systematic manner which are clinically meaningless and bear little resemblance to our clinical concept of atopic dermatitis. The UK Atopic Dermatitis Working Party believes that what is defined as a case of AD by the UK criteria is an entity which is worthy of measurement, reflecting a 'typical average case of AD'. That the criteria may miss the occasional mild cases of inactive AD is not a bad thing as most population surveys are interested in quantifying the distribution of *clinically important* as opposed to subclinical disease. Further studies examining the severity threshold of cases defined by the criteria, such as by measuring disability (Finlay & Khan, 1994), may be useful in this respect. It would be very easy to define 'definite AD' by making the diagnostic criteria more stringent, but this might exclude many cases of mild yet symptomatic diseases, which may form the bulk of community cases. It is recommended that researchers therefore stick to a binary as opposed to ordered categorical classification, and accept that the dividing line will always represent some form of compromise between excluding other itchy dermatoses and asymptomatic cases.

Adults and infants

Some modification of diagnostic criteria for AD may be necessary for young children (Williams et al.,

1994c). Since early onset and inhalant allergy are likely to be less useful in the young child, early onset are omitted, and personal history of atopic disease is replaced by family history of atopic disease for children under four years of age. This scheme resulted in a sensitivity of 85% and specificity of 96% when applied to the 38 children aged four years and under in the hospital paediatric validation study (Williams et al., 1994c).

The author is less confident about the validity of the UK criteria in the first year of life. Although most children at this age were correctly classified, numbers were small, and validation against physician's diagnosis is perhaps not so useful due to the widespread disagreement between experts of what constitutes a case of AD at this age (Yates, Kerr & MacKie, 1983). One approach of describing AD in the first year of life is simply to focus on recording the prevalence of symptoms such as itchy rash or signs such as flexural dermatitis, analogous to similar conventions in asthma research. Further research using longitudinal designs might then delineate which features best discriminate those individuals who later develop typical AD, although it does not overcome the problem of saying that those who do clear did not originally have AD.

Based on our own data and other studies which have tried to separate seborrhoeic dermatitis of infancy from AD (Yates et al., 1983), we suggest that in order to be classified as a case of AD, children under the age of one year should have a history of scratching or rubbing plus three or more of: history of involvement of outer arms or legs, family history of atopic disease in first degree relatives, history of a general dry skin, and visible dermatitis on the cheeks or outer arms or legs with absence of axillary involvement.

Although the effect of potential confounding by age on the usefulness of the six diagnostic criteria has been thoroughly explored in the development work (*a*) by performing separate regression analyses in children and adults, (*b*) by looking for interaction between the criteria and a dummy variable for 'age under 16', and (*c*) by separate analysis of adult and paediatric data in the hospital validation study, further testing of the performance of the criteria in adults in a community setting is still desirable because of the low numbers of adults with AD in our study.

Applicability to other ethnic groups

Although clinical experience suggests that AD in Black children can appear very different in its propensity to follicular lichenification, extensor involvement, later onset and lower frequency of personal or family history of atopy, the UK diagnostic criteria have performed well in Afro-Caribbean children in our community validation study in London and in another study in Jamaica (Williams et al., 1995b; Burrell-Morris et al., 1997). Another study has found that the physical features of atopic dermatitis in Black children are very similar to those in Whites (Macharia, Anabwani & Owili, 1993). It is important to appreciate that some cultures may not have a direct translation of the word 'itching', although recognition of the word *scratching* is universal – hence its inclusion in the wording of the major diagnostic criterion.

Use of the criteria in other communities

In countries where there is a high prevalence of other skin diseases which could be confused with atopic dermatitis, such as scabies or onchocerciasis, it seems prudent to stipulate that *the eruption must lack specific features of that dermatosis.* In studies of atopic dermatitis in areas where scabies is endemic, it would be wise to stipulate the addition of 'absence of burrows or finger web lesions' as a necessary major criterion in these circumstances. This presupposes that those conducting the examination are capable of identifying burrows, but if the disease is particularly prevalent, it is highly likely that nurses and health workers will be very familiar with the signs. In a study of scabies off the coast of Panama for instance, mothers of children were so adept at spotting scabies burrows and extracting mites that they were employed as survey helpers (Taplin et al., 1991).

It is also important that the criteria are tested in tropical countries where the appearance of a 'typical' case of AD may be altered by environmental factors such as UV light and infection. It should also not be assumed that some of the key words used in the criteria will retain their meaning when translated into other languages (Williams, 1999). Any translation of the questions should be performed by a person with good knowledge of local terms, such as a schoolteacher, and the translated version should be translated back into English by another independent person to ensure that the meaning of the questions is not grossly altered (Asher et al., 1995). Further validation studies of the UK refinement of Hanifin and Rajka's criteria for AD are currently in progress in China, Germany and India.

Where do other 'variants' of atopic dermatitis fit in?

When discussing the diagnostic criteria with other dermatologists, the author is often asked how other dermatological conditions which have been considered as possible variants of atopic dermatitis – such as dyshidrotic eczema, discoid eczema in children, juvenile plantar dermatosis and follicular and papular forms (Wüthrich, 1991) – fit in with the criteria. The answer is that the criteria will not provide an easy way of saying whether these conditions are truly variants of atopic dermatitis. The criteria derived in our studies were only designed to discriminate between typical mild to moderate AD and other inflammatory conditions, as opposed to determining the degree of 'atopic dermatitis' in other purported atopic dermatitis variants. Thus, it would be quite wrong to say that an individual with an unusual pattern of dermatitis 'definitely does not have atopic dermatitis' simply because he/she does not fulfil the UK criteria for AD. It would be accurate, however, to state that such an individual has a 97% probability of not having 'typical atopic dermatitis'. The author accepts that vesicles on the sides of the fingers in summer months in someone predisposed to atopy, discoid eczema in a child and late-onset eczematous erythroderma with high IgE levels in an adult, may all be related to atopic dermatitis but their precise relationship to AD would require a special study such as cluster analysis or numerical taxonomy, preferably backed by genetic marker studies.

Dangers of suggesting a disease definition

It is possible that the mere proposal of a disease definition can create a spurious impression of understanding that disease which could stagnate further research into disease aetiology. This is unlikely to occur providing the limitations of our definition are recognized. The author feels that the advent of a definition for AD that is designed for use in population studies is likely to stimulate rather than stifle further studies of disease aetiology.

Will the criteria change again in five years?

One must consider the possibility that the newly proposed criteria will not last very long. This does not unduly concern the author, providing that they are replaced by something better. The author recognizes that the criteria as proposed today are but a transient step in the process of progressive nosology (Kendell, 1975). Thus if a more rational basis for the classification of atopic dermatitis is found in the next 20 years, then the current definition based on a clinical syndrome might well lose its value. As Kendell (1975) commented, 'to the contemporary medical research worker, if not to every practising clinician, diseases are little more than convenient working concepts based on a variety of different defining criteria, anatomical, physiological or behavioural, and liable to change their defining characteristics, or even to be abandoned altogether, with advances in knowledge'.

The emergence of many similar 'rival' criteria based on arbitrary arrangements of clinical features alone would not be useful, however, unless they were shown to produce marked benefits over the UK criteria when put to the test in independent validation studies. Even in the absence of 'rival' diagnostic criteria, it is likely that the criteria will produce a number of 'boundary disputes'. Difficulties in establishing international agreement of diagnostic criteria are more likely to be encountered when defining the boundary or outer rim of what separates a condition from other adjacent categories as opposed to agreeing on what constitutes the core of typical clinical features. Thus, one group might insist that all subjects with AD must be atopic as defined by objective tests of immediate hypersensitivity, or that visible 'eczematous' skin changes must be visible in all subjects. Providing these modifications are explicit, and that the individual elements of the diagnostic criteria are recorded separately, then most of these 'boundary disputes' are unlikely to be insurmountable. Indeed, the different nature of the many types of study designs available to researchers means that some modification of the criteria for the purposes of a particular study is inevitable.

It should be pointed out that even if a genetic basis for atopic dermatitis is discovered in the future, there will always be a need to provide an adequate description of the disease phenotype with well defined clinical criteria. The UK diagnostic criteria for atopic dermatitis may be useful for ensuring a degree of comparability of subjects in future epidemiological surveys. The author views the diagnostic criteria for atopic dermatitis as an evolving instrument, and welcomes modifications and improvements in the light of further knowledge.

Conclusions

This chapter has challenged the way we think about defining atopic dermatitis for epidemiological studies. Having stated the desirable properties of diagnostic criteria for epidemiological studies, the development of a refined set of simple criteria has been described. These appear to work well, but more testing is needed in other communities. The validity of these criteria in infants and in adults is still not known, and a satisfactory definition of an incident case of AD is still lacking.

Although other definitions will undoubtedly emerge for AD, the key issue in epidemiological studies is the need to compare results from many studies from around the world. For this, *standardization* is of paramount importance. It is better to have a less than perfect disease definition of known validity and repeatability than a definition that is claimed to be better but which is of unknown validity.

The point of defining a disease is to improve our understanding of the disease and to improve our predictive abilities (Burton, 1981), whether this be in relation to its causes and distribution, natural history, biology or treatment. As described in this chapter, even within the sphere of epidemiology, there may be a range of requirements for disease definition with different degrees of precision, depending on the nature of the study. Disease definition in epidemiology should be viewed as an instrument or tool of known validity which is only important in relation to the biological or social question that is being addressed.

Summary of key points

- Atopic dermatitis (AD) should be viewed as a multidimensional phenomenon.
- It is unclear at present if *any* individual could develop AD under the right adverse circumstances, or whether genetic predisposition is a prerequisite for disease expression.
- Despite its limitations, a binary definition for AD is most readily understood by clinicians and epidemiologists throughout the world.
- Data-driven post hoc subcategories of AD are only useful if they are shown to increase our predictive ability on factors such as prognosis or responsiveness to treatment.
- Because many individuals with AD have normal IgE responsiveness, the word 'atopy' when used in the term 'atopic dermatitis' does not have a precise meaning.
- Other mechanisms such as altered nonspecific reactivity or T-lymphocyte dysfunction may be just as important in the pathogenesis of AD as IgE hyper-responsiveness.
- The terms 'atopic eczema' and 'atopic dermatitis' are synonymous.

- Although the term 'atopic dermatitis' may have a scientific and objective ring to it, it may not increase our predictive ability much more than the phrase 'itchy red rash in the skin folds'.
- Standardized diagnostic criteria are essential if valid comparisons are to be made between groups of people.
- Disease definitions have meaning only in context to the biological question which is being asked.
- A good disease definition is valid, repeatable, easy to use, applicable to a wide range of situations, acceptable to the population and contains elements that are coherent with prevailing clinical concepts.
- The Hanifin, Lobitz and Rajka diagnostic criteria represented a major milestone in summarizing the clinical concept of AD. However, because of their unknown validity and complexity, they are not suitable for epidemiological studies.
- A UK refinement of the Hanifin, Lobitz and Rajka diagnostic criteria has been developed for use in epidemiological studies. These criteria have good repeatability and contain elements which allow comparability with older studies.
- The UK criteria have a sensitivity of 80% and 74% and a specificity of 97% and 97% when tested against a dermatologist's diagnosis in population studies in the UK and Romania, respectively.
- Different arrangements of the UK criteria with different specificities may be used for different types of study requirements.
- Misclassification of disease is unlikely to obscure clinically important prevalence differences for disease prevalences above 5%.
- The validity of the UK diagnostic criteria in infants and in adults needs further study.
- There is currently no accepted method for defining an incident case of AD.
- It is better to have a less than perfect disease definition of known validity and repeatability than a definition that is claimed to be better with unknown validity.
- Disease definition is an evolutionary process which should be modified in the light of new knowledge.

- The possibility that what we recognize as the clinical syndrome of AD today will be subsequently shown to be caused by three or four different agents does not imply that older diagnostic criteria are 'wrong', providing they measure something useful or that they are instrumental in stimulating further research.

References

Abrams, P. (1994). New words for old: lower urinary tract symptoms for 'prostatism'. *Br Med J*, **308**, 929–30.

Ackerman, A.B. (1982). A plea to expunge the word 'eczema' from the lexicon of dermatology and dermatopathology. *Am J Dermatopath*, **4**, 315–26.

Asher, M.I., Keil, U., Anderson, H.R. et al. (1995). International study of asthma and allergies in childhood (ISAAC): rationale and methods. *Eur Resp J*, **8**, 483–91.

Bakke, P., Gulsvik, A. & Eide, G.E. (1990). Hay fever, eczema and urticaria in southwest Norway. *Allergy*, **45**, 515–22.

Barbee, R., Kaltenborn, W., Lebowitz, M. & Burrows, B. (1987). Longitudinal changes in allergen skin test reactivity in a community population sample. *J Allergy Clin Immunol*, **79**, 16–24.

Barker, D.J.P. & Rose, G. (1979). *Epidemiology in Medical Practice*, 2nd edn. Edinburgh: Churchill Livingstone.

Barrows, H.S., Norman, G.R., Neufield, V.R. & Feightner, J.W. (1982). The clinical reasoning of randomly selected physicians in general medical practice. *Clin Invest Med*, **5**, 49–55.

Bos, J.D., Wierenga, E.A., Smitt, J.H.S. et al. (1992). Immune dysregulation in atopic eczema. *Arch Dermatol*, **128**, 1509–12.

Burrell-Morris, C.E., LaGrenade, L., Williams, H.C. & Hay, R.J. (1997). The prevalence of atopic dermatitis in Black Caribbean children in London and Kingston, Jamaica. *Br J Dermatol*, **137** (Suppl. 50), 22.

Burton, J.L. (1981). The logic of dermatological diagnosis. *Clin Exp Dermatol*, **6**, 1–21.

Buser, K., von Bohlen, F., Werner, P. et al. (1993). The prevalence of neurodermatitis among schoolchildren in the Hannover administrative district. *Dtsh Med Wschr*, **118**, 1141–5.

Champion, R.H & Parish, W.E. (1986). Atopic dermatitis. In: Rook, A.J., Wilkinson, D.S. & Ebling, F.J.G. (eds.) *Textbook of Dermatology*, 4th edn. Oxford: Blackwell Scientific.

Coca, A.F. & Cooke, R.A. (1923). On the classification of the phenomena of hypersensitiveness. *J Immunol*, **8**, 163–82.

Coombs, R.R.A. & Gell, P.G.H. (1963). The classification of allergic reactions underlying disease. In: Gell, P.G.H. & Coombs, R.R.A. (eds.) *Clinical Aspects of Immunology*. Philadelphia: Davis.

David, T.J. (1991). Conventional allergy tests. *Arch Dis Childh*, **66**, 281–2.

de Dombal, F.T., Horrocks, J.C., Staniland, J.R. & Guillou, P.J. (1972). Pattern recognition: a comparison of the performance of clinicians and non-clinicians – with a note on the performance of a computer-based system. *Methods Inf Med*, **11**, 32.

Diepgen, T.L. & Fartasch, M. (1991). Stigmata and signs of atopic eczema. In: Ring, J. & Pryzbilla, B. (eds.) *New Trends in Allergy*, 3rd edn. pp. 222–9. Berlin: Springer-Verlag.

Diepgen, T.L. & Fartasch, M. (1992). Recent epidemiological and genetic studies in atopic dermatitis. *Acta Derm Venereol (Stockh)*, Suppl. 176, 13–18.

Diepgen, T.L., Fartasch, M. & Hornstein, O.P. (1989). Evaluation and relevance of atopic basic and minor features in patients with atopic dermatitis and in the general population. *Acta Dermatol Venereol (Stockh)*, Suppl. 144, 50–54.

Diepgen, T.L., Sauerbrei, W. & Fartasch, M. (1994). Evaluation and validation of diagnostic models of atopic dermatitis. *J Invest Dermatol*, **102**, 619 (abstract).

Dotterud, L.K., Kvammen, B., Lund, E. & Falk, E.S. (1995). Prevalence and some clinical aspects of atopic dermatitis in the community of Sør-Varanger. *Acta Derm Venereol (Stockh)*, **75**, 50–3.

Edenharter, G., Bergmann, R.L., Bergmann, K.E. & Wahn, U. (1998). Definition of atopic dermatitis (AD) in infants at 5 years: combining atopic symptoms and signs with atopic biomarkers. *Proceedings of the EDEN Congress*, Bamberg, Germany, May 2–4, 1998.

Fartasch, M. & Diepgen, T.L. (1994). Atopic diathesis and occupational dermatoses. *J Invest Dermatol*, **102**, 620.

Finlay, A.Y. & Khan, G.K. (1994). The Dermatology Life Quality Index: a simple practical measure for routine clinical use. *Clin Exp Dermatol*, **19**, 210–16.

Freiman, J.A., Chalmers, T.C., Smith, H. & Kuebler, R.R. (1978). The importance of beta, the type 2 error and sample size in the design and interpretation of the randomized controlled trial. *N Engl J Med*, **299**, 690–4.

Gelmetti, C. (1992). Extracutaneous manifestations of atopic dermatitis. *Ped Dermatol*, **9**, 380–2.

Gerber, L.M., Wolf, A.M., Braham, R.L. & Alderman, M.H. (1982). Effects of sample selection on the coincidence of hypertension and diabetes. *J Am Med Ass*, **247**, 43–6.

Hanifin, J.M. (1983). Clinical and basic aspects of atopic dermatitis. *Sem Dermatol*, **2**, 5–19.

Hanifin, J.M. (1992a). Atopic dermatitis. In: Marks, R. (ed.) *Eczema*, pp. 77–101. London: Martin Dunitz.

Hanifin, J.M. (1992b). Atopic dermatitis. In: Moschella, S.L. & Hundey, H.J. (eds.) *Dermatology*, 3rd edn., pp. 441–64. Philadelphia: Saunders.

Hanifin, J.M. & Lobitz, W.C. Jr. (1977). Newer concepts in atopic dermatitis. *Arch Dermatol*, **113**, 663–70.

Hanifin, J.M. & Rajka, G. (1980). Diagnostic features of atopic dermatitis. *Acta Derm Venereol (Stockh)*, Suppl. 92, 44–7.

Hardin, G. (1956). Meaninglessness of the word protoplasm. *Sci Monthly*, **82**, 112–20.

Imayama, S., Hashizume, T., Miyahara, H. et al. (1992). Combination of patch test and IgE for dust mite antigens differentiates 130 patients with atopic eczema into four groups. *J Am Acad Dermatol*, **27**, 531–8.

Kang, K. & Tian, R. (1987). Atopic dermatitis. An evaluation of clinical and laboratory findings. *Int J Dermatol*, **26**, 27–32.

Kanwar, A.J., Dhar, S. & Kaur, S. (1991). Evaluation of minor clinical features of atopic dermatitis. *Ped Dermatol*, **8**, 114–16.

Kendell, R.E. (1975). *The Role of Diagnosis in Psychiatry*. Oxford: Blackwell Scientific.

Kennedy, R.H., Bourne, W.M. & Dyer, J.A. (1986). A 48-year clinical and epidemiologic study of keratoconus. *Am J Ophthalmol*, **101**, 267–73.

Kim, K.H., Chung, J.H. & Park, K.C. (1993). Clinical evaluation of minor clinical features of atopic dermatitis. *Ann Dermatol*, **5**, 9–12.

Leung, D.Y.M. & Geha, R.S. (1986). Immunoregulatory abnormalities in atopic dermatitis. *Clin Rev Allergy*, **4**, 67–86.

Macharia, W.M., Anabwani, G.M. & Owili, D.M. (1993). Clinical presentation of atopic dermatitis in Negroid children. *Afr J Med Sci*, **22**, 41–4.

Mevorah, B., Frank, E., Wietlisbach, V. & Carrel, C-F. (1988). Minor clinical features of atopic dermatitis. *Dermatologica* **177**, 360–4.

Miller, G.A. (1956). The magical number seven plus or minus two: some limits on our capacity for processing information. *Psych Rev*, **63**, 81–97

Neame, R.L., Berth-Jones, J. & Graham-Brown, R. (1993). A population based prevalence study of atopic dermatitis in the UK. *J Invest Dermatol*, **100**, 543.

Neufield, V.R., Norman, G.R., Feightner, J.W. & Barrows, H.S. (1981). Clinical problem-solving by medical students: a cross-sectional and longitudinal analysis. *Med Ed*, **15**, 315–22.

Ogawa, H. & Yoshiike, T. (1993). A speculative view of atopic dermatitis: barrier dysfunction in pathogenesis. *J Dermatol Sci*, **5**, 197–204.

Oldham, P.D., Pickering, G., Fraser Roberts, J.A. & Sowry, G.S.C. (1960). The nature of essential hypertension. *Lancet* **1**, 1085–93.

Pearce, J.M.S. (1994). New diagnoses for old diseases: dangers and distractions. *Q J Med*, **87**, 253–8.

Popescu, C.M., Popescu, R., Williams, H.C. & Forsea, D. (1998). Community validation of the UK diagnostic criteria for atopic dermatitis in Romanian schoolchildren. *Br J Dermatol*, **138**, 436–42.

Pye, R.J. (1986). Bullous eruptions. In: Rook, A.J., Wilkinson, D.S. & Ebling, F.J.G. (eds.) *Textbook of Dermatology*, 4th edn. Oxford: Blackwell Scientific.

Rajka, G. (1975). The clinical aspects of atopic dermatitis. In: *Atopic Dermatitis*. London: Saunders.

Ring, J. (1991). Atopy: condition, disease or syndrome? In: Ruzicka, T., Ring, J. & Pryzbilla, B. (eds.) *Handbook of Atopic Eczema*. London: Springer-Verlag.

Roth, H.L. (1987). Atopic dermatitis revisited. *Int J Dermatol*, **26**, 139–49.

Rothe, M.J. & Grant-Kels, J.M. (1996). Diagnostic criteria for atopic dermatitis. *Lancet*, **348**, 769–70.

Rudzki, E., Samochocki, Z., Rebandel, P. et al. (1994). Frequency and significance of the major and minor features of Hanifin and Rajka among patients with atopic dermatitis. *Dermatology*, **189**, 41–6.

Sackett, D.L., Haynes, R.B., Guyatt, G.H. & Tugwell, P. (1991). *Clinical Epidemiology*, 2nd ed. Boston: Little, Brown.

Scadding, J.G. (1963). Meaning of diagnostic terms in bronchopulmonary disease. *Br Med J*, **2**, 1425–30.

Schultz Larsen, F. & Hanifin, J.M. (1992). Secular change in the occurrence of atopic dermatitis. *Acta Derm Venereol (Stockh)*, Suppl. 176, 7–12.

Sehgal, V.N. & Jain, S. (1993). Atopic dermatitis: clinical criteria. *Int J Dermatol*, **32**, 628–37.

Seymour, J.L., Keswick, B.H., Hanifin, J.M., Jordan, W.P. & Milligan, M.C. (1987). Clinical effects of diaper types on the skin of normal infants with atopic dermatitis. *J Am Acad Dermatol*, **17**, 988–97.

Sibbald, B. (1986). Genetic basis of asthma. *Sem Resp Med*, **7**, 307–15.

Sugiura, H., Uchiyama, M., Omoto, M. et al. (1997). Prevalence of infantile and early childhood eczema in a Japanese population: comparison with the disease frequency examined 20 years ago. *Acta Derm Venereol (Stockh)*, **77**, 52–3.

Sulzberger, M.B. (1983). Historical notes on atopic dermatitis: its names and nature. *Sem Dermatol*, **2**, 1–4.

Svensson, Å., Edman, B. & Möller, H. (1985). A diagnostic tool for atopic dermatitis based on clinical criteria. *Acta Derm Venereol (Stockh)*, Suppl. 114, 33–40.

Tada, J., Toi, Y., Akinyama, H. & Arata, J. (1994). Infra-auricular fissures in atopic dermatitis. *Acta Derm Venereol (Stockh)*, **74**, 129–31.

Taplin, D., Porcelain, S.L., Meinking, T.L. et al. (1991). Community control of scabies: a model based on use of permethrin cream. *Lancet*, **337**, 1016–18.

Turner, K.J. (1987). Epidemiology of atopic disease. In: Lessof,

M.H., Lee, T.H. & Kemeny, D.M. (eds.) *Allergy: An International Textbook*, pp. 337–45. London: John Wiley.

Visscher, M.O., Hanifin, J.M. & Bowman, W.J. (1989). Atopic dermatitis and atopy in non-clinical populations. *Acta Dermatol Venereol (Stockh)*, Suppl. 144, 34–40.

Wells, C.K., Feinstein, A.R. & Walter, S.D. (1990). A comparison of mathematical multivariate models for predicting survival – III. Accuracy of predictors in generating and challenge sets. *J Clin Epidemiol*, 43, 361–72.

Williams, H.C. (1992). Is the prevalence of atopic dermatitis increasing? *Clin Exp Dermatol*, 17, 385–91.

Williams, H.C. (1994). Epidemiology of atopic eczema. *Curr Med Lit Allergy*, 2, 3–7.

Williams, H.C. (1997a). Atopic dermatitis. In: Williams, H.C. & Strachan, D.P. (eds.) *The Challenge of Dermato-epidemiology*, pp. 125–44. Boca Raton: CRC Press.

Williams, H.C. (1997b). Defining cases. In: Williams, H.C. & Strachan, D.P. (eds.), *The Challenge of Dermato-epidemiology*, pp. 113–23. Boca Raton: CRC Press.

Williams, H.C. (1997c). So how do I define atopic eczema? – a practical manual for researchers. Department of Dermatology, University of Nottingham.

Williams, H.C. (1999). Diagnostic criteria for atopic dermatitis. Where do we go from here? *Arch Dermatol*, 135, 583–6.

Williams, H.C., Burney, P.G.J., Hay, R.J. et al. (1994a). The UK working party's diagnostic criteria for atopic dermatitis. I: Derivation of a minimum set of discriminators for atopic dermatitis. *Br J Dermatol*, 131, 383–96.

Williams, H.C., Burney, P.G.J., Strachan, D. et al. (1994b). The UK working party's diagnostic criteria for atopic dermatitis II: Observer variation of clinical diagnosis and signs of atopic dermatitis. *Br J Dermatol*, 131, 397–405.

Williams, H.C., Burney, P.G.J., Pembroke, A.C. et al. (1994c). The UK working party's diagnostic criteria for atopic dermatitis. III: Independent hospital validation. *Br J Dermatol*, 131, 406–16.

Williams, H.C., Forsdyke, H., Boodoo, G. et al. (1995a). A protocol for recording the sign of visible flexural dermatitis. *Br J Dermatol*, 133, 941–9.

Williams, H.C., Pembroke, A.C., Forsdyke, H. et al. (1995b). London-born black Caribbean children are at increased risk of atopic dermatitis. *J Am Acad Dermatol*, 32, 212–17.

Williams, H.C., Forsdyke, H. & Pembroke, A.C. (1996a). Infraorbital crease, ethnic group and atopic dermatitis. *Arch Dermatol*, 132, 51–4.

Williams, H.C., Pembroke, A.C., Burney, P.G.F. et al. (1996b). Community validation of the UK working party's diagnostic criteria for atopic dermatitis. *Br J Dermatol*, 135, 12–17.

Williams, H.C., Robertson, C.F., Stewart, A.W. et al. (1999). Worldwide variations in the prevalence of symptoms of atopic eczema in the International Study of Asthma and Allergies in Childhood. *J Allergy Clin Immunol*, 103, 125–38.

Wüthrich, B. (1991). Minimal forms of atopic eczema. In: Ruzicka, T., Ring, J. & Przybilla, B. (eds.), *Handbook of Atopic Eczema*, pp. 46–53. Berlin: Springer-Verlag.

Wüthrich, B. & Schudel, P. (1983). Die Neurodermatitis atopica nach dem Kleinkindesalter. *Z Hautkr*, 58, 1013–23.

Yates, V.M., Kerr, R.E.I. & MacKie, R.M. (1983). Early diagnosis of infantile seborrhoeic dermatitis and atopic dermatitis – clinical features. *Br J Dermatol*, 108, 633–8.

2

The pathophysiology and clinical features of atopic dermatitis

Clive B. Archer

Introduction

Atopic dermatitis (AD) is a common and fascinating inflammatory skin disease, frequently seen in patients with a personal or family history of atopic diseases, including asthma, allergic rhinitis or atopic dermatitis itself. As discussed in Chapter 1, AD is sometimes referred to as atopic eczema or infantile eczema, and here the terms 'dermatitis' and 'eczema' are used synonymously to describe skin inflammation characterized by erythema and scaling, and sometimes accompanied by vesiculation and crusting. The characteristic feature histologically is epidermal intercellular oedema (spongiosis, spongiotic microvesiculation), and the eruption of AD is usually extremely itchy.

Earlier studies showed the prevalence of AD to be 2% in the United States (Johnson, 1977) and 3% in England (Walker & Warin, 1956), but most recent studies suggest an increased prevalence. Kay et al. (1994) reported a lifetime prevalence of 20% in a UK population and, in a twin study, Schultz Larsen (1993) found a cumulative incidence rate up to seven years of age of 3% for twins born between 1960 and 1964, compared with 12% for those born between 1975 and 1979. Although AD can occur for the first time in adulthood, it begins in the first year of life in about 60% of cases, asthma and allergic rhinitis occurring after infancy (Rajka, 1975). Differences in climate and in exposure to environmental allergens, or genetic susceptibility to such factors, have been put forward to explain apparent differences in prevalence of AD in different racial or socioeconomic groups (Sladden et al., 1991; Jaafar & Pettit, 1993; Williams, Strachan & Hay, 1994; Williams et al., 1995). The disease generally runs a chronic relapsing course with a tendency to gradual improvement. Atopic dermatitis clears in about 40% of patients (Roth & Kierland, 1964; Musgrove & Morgan, 1976), being more likely to persist in those who are severely affected (Musgrove & Morgan, 1976).

Atopic dermatitis results from an interaction between genetic and environmental influences, trigger factors including irritants (e.g. detergents, house dust) and allergic factors (e.g. cow's milk, house dust mite). The importance of genetic factors has been confirmed by clinical studies (Uehara & Kimura, 1993; Diepgen & Fartasch, 1992; Dold et al., 1992; Schultz Larsen, 1993), although a specific gene abnormality (or, more likely, abnormalities) has not yet been determined. In 1989, Cookson et al. reported linkage between immunoglobulin E responses underlying asthma and rhinitis and chromosome 11q, but Coleman et al. (1993) were unable to establish linkage to chromosome 11q13 and AD. The aim of this chapter is to consider the pathophysiological mechanisms in AD at a cellular level before discussing the wide range of clinical features which may vary, depending on the age of the affected individual.

Pathophysiological mechanisms

Altered reactivity to a number of environmental stimuli is an important feature of atopy. The primary abnormality in AD may be genetic, immunological or biochemical, and these disciplines should not be considered in isolation. There is much experimental evidence for immune dysfunction in AD (for a review, see Leung, 1995), and we have some understanding of the cell regulatory mechanisms which underlie them. It has proved difficult to distinguish those abnormalities of relevance to AD per se as opposed to atopy in general, including asthma and allergic rhinitis.

Immunopathogenesis

Immunoglobulin E seems to play an important role in the pathogenesis of AD, having been implicated both in observations of immediate hypersensitivity and altered cell mediated immunity. Serum IgE levels are elevated in most patients with AD, the degree of elevation correlating with the severity of the disease (Juhlin et al., 1969; Stone, Muller & Gleich, 1973; Hoffman et al., 1975; Sampson & Albergo, 1984; Archer, 1986a). However, the fact that serum IgE levels are raised in around 80% of patients with AD does not explain the aetiology of the disease phenotype in those 20% of patients with normal IgE levels. Furthermore, the lesions of AD are not wheal and flare responses, suggesting that the clinical disease is not merely dependent on IgE-mediated mast cell degranulation. Positive immediate skin test responses to specific allergens do not always reflect clinical relevance, and patients in whom the AD burns itself out often continue to have positive skin test responses.

The mechanisms whereby allergens play a role in the pathogenesis of AD are complex. From a clinical point of view, in most patients under the care of dermatologists, irritant factors probably play a more important exacerbating role than allergic mechanisms, but recent evidence points to a role for food allergens (at least in a subset of patients), inhalant allergens and *Staphylococcus aureus*-secreted toxins, termed superantigens.

Most patients with AD, particularly older children and adults, are not allergic to foods. The occurrence of food allergy is likely to vary according to the age

and clinical features of the study population which, in turn, will depend on the special interests of clinicians and researchers. Early studies showed no advantage of soya milk or breast feeding in the prevention of atopic diseases (Halpern et al., 1973; Kjellman & Johanssen, 1979). More recent allergen avoidance studies in high-risk infants and their mothers have been conflicting (Hide et al., 1994; Sigurs, Hattevig & Kjellman, 1992; Falth-Magnusson & Kjellman, 1992), but at present it seems that strict avoidance of food allergens in infancy may delay, if not prevent, the onset of AD. In a large tertiary referral group of patients with AD and possible food allergy, Jones & Sampson (1993) found that 80% had a reaction to at least one food in a double-blind placebo-controlled food challenge, 75% of the food reactions involving the skin. Skin reactions occurred within two hours as itching, erythema or morbilliform rashes. Although some of the reactions resolved in three hours, others had itchy, macular reactions six to eight hours after challenge and, in some, repeated skin reactions led to scratching and the development of eczema. Cow's milk, eggs, peanuts, soy and wheat accounted for around 75% of positive food challenge results. With regard to therapy, a double-blind cross-over study showed that an antigen avoidance diet (excluding cow's milk, cow's milk products and eggs) was beneficial in a group of children with AD (Atherton et al., 1978).

The implication of inhalant allergens in the pathogenesis of AD is controversial. Mitchell et al. (1982) showed that patch testing of abraded skin with mite extract caused an eczematous rash, apparently not due to irritant effects. Subsequently, positive patch tests to inhalant allergens were reported in non-abraded skin of patients with AD (Clark & Adinoff, 1989), and the application to eczematous skin of mite antigen in anticipated environmental concentrations was shown to exacerbate AD (Norris, Schofield & Camp, 1988). Furthermore, avoidance of those inhalant allergens yielding positive patch tests or immediate hypersensitivity reactions has been reported to lead to clinical improvement of AD (Platts-Mills et al., 1991), although strict inhalant allergen avoidance measures are not presently routinely employed in the management of most cases of AD. IgE antibody to specific inhalant allergens has been found in some patients with AD, and IL-4-secreting T-cells which recognize *Dermatophagoides pteronyssimus* have been isolated from lesional skin (Van der Heijden et al., 1991; Van Reijsen et al., 1992).

Patients with AD have an increased tendency to develop bacterial, viral and fungal infections (Lacour & Hauser, 1993). It seems that *Staphylococcus aureus*, ubiquitous on the skin of patients with AD, exacerbates the inflammatory process by secreting toxins. These superantigens stimulate activation of T-cells and macrophages (Leung et al., 1993; Kotzin et al., 1993). Basophils from patients with AD who produce IgE antistaphylococcal toxin, release histamine on exposure to the specific exotoxin, in contrast to the lack of resonse in basophils from normal subjects or patients with AD who do not have IgE antitoxin (Leung et al., 1993). Other infectious agents, such as pityrosporum yeasts, may exacerbate AD, *Pityrosporum ovale* IgE antibodies having been found commonly in patients with AD, particularly in those with eczema of the head and neck (Kieffer et al., 1990).

Immunoregulatory dysfunction

There is much evidence to suggest immunoregulatory dysfunction in AD. Decreased peripheral blood CD8+ suppressor/cytotoxic T-cell number and function (Leung, Rhodes & Geha, 1981; Leung et al., 1983) is accompanied by evidence of cellular activation, serum levels of soluble IL-2 receptor being elevated in AD (Colver, Symonds & Duff, 1989). B-cells and monocytes from patients with AD express increased levels of CD23, low-affinity IgE receptor. IL-4 plays an important role in the induction of IgE synthesis and expression of CD23 on these cells, and AD lymphocytes secrete increased amounts of IL-4, expressing high levels of IL-4 receptor (Rousset et al., 1991; Renz et al., 1992).

The T-cells in a conventional delayed type hypersensitivity reaction are the Th1 type which secrete IFN-γ and therefore induce the expression of HLA-DR on keratinocytes (Tsicopoulous et al., 1992).

However, in lesional skin of AD, TH2 cells predominate and lesional keratinocytes do not express HLA-DR (Barker & MacDonald, 1987). Circulating mononuclear leukocytes (MNLs) from patients with AD have also been shown to produce less interferon-γ (IFN-γ) in response to a number of stimuli (Reinhold et al., 1988; Mosmann et al., 1986). IFN-γ usually inhibits IgE synthesis and the proliferation of TH2 lymphocytes (Jujo et al., 1992; Gajewski & Fitch, 1988), and the decreased IFN-γ production in AD along with the concomitant activation of IL-4 and IL-5, the characteristic TH2 cytokine profile (in contrast to the TH1 cytokine profile), is thought to play a central role in the pathogenesis of AD.

A number of studies have demonstrated increased numbers of allergen-specific T-cells producing increased IL-4 and IL-5 but little IFN-γ in peripheral blood and skin lesions of patients with AD (Wierenga et al., 1990; Van der Heijden et al., 1991; Van Reijsen et al., 1992; Chan et al., 1993). In addition, IL-4 inhibits IFN-γ production and downregulates the differentiation of TH1 cells (Vercelli et al., 1990). Monocytes from patients with AD have also been shown to secrete increased levels of IL-10 and prostaglandin E2 (Vercelli et al., 1990; Chan et al., 1993), both of which inhibit IFN-γ production. The cytokine profile may vary depending on whether the lesions are acute or chronic, there being some evidence for a predominance of IL-4 mRNA expression in early lesions (present for <3 days) of AD, whereas persistent lesions (present for >2 weeks) are associated with increased IL-5 mRNA and eosinophil infiltration (Hamid, Boguniewicz & Leung, 1994), better demonstrated by immunostaining for major basic protein than by routine histological techniques (Leiferman et al., 1985).

Thus, IgE-mediated mechanisms in AD may be immediate or delayed. Selected patients with AD exhibit increased plasma histamine levels after positive oral food challenges compared with placebo (Sampson & Jolie, 1984), and higher spontaneous histamine release from basophils (easier to study than mast cells) has been found in children with food sensitivity associated with AD (Sampson, Broadbent & Bernhisel-Broadbent, 1989).

Langerhans cells and macrophages in skin lesions from AD patients bear IgE antibody on their surfaces (Leung et al., 1987; Bruijnzeel-Koomen et al., 1986). Binding of IgE to Langerhans cells occurs through both high-affinity and low-affinity IgE receptors (Bieber et al., 1992; Vercelli et al., 1988). Patients with AD also have circulating autoantibodies to IgE, which can activate macrophages bearing IgE (Quinti et al., 1986). The activation of IgE-bearing Langerhans cells and macrophages of antigens and autoantibodies to IgE may therefore contribute to the inflammatory skin lesions in AD. Perpetuation of the lesions by scratching seems to be associated with release of keratinocyte-derived cytokines (Nickoloff & Naidu, 1994), including IL-1, tumour necrosis factor (TNF)-α and IL-4 which, via cell adhesion molecules, induce infiltration with lymphocytes, macrophages and eosinophils. In addition, inflammatory mediators derived from these cells or mast cells, such as histamine and platelet activating factor, are likely to play a role (Archer et al., 1984; Markey et al., 1990) (Figure 2.1).

Cell regulatory abnormalities

It has long been understood that cyclic nucleotides play an important role in cell regulation, and cyclic adenosine monophosphate (cyclic AMP) is a modulator of inflammation and immune responses (Bourne et al., 1974). The subject of cyclic nucleotide metabolism in AD has been extensively reviewed (Archer, 1987). Other cell regulatory mechanisms include the calcium–calmodulin system (Tomlinson et al., 1984; Rassmussen & Goodman, 1977), the phosphoinositide system (Berridge, 1984; Nishizuka, 1984), and the IL-4/IFN-γ system (Chan, Li & Hanifin, 1993).

Peripheral blood mononuclear leukocytes have frequently been studied, partly for convenience, but the relevance of these bone marrow-derived cells to the pathogenesis of AD has been emphasized by the findings that bone marrow transplantation for other indications can either confer a state of atopy (Saarinen, 1984; Tucker, Barnetson & Eden, 1985), or induce clearance of AD in patients with immunodeficiency disorders followed for up to five years (Saurat, 1985).

Cyclic AMP generally inhibits cellular activation, e.g. mast cell secretion, so that impaired cyclic AMP production might lead to increased activation of a number of cell types. Leukocytes from patients with AD have shown impaired beta-adrenoceptor effects on secretory responses and on cyclic AMP responses (Reed, Busse & Lee, 1976), a reduced affinity of beta-adrenoceptor binding sites (Pochet, Delespesse & Demaubeuge, 1980), and an increased ratio of alpha- to beta-adrenoceptor binding sites (Szentivanyi et al., 1980). Differences between cells from patients with AD and those from normal subjects have commonly been observed, although others have failed to confirm abnormal beta-adrenoceptor numbers of peripheral blood leukocytes (Galant et al., 1979; Ruoho, DeClerque & Busse, 1980).

In some studies, normal reactivity to prostaglandin E1 in leukocytes has accompanied reduced reactivity to beta-adrenoceptor stimulation (Reed, Busse & Lee, 1976). However, the selectivity of this impaired reactivity can be disputed, since it has been independently reported that cyclic AMP responses of MNLs are reduced in AD, not only to beta-adrenoceptor stimulants, but also to histamine (Busse & Lantis, 1979) and to prostaglandin E1 (Parker, Kennedy & Eisen, 1977). In one series of experiments, Archer et al. (1983) found that MNLs from patients with AD exhibited impaired cyclic AMP responses to prostaglandin E2 and histamine, as well as to isoprenaline, implying that impaired reactivity if not confined to the beta-adrenoceptor, as suggested by Szentivanyi (1968), but lies at a site common to all three agonists. In the same study, differences between cells from atopic and control groups were exaggerated by the omission of a potent phosphodiesterase inhibitor, providing indirect evidence consistent with the suggestion that nonselective impairment of responses may be secondary to increased cyclic AMP-phosphodiesterase activity observed in MNLs in AD (Grewe, Chan & Hanifin, 1982) (Figure 2.2).

Increased MNL cyclic AMP phosphodiesterase

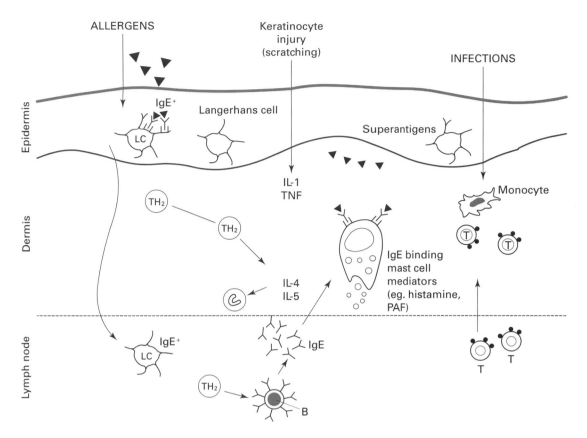

Fig. 2.1. In atopic dermatitis, it is proposed that prolonged exposure of the skin to allergens or superantigens leads to TH2 cell stimulation, allergen-specific IgE production, mast cell degranulation, eosinophil infiltration and inflammatory changes secondary to scratching

activity in AD may, in part, be due to *in vivo* desensitization due to chronic exposure to circulating histamine and other mediators (Safko et al., 1981; Chan et al., 1982). MNL adrenoceptor function will also partly depend on circulating adrenaline levels, but there is no evidence for desensitization at the level of the adrenal medulla in AD, since adrenaline responses to intravenous histamine infusions are not significantly different from normal responses (Archer et al., 1987).

Some of the studies on impure MNL populations have been repeated following isolation of monocytes and lymphocytes, and elevated phosphodieste-

rase activity has been reported to reside predominantly in the monocyte fraction (Holden, Chan & Hanifin, 1986), although Cooper, Chan & Hanifin (1985), in studies carried out in the same laboratory, also demonstrated elevated phosphodiesterase activity in the lymphocyte fraction. Whether elevated MNL phosphodiesterase activity in AD is a primary or secondary event is debatable, but elevated levels in the cord blood of neonates from atopic parents (Heskel et al., 1984) do not seem to be a sufficiently specific finding for this biochemical abnormality to be considered a genetic marker for atopy.

However, increased phosphodiesterase activity could underlie defective immune regulation in AD, since increased synthesis of IgE and increased histamine release by atopic leukocytes (presumably basophils) in culture have been shown to correlate with elevated phosphodiesterase activity in the same

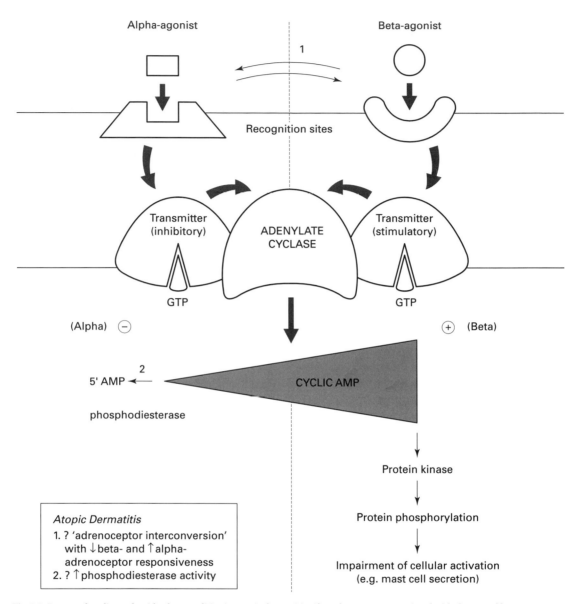

Fig. 2.2. Proposed cyclic nucleotide abnormalities in atopic dermatitis. Altered responses associated with decreased beta-adrenoceptor and increased alpha-adrenoceptor numbers and increased cyclic AMP phosphodiesterase activity would result in impaired cyclic AMP responses and unimpaired cellular activation (for example, increased mast cell secretion) (Archer, 1986a)

cells (Butler et al., 1983; Cooper et al., 1985). Cooper et al. (1985) further demonstrated that a phosphodiesterase inhibitor significantly reduced both the increased cyclic AMP-phosphodiesterase activity and the raised spontaneous IgE synthesis in vitro of MNLs from patients with AD. It has been suggested that altered cyclic nucleotide metabolism in T-helper lymphocytes in AD could result in abnormalities of T-cell immunoregulation (Cooper et al., 1983). Alternatively, impaired monocyte control of T-lymphocyte activation might be a consequence of abnormal monocyte cyclic nucleotide metabolism.

With regard to the calcium–calmodulin and phosphoinositide cell regulatory systems, there have been relatively few published studies in AD. The second messengers of the phosphoinositide system, diacylglycerol and inositol 1,4,5-triphosphate, are responsible for the activation of protein kinase C and mobilization of calcium ions, respectively. There is some evidence of aberrant protein kinase A and protein kinase C activity in the MNLs of patients with AD (Trask et al., 1985). In addition, there is likely to be some degree of interaction between the phosphoinositide and cyclic nucleotide cell regulatory systems.

The increased production of IgE by B lymphocytes in AD can be corrected in vitro by exposure of cells to the cyclic AMP-phosphodiesterase inhibitor, Ro 20-1724 (Cooper et al., 1985). As discussed above, B-cell IgE synthesis is also regulated by cytokines, increased IL-4 from T-cells in AD being associated with increased synthesis of IgE and decreased production of IFN-γ (Vercelli et al., 1990; Delprete et al., 1988). Evidence for interaction between the cyclic nucleotide cell regulatory system and cytokine-mediated immune dysregulation in AD has been put forward by Chan, Li & Hanifin (1993). Increased IL-4 production was demonstrated in 24 h cultures of MNLs and purified T-cells from patients with AD, there being a strong correlation between phosphodiesterase activity and IL-4 production in the atopic MNL fraction. IL-4 production in MNLs from patients with AD, but not normal subjects, could be reduced by the phosphodiesterase inhibitor, Ro 20-1724, this inhibitory effect acting primarily on the monocyte fraction and correlating with increased levels of cyclic AMP. This mechanism, and the apparent increased sensitivity of the phosphodiesterase isoform in AD (Chan & Hanifin, 1993; Chan, Li & Hanifin, 1993), may prove useful in the development of future drug therapy for AD.

Clinical features of atopic dermatitis

The diagnosis of AD depends on the history and physical examination, in conjunction with a personal and family history of atopy. Adjunctive immunological tests, such as total serum IgE level, immediate (type I) skin test reactivity, and radioallergosorbent tests (RASTs), have limited usefulness (Archer, 1986b).

In AD the skin in usually dry and extremely itchy. Scratching makes the eczema worse and produces lichenification, in which there is epidermal thickening and increased skin markings. The severity fluctuates with time and secondary bacterial infection, usually with *Staphylococcus aureus*, can be recognized as exudation and crusting. The severity of the disease can vary enormously, ranging from a child with the occasional dry, scaly patch of eczema, easy to treat with emollients, to a debilitating disease, much of the body being covered by excoriated, bleeding, infected lesions, and the patient severely distressed by the uncontrollable desire to tear at the skin. At whatever age of presentation, AD can dramatically affect quality of life and its high prevalence makes it an important health care issue.

In infancy, AD is typically manifested at three to six months by a red, sometimes scaly, rash on the cheeks (Figure 2.3). The wrists, extensor aspects of the legs (Figure 2.4), arms and neck are also frequently involved, and peri-auricular (often infra-auricular) fissures are common. In severe cases, weeping lesions, secondary bacterial infection and crusting may be present. The skin lesions may clear in a few months but relapse often occurs, for instance, during teething.

Older children and adults characteristically have a red, scaly eruption with a distribution on the flexural surfaces, particularly affecting the antecubital and

Table 2.1. A classifiction of the eczemas

Endogenous	Exogenous
Atopic dermatitis	Irritant dermatitis
Seborrhoeic dermatitis	Allergic contact dermatitis
Discoid eczema	Infective eczema
Asteatotic eczema	Photodermatitis
Pompholyx	Drug-induced eczema
Varicose (venous) eczema	

the popliteal fossae (Figures 2.5 and 2.6). A detailed analysis of skin lesion distribution in AD in relation to childhood age was reported by Aoki et al. (1992). As mentioned above repeated rubbing and scratching by the patient leads to lichenification (Figures 2.7 and 2.8), although this finding is not specific to AD. Vesicle formation is uncommon, although the histological finding of spongiosis is seen frequently.

Other typical sites of involvement are the eyelids, neck, forehead, and chest. Skin that clinically seems to be unaffected often appears dry and, during remissions, skin lesions may be absent. In black skin, close inspection of the skin may reveal erythema with epidermal changes, such as scaling, and the distribution of the eruption may be as in white skin. However, the predominant colour changes are often those of postinflammatory hyperpigmentation (Figure 2.8) and hypopigmentation, and the elbows, knees and extensor aspects of the limbs can be involved in the so-called 'reverse pattern' of AD (Figure 2.9). Perifollicular accentuation refers to the follicular papular appearance more commonly noted in patients with black skin or Orientals who have AD (Figure 2.10).

The distribution and pattern of eczema is often atypical and nonspecific, and definitive diagnosis is difficult. Before making a diagnosis of 'unclassified endogenous eczema', however, the many other forms of dermatitis should be considered (Table 2.1).

Diagnostic criteria

The criteria for the diagnosis of AD (Hanifin & Lobitz, 1977; Hanifin & Rajka, 1980) were initially

Table 2.2. Diagnostic criteria for atopic dermatitis in children and adults* (Modified from Hanifin & Rajka, 1980)

Major criteria
Pruritus
Flexural eczema and lichenification
Chronic relapsing course
Personal or family history of atopic disease

Minor criteria
Dry skin (xerosis)/ichthyosis vulgaris/hyperlinear palms
Immediate (type 1) skin test reactivity, elevated radioallergosorbent tests
Elevated total serum IgE
Tendency towards skin infection (*Staphylococcus aureus*, herpes simplex)
Tendency toward nonspecific hand or foot dermatitis
Infraorbital fold (of Dennie–Morgan)
Periocular darkening
Pityriasis alba
Itch when sweating
Intolerance of irritants
Perifollicular accentuation
Food allergies (e.g. urticarial reactions)

*A patient should have at least three major criteria accompanied by at least three minor ones.

drawn up to unify the concept of AD held by nondermatological researchers, but these criteria can be particularly helpful where the pattern of eczema is nonspecific. A modified form of the diagnostic criteria for patients over one year of age is shown in Table 2.2 (Archer & Hanifin, 1987). For definitive diagnosis, it has been suggested that the patient exhibit at least three of the major criteria, accompanied by at least three of the minor criteria.

The diagnosis of AD in infancy can be particularly difficult. Eczema is common in this age group, and it may be impossible to distinguish AD from seborrhoeic dermatitis. Facial eczema and involvement of the forearms and shins may help to distinguish AD in infancy from seborrhoeic dermatitis (Yates, Kerr & MacKie, 1983). Most dermatologists consider these two disorders in infancy to be separate entities (Rajka, 1975; Moller, 1981; Yates, Kerr & MacKie, 1983; Yates et al., 1983), although this has been dis-

Table 2.3. Diagnostic criteria in infants*

Major criteria
Family history of atopic disease
Evidence of pruritic dermatitis
Typical facial or extensor eczema and lichenification

Minor criteria
Dry skin (xerosis)/ichthyosis vulgaris/hyperlinear palms
Perifollicular accentuation
Chronic scalp scaling
Periauricular fissures

---

*An infant should have at least two major criteria or one major criterion plus one minor one.

puted (Vickers, 1980). Follow-up of infants with presumed AD may be necessary to confirm the diagnosis. In 1987, Archer & Hanifin suggested diagnostic criteria for AD in infancy, suggesting that the diagnosis of AD in this age group should depend on the presence of at least two of the major criteria, or one major criterion and one minor criterion listed in Table 2.3.

As discussed in detail in Chapter 1, Williams et al. reported in 1994 on the UK Working Party's Diagnostic Criteria for Atopic Dermatitis (Williams et al., 1994a, 1994b, 1994c), having systematically assessed the validity of the lengthy Hanifin & Rajka concensus criteria (1980). We determined a set of minimum discriminators for the diagnosis of AD, and our proposed diagnostic guidelines are as follows:

The patient must have:
An *itchy* skin disorder (or parental report of scratching or rubbing in a child), plus three or more of the following:

(1) History of the involvement of the skin creases such as folds of elbows, behind the knees, fronts of ankles or around the neck (including cheeks in children under 10).
(2) A personal history of asthma or hay fever (or history of atopic disease in a first-degree relative in children under 4).
(3) A history of general dry skin in the last year.

(4) Visible flexural eczema (or eczema involving the cheeks or forehead and outer limbs in children under 4).
(5) Onset under the age of 2 (not used if child is under 4).

These simplified and evaluated diagnostic criteria are more specific than the Hanifin & Rajka consensus criteria (1980) (93% compared with 78%), with only a slight fall in sensitivity (88% from 93%) (Williams et al., 1994c). It is of interest that, of the four major criteria suggested by Hanifin & Rajka (1980), i.e. pruritus, typical morphology and distribution, personal or family history of atopy, and chronicity, three are included in the six features derived from the UK Working Party's study (Williams et al., 1994a). The improved discrimination of the UK Working Party's diagnostic criteria for AD, along with the language of the criteria, should prove to be of great value in future studies of this capricious disease, whether carried out by dermatologists or nondermatologists.

Specific clinical features

Pruritus is an essential clinical feature of the disorder although, of course, it alone does not distinguish AD from other forms of eczema. About 50% of patients have a history of other atopic manifestations, such as asthma and allergic rhinitis, the incidence increasing with age. Around 70% have a family history of atopy (Hanifin & Rajka, 1980). Atopic dermatitis has nonspecific histological features which cannot be relied upon to distinguish it from other forms of eczema. Furthermore, biopsy of skin lesions in AD will not always reveal eczematous histological results; for example, there may be evidence of excoriation only.

Generalized dry skin (xerosis) is a helpful clinical sign of AD, and the disease is sometimes associated with ichthyosis vulgaris. Histological studies of the dry skin in AD have also revealed features of mild eczema (Finlay et al., 1980; Uehara, 1985). Hyperlinear palms are seen in patients with ichthyosis vulgaris, 50% of whom have atopic features (Rajka, 1975).

Immediate (type I) skin test reactivity (prick tests), RASTs, and elevated total serum IgE level are considered minor diagnostic criteria for AD. Immediate skin test reactivity is nonspecific, and routine skin testing in patients with AD can be misleading. Patients with AD usually have multiple positive skin test responses and may become convinced that apparent allergies are the cause of the eczema. Allergen avoidance is time-consuming and its value in treating the *majority* of patients with AD remains unproven (Halbert, Weston & Morrelli, 1995). The antigen battery used in skin testing is variable and the interpretation of results controversial. Allergists sometimes regard two or more positive wheal responses as significant but, in the presence of a negative control, even one positive wheal could be interpreted as being significant. Negative skin test responses, however, can help exclude a diagnosis of AD in a patient with nonspecific eczema.

Elevated total serum IgE levels are detected in a variety of skin diseases and in the hyperimmunoglobulin E syndrome (O'Loughlin et al., 1977), and normal total serum IgE levels can occur in up to 20% of patients with AD (Juhlin et al., 1969; Stone, Muller & Gleich, 1973; Hoffman et al., 1975; Sampson & Albergo, 1984). Whereas obtaining a clear-cut increase in total serum IgE (for example, more than 1000 units/ml in adults) and positive skin tests might be useful in diagnosing atypical AD, a normal total serum IgE level is not helpful.

Colonization of lesions of AD with *Staphylococcus aureus* is a common complication. Although rarely found in significant numbers on the skin of normal individuals, this organism appears to be universally present on patients who are experiencing exacerbations of AD. Infected areas of skin may resemble impetigo, a situation referred to as impetiginized eczema. Many patients with AD have staphylococcal infections (Hanifin & Rogge, 1977). In one study staphylococcal folliculitis was recorded in 16 of 45 patients who were admitted for hospital treatment (White & Noble, 1986). Herpes simplex lesions occur quite frequently on the skin of patients who have AD. The lesions are characteristically monomorphic and, in the presence of much scratching, one often

does not see vesicles. Clinically, the diagnosis can be difficult to distinguish from staphylococcal infection. Herpes simplex lesions on the skin of patients with AD may represent a relatively minor problem or, as extensive eczema herpeticum, can present with a very ill child, having systemic involvement and perhaps herpes encephalitis. As discussed above, altered cell-mediated immunity in AD is associated with an increased occurrence of superficial fungal infections (Jones, Reinhardt & Rinaldi, 1973; Kieffer et al., 1990).

Hand and foot dermatitis frequently occurs in patients with AD (Agrup, 1969). It can be difficult to decide, however, whether hand dermatitis in a patient with a history of AD but no other active lesions, represents atopic hand dermatitis or incidental irritant dermatitis. Since reactivity to irritants and AD are interrelated, some dermatologists would always diagnose atopic hand dermatitis in this situation. 'Protein contact dermatitis', particularly in patients with AD, is a cause of occupational dermatitis in food handlers (Janssens et al., 1995). Young children may have food allergies, usually urticarial reactions such as perioral contact urticaria in response to eggs and fish. From a clinical point of view, definite worsening of dermatitis in response to foods is unusual, but in one study, Oranje et al. (1992) reported the gradual development of an eczematous reaction at such 'food immediate-contact hypersensivity' sites.

More than 70% of patients with AD have a single infraorbital fold (of Dennie-Morgan), the more specific double fold occurring less frequently (Hanifin & Rajka, 1980). Periocular darkening of the skin (allergic shiners) is characteristic of a number of atopic disorders. Pityriasis alba, an eczematous condition with postinflammatory hypopigmentation, usually occurs on sun-exposed areas. It is common in patients with AD but may be seen in other individuals. Generally, hypopigmentation associated with AD results from the inflammatory disease and not the topical treatments, a misconception occasionally held by patients or their parents.

The following findings have also been associated with AD: nipple eczema, cheilitis, recurrent con-

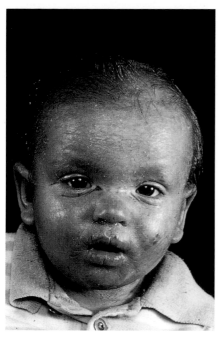

Fig. 2.3. Atopic dermatitis of infancy, with typical involvement of the face

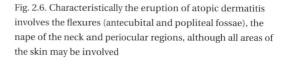

Fig. 2.5. Excoriated lesions of atopic dermatitis affecting the antecubital fossae

Fig. 2.4. Characteristic extensor involvement in infantile atopic dermatitis, with prominent post-inflammatory hyper-pigmentation in a Black child

Fig. 2.6. Characteristically the eruption of atopic dermatitis involves the flexures (antecubital and popliteal fossae), the nape of the neck and periocular regions, although all areas of the skin may be involved

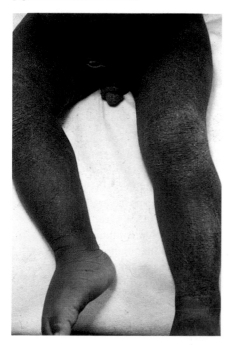

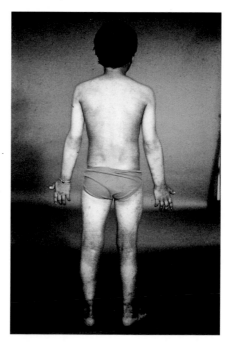

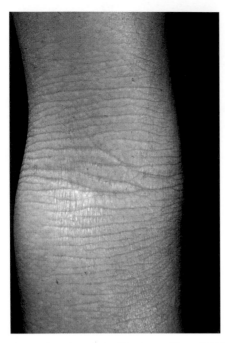

Fig. 2.7. Prominent lichenification (epidermal thickening with increased skin markings) in atopic dermatitis, as a result of rubbing and scratching

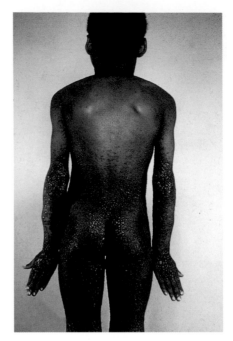

Fig. 2.9. 'Reverse pattern' of atopic dermatitis in black skin, showing thick lichenified lesions, particularly over the elbows and extensor surfaces

Fig. 2.8. Atopic dermatitis, showing post-inflammatory hyperpigmentation and lichenification of the popliteal fossae in a patient with deeply pigmented skin

Fig. 2.10. Follicular pattern of atopic dermatitis in black skin, the eczematous lesions being accentuated around hair follicles. Close inspection shows grey scales overlying areas of post-inflammatory hyperpigmentation

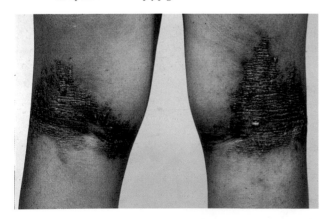

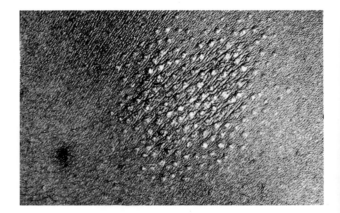

junctivitis, keratoconus, anterior subcapsular cataracts, facial pallor or erythema, anterior neck folds, all influenced by environmental and emotional factors, and white dermographism or delayed blanch in response to cholinergic agents (Hanifin & Rajka, 1980). The clinical variants of AD have been reviewed by Wüthrich (1991). However, in a study of the frequency of minor criteria in children with AD and unaffected children, nipple eczema, cheilitis, recurrent conjunctivitis, anterior neck folds, and perifollicular accentuation were no more common in the atopics compared with the control group (Kanwar, Dhar & Kaur, 1991). Diffuse scaling and peri-auricular (infra-auricular) fissures (Kanwar, Dhar & Kaur, 1991; Tada et al., 1994) seem to be justifiable minor diagnostic criteria and one group's findings endorsed the association of infraorbital folds and anterior neck folds with AD (Rudzkia et al., 1994), although prominent infraorbital folds are common in black children in the absence of AD (Williams & Pembroke, 1996).

Conclusions

Atopic dermatitis is a common skin disease which is frequently, but not always, associated with a personal or family history of atopic diseases, including asthma, allergic rhinitis and AD itself. The clinical features are sometimes characteristic but, as will be appreciated from the preceding account, the clinical expression of the disease can be extremely variable in site, morphology and time. In particular, the clinical severity and natural history of AD differs enormously between individuals.

It is broadly accepted that AD results from an interaction between genetic and environmental influences although, in contrast to findings in a specific subgroup of individuals with atopy, the precise genetic abnormality in AD, has not yet been established. It is my belief that AD is likely to represent the phenotypic expression of a number of genetic abnormalities. The relative importance of the roles played by irritant factors and allergens in the pathophysiology of atopic disorders seems to vary, depending on which target organ is predominantly involved. For many years, allergic mechanisms were considered to be less important in AD than in asthma, for example, but there is presently much evidence to suggest that immune dysregulation is central to the development and exacerbation of skin lesions in AD.

Future therapeutic measures might include those based on pharmacology or others, such as allergen avoidance. There is no shortage of potential targets for drug therapy and, as with other complex disorders, agents with defined but relatively nonselective mechanisms of action are likely to be more successful than selective agents. Nevertheless, selective agents are necessary in the context of research to determine the importance of a particular pathophysiological mechanism to the overall disease process.

In terms of health care, AD deserves much attention since it is such a common and often debilitating problem. The prevalence of AD appears to have increased over the past 30 years. It is important to continue to question the role of genetic factors, race, socioeconomic status and exposure to irritants (including pollutants such as cigarette smoke) and allergens (such as dietary antigens, inhalant antigens and bacterial superantigens).

Summary of key points

- Atopic dermatitis (AD) results from an interaction between genetic and environmental influences.
- Pathophysiological mechanisms in AD at a cellular level are complex.
- The importance of genetic factors has been confirmed by clinical studies, although a specific gene abnormality (or abnormalities) has not yet been determined.
- Environmental trigger factors include irritants (e.g. detergents, house dust, cigarette smoke) and allergic factors (e.g. cow's milk, house dust mite, bacterial superantigens).
- There is much experimental evidence for immune dysfunction in AD, which may be considered in relation to: immunoglobulin E; food allergens, inhalant allergens, superantigens; immediate hypersensitivity; cell-mediated immunity; IgE-

bearing Langerhans cells and macrophages; TH2 cytokine profile.

- Cell regulatory abnormalities in AD include impaired mononuclear leukocyte (MNL) cyclic AMP responsiveness, predominantly due to increased MNL cyclic AMP-phosphodiesterase activity, possible phosphoinositide system abnormalities, and cytokine (IL-4/IFN-γ)-mediated immune dysregulation.
- The clinical features of AD are often characteristic but can be extremely variable. The diagnosis of AD is discussed in the context of children and adults, infants, and the UK Working Party's Diagnostic Criteria.
- Since the prevalence of AD appears to have increased, it is important to continue to question the role of genetic factors, race, socioeconomic status, and exposure to irritants and allergens.

Acknowledgment

Figures 2.3 to 2.10 are reproduced from *Black and White Skin Diseases: An Atlas and Text*, by Archer, C.B. and Robertson, S.J. (1995), with kind permission from Blackwell Scientific Publications.

References

Agrup, G. (1969). Hand eczema and other hand dermatoses in South Sweden. *Acta Derm Venereol (Stockh)*, **49** Suppl. 61, 58–9.

Aoki, T., Fukuzumi, T., Adachi, J., Endo, K. & Kojima, M. (1992). Re-evaluation of skin lesion distribution in atopic dermatitis. *Acta Derm Venereol (Stockh)*, Suppl. 176, 19–23.

Archer, C.B. (1986a). Adrenoceptor function in atopic dermatitis. MD Thesis, London.

Archer, C.B. (1986b). Atopic dermatitis – an obvious diagnosis? *Clin Exp Dermatol*, **11**, 1–3.

Archer, C.B. (1987). Cyclic nucleotide metabolism in atopic dermatitis. *Clin Exp Dermatol*, **12**, 424–31.

Archer, C.B. & Hanifin, J.M. (1987). Recognizing atopic dermatitis. *Diagnosis*, **3**, 91–6.

Archer, C.B., Morley, J. & MacDonald, D.M. (1983). Impaired lymphocyte cyclic adenosine monophosphate responses in atopic eczema. *Br J Dermatol*, **109**, 559–64.

Archer, C.B., Page, C.P., Paul, W., Morley, J. & MacDonald, D.M.

(1984). Inflammatory characteristics of platelet activating factor (PAF-acether) in human skin. *Br J Dermatol*, **110**, 45–50.

Archer, C.B., Dalton, N., Turner, C. & MacDonald, D.M. (1987). Investigation of adrenomedullary function in atopic dermatitis. *Br J Dermatol*, **116**, 793–800.

Atherton, D.J., Sewell, M., Soothill, J.F. & Wells, R.S. (1978). A double-blind controlled cross-over trial of an antigen-avoidance diet in atopic eczema. *Lancet*, **1**, 401–3.

Barker, J.N.W.N. & MacDonald, D.M. (1987). Epidermal class II human lymphocyte antigen expression in atopic dermatitis: a comparison with experimental allergic contact dermatitis. *J Am Acad Dermatol*, **16**, 1175–9.

Berridge, M.J. (1984). Inositol triphosphate and diacylglycerol as second messengers. *Biochemical J*, **220**, 345–60.

Bieber, T., de la Salle, H., Wollenberg, A. et al. (1992). Human epidermal Langerhans cells express the high affinity receptor for immunoglobulin E (FceRI). *J Exp Med*, **175**, 1285–90.

Bourne, H.R., Lichtenstein, L.M., Melmon, K.L., Henney, C.S., Weinstein, Y. & Shearer, G.M. (1974). Modulation of inflammation and immunity by cyclic AMP. Receptors for vasoactive hormones and mediators of inflammation regulate many leukocyte functions. *Science*, **184**, 19–28.

Bruijnzeel-Koomen, C., van Wichen, D.F., Toonstra, J., Berrens, L. & Bruijnzeel, P.L.B. (1986). The presence of IgE molecules on epidermal Langerhans cells in patients with atopic dermatitis. *Arch Derm Res*, **287**, 199–205.

Busse, W.W. & Lantis, S.D.H. (1979). Impaired H2 histamine granulocyte release in active atopic eczema. *J Invest Dermatol*, **73**, 184–7.

Butler, J.M., Chan, S.C., Stevens, S.R. & Hanifin, J.M. (1983). Increased leukocyte histamine release with elevated cyclic AMP-phosphodiesterase activity in atopic dermatitis. *J Allergy Clin Immunol*, **71**, 490–7.

Chan, S.C. & Hanifin, J.M. (1993). Differential inhibitor effects on phosphodiesterase isoforms in atopic and normal leukocytes. *J Lab Clin Med*, **121**, 44–51.

Chan, S.C., Grewe, S.R., Stevens, S.R. & Hanifin, J.M. (1982). Functional desensitization due to stimulation of cyclic AMP-phosphodiesterase in human mononuclear leukocytes. *J Cyclic Nucleotide Res*, **8**, 211–24.

Chan, S.C., Li, S-H. & Hanifin, J.M. (1993). Increased interleukin-4 production by atopic mononuclear leukocytes correlates with increased cyclic adenosine monophosphate-phosphodiesterase activity and is reversible by phosphodiesterase inhibition. *J Invest Dermatol*, **100**, 681–4.

Chan, S.C., Kim, J.W., Henderson, W.R. & Hanifin, J.M. (1993). Altered prostaglandin E2 regulation of cytokine production in atopic dermatitis. *J Immunol* **151**, 3345–52.

Clark, R.A. & Adinoff, A.D. (1989). The relationship between positive aeroallergen patch test reactions and aeroallergen exacerbations of atopic dermatitis. *Clin Immunol Immunopathol*, **53**, 132–40.

Coleman, R., Trembath, R.C. & Harper, J.L. (1993). Chromosome 11q13 and atopy underlying atopic eczema. *Lancet*, **341**, 1121–2.

Colver, G.B., Symonds, J.A. & Duff, G.W. (1989). Soluble IL-2 receptor in atopic eczema. *Br Med J*, **298**, 1426–8.

Cookson, W.O.C.M., Sharp, P.A., Faux, J.A. et al. (1989). Linkage between immunoglobulin E responses underlying asthma and rhinitis and chromosome 11q. *Lancet*, **1**, 1292–5.

Cooper, K.D., Kazmierowski, J.A., Wuepper, K.D. & Hanifin, J.M. (1983). Immunoregulation in atopic dermatitis: functional analysis of T-B cell interactions and the enumeration of Fc receptor bearing T cells. *J Invest Dermatol*, **80**, 139–45.

Cooper, K.D., Chan, S.C. & Hanifin, J.M. (1985). Lymphocyte and monocyte localization of altered adrenergic receptors, cAMP responses, and cAMP phosphodiesterase in atopic dermatitis. A possible mechanism for abnormal radiosensitive helper T-cells in atopic dermatitis. *Acta Derm Venereol (Stockh)*, Suppl. 114, 41–7.

Cooper, K.D., Kang, K., Chan, S.C. & Hanifin, J.M. (1985). Phosphodiesterase inhibition by Ro 20-1724 reduces hyper-IgE synthesis by atopic dermatitis cells *in vitro*. *J Invest Dermatol*, **84**, 477–82.

Delprete, G., Maggi, E., Parronchi, P., Chretien, I., Tiri, A., Macchia Ricci, M., Bancbereau, J., De Vries, J. & Romagnani, S. (1988). IL-4 is an essential factor for the IgE synthesis induced in vitro by human T cell clones and their supernatants. *J Immunol*, **140**, 4193–8.

Diepgen, T.L. & Fartasch, M. (1992). Recent epidemiological and genetic studies in atopic dermatitis. *Acta Derm Venereol (Stockh)*, Suppl. 176, 13–18.

Dold, S., Wjst, M., von Mutius, E. et al. (1992). Genetic risk for asthma, allergic rhinitis, and atopic dermatitis. *Arch Dis Child*, **67**, 1018–22.

Falth-Magnusson, K. & Kjellman, N.I. (1992). Allergy prevention by maternal elimination diet during late pregnancy – a 5-year follow-up of a randomized study. *J Allergy Clin Immunol*, **89**, 709–13.

Finlay, A.Y., Nicholls, S., King, C.S. et al. (1980). The 'dry' non-eczematous skin associated with atopic eczema. *Br J Dermatol*, **103**, 249–56.

Gajewski, T.F. & Fitch, F.W. (1988). Anti-proliferative effect of IFN-γ in murine regulation. *J Immunol*, **140**, 4243–52.

Galant, S.P., Underwood, S., Allred, S. & Hanifin, J.M. (1979). Beta-adrenergic receptor binding on polymorphonuclear leukocytes in atopic dermatitis. *J Invest Dermatol*, **72**, 330–2.

Grewe, S.R., Chan, S.C. & Hanifin, J.M. (1982). Elevated leukocyte cyclic AMP-phosphodiesterase in atopic disease: a possible mechanism of cyclic AMP agonist hyporesponsiveness. *J Allergy Clin Immunol*, **70**, 452–7.

Halbert, A.R., Weston, W.L. & Morrelli, S.G. (1995). Atopic dermatitis: is it an allergic disease? *J Am Acad Dermatol*, **33**, 1008–18.

Halpern, S.R., Sellars, W.A., Johnson, R.B., Anderson, D.W., Saperstein, S. & Reisch, J.S. (1973). Development of childhood allergy in infants fed breast, soy or cow's milk. *J Allergy Clin Immunol*, **51**, 139–51.

Hamid, Q., Boguniewicz, M. & Leung, D.Y.M. (1994). Differential *in situ* cytokine gene expression in acute vs. chronic atopic dermatitis. *J Clin Invest*, **94**, 870–6.

Hanifin, J. M. (1977). Type I hypersensitivity diseases of the skin: divergent aspects of urticaria and atopic dermatitis. *Ann Allergy*, **39**, 153–60.

Hanifin, J.M. & Lobitz, W.C. Jr. (1977). Newer concepts in atopic dermatitis. *Arch Dermatol*, **113**, 663–70.

Hanifin, J.M. & Rogge, J.L. (1977). Staphylococcal infections in patients with atopic dermatitis. *Arch Dermatol*, **113**, 1383–6.

Hanifin, J.M. & Rajka, G. (1980). Diagnostic features of atopic dermatitis. *Acta Derm Venereol (Stockh)*, Suppl. 92, 44–7.

Heskel, N.S., Chan, S.C., Thiel, M.L., Stevens, S.R., Casperson, L.S. & Hanifin, J.M. (1984). Elevated umbilical cord blood leukocyte cyclic adenosine monophosphate–phosphodiesterase activity in children with atopic parents. *J Am Acad Dermatol*, **11**, 422–6.

Hide, D.W., Matthews, S. Matthews, L. et al. (1994). Effect of allergen avoidance in infancy on allergic manifestations at age two years. *J. Allergy Clin Immunol*, **93**, 842–6.

Hoffman, D.R., Yamamoto, F.Y., Geller, B. & Haddad, Z. (1975). Specific IgE antibodies in atopic eczema. *J Allergy Clin Immunol*, **55**, 256–67.

Holden, C.A., Chan, S.C. & Hanifin, J.M. (1986). Monocyte localization of elevated cAMP phosphodiesterase activity in atopic dermatitis. *J Invest Dermatol*, **87**, 372–6.

Jaafar, R.B. & Pettit, J.H.S. (1993). Atopic eczema in a multiracial country (Malaysia). *Clin Exp Dermatol*, **18**, 496–9.

Janssens, V., Morren, M., Dooms-Goossens, A. et al. (1995). Protein contact dermatitis: myth or reality? *Br J Dermatol*, **132**, 1–6.

Johnson, M.L. (1977). Prevalence of dermatologic disease among persons in numbers 1–74 years of age: United States. Vital and Health statistics of the National Center for Health Statistics. Jan 26: 4.

Jones, S.M. & Sampson, H.A. (1993). The role of allergens in atopic dermatitis. *Clin Rev Allergy*, **11**, 471–90.

Jones, H.E., Reinhardt, J.H. & Rinaldi, M.G. (1973). A clinical, mycological and immunological survey for dermatophytosis. *Arch Dermatol*, **107**, 217–22.

Juhlin, L., Johansson, G.O., Bennich, H. et al. (1969). Immunoglobulin E in dermatoses: levels in atopic dermatitis and urticaria. *Arch Dermatol*, **100**, 12–16.

Jujo, K., Renz, H., Abe, J., Gelfand, E.W. & Leung, D.Y.M. (1992). Decreased gamma interferon and increased interleukin-4 production promote IgE synthesis in atopic dermatitis. *J Allergy Clin Immunol*, **90**, 323–30.

Kanwar, A.J., Dhar, S. & Kaur, S. (1991). Evaluation of minor clinical features of atopic dermatitis. *Pediatr Dermatol*, **8**, 114–116.

Kay, J., Gawkrodger, D.J., Mortimer, M.J. et al. (1994). The prevalence of childhood atopic eczema in a general population. *J Am Acad Dermatol*, **30**, 35–9.

Kieffer, M., Bergbrant, I-M., Faergemann, J. et al. (1990). Immune reactions to *Pityrosporum ovale* in adult patients with atopic and seborrhoeic dermatitis. *J Am Acad Dermatol*, **22**, 739–42.

Kjellman, N.I. & Johanssen, S.G.O. (1979). Soy versus cow's milk in infants with bi-parental history of atopic disease: development of atopic disease in immunoglobulins from birth to four years of age. *Clin Allergy*, **9**, 347–58.

Kotzin, B.L., Leung, D.Y.M., Kappler, J. & Marrack, P. (1993). Superantigens and human disease. *Adv Immunol*, **54**, 99–166.

Lacour, M. & Hauser, C. (1993). The role of microorganisms in atopic dermatitis. *Clin Rev Allergy*, **11**, 491–522.

Leiferman, K.M., Ackerman, S.J., Sampson, H.A., Haugen, H.S., Venecie, P.Y. & Cleich, G.J. (1985). Dermal deposition of eosinophil granule major basic protein in atopic dermatitis: comparison with onchocerciasis. *N Engl J Med*, **313**, 282–5.

Leung, D.Y.M. (1995). Atopic dermatitis: the skin as a window into the pathogenesis of chronic allergic diseases. *J Allergy Clin Immunol*, **96**, 302–19.

Leung, D.Y.M., Rhodes, A.R. & Geha, R.S. (1981). Enumeration of T-cell subsets in atopic dermatitis using monoclonal antibodies. *J Allergy Clin Immunol*, **67**, 450–5.

Leung, D.Y.M., Wood, N., Dubey, D., Rhodes, A.R. & Geha, R.S. (1983). Cellular basis of defective cell-mediated lympholysis in atopic dermatitis. *J Immunol*, **130**, 1678–82.

Leung, D.Y.M., Schneeberger, E.E., Siraganian, R.P., Geha, R.S. & Bhan, A.K. (1987). The presence of IgE on monocytes/macrophages infiltrating into the skin lesion of atopic dermatitis. *Clin Immunol Immunopathol*, **42**, 328–37.

Leung, D.Y.M., Harbeck, R., Bina, P. Hanifin, J.M., Reiser, R.F. & Sampson, H.A. (1993). Presence of IgE antibodies to staphylococcal exotoxins on the skin of patients with atopic dermatitis: evidence for a new group of allergens. *J Clin Invest*, **92**, 1374–80.

Markey, A.C., Barker, J.N.W.N., Archer, C.B., Guinot, P., Lee, T.H. & MacDonald, D.M. (1990). Platelet activating factor-induced clinical and histopathological responses in atopic skin and their modification by the platelet activating factor antagonist BN 52063. *J Am Acad Dermatol*, **23**, 263–8.

Mitchell, E.B., Crow, J., Chapman, M.D., Jouhal, S.S., Pope, F.M. & Platts-Mills, T.A.E. (1982). Basophils in allergen-induced patch test sites in atopic dermatitis. *Lancet*, **1**, 127–30.

Moller, H. (1981). Clinical aspects of atopic dermatitis in childhood. *Acta Derm Venereol (Stockh)*, Suppl. 95, 25–8.

Mosmann, T.R., Cherwinski, H., Bond, M.W., Giedlin, M.H. & Coffman, R. (1986). Two types of murine helper T-cell clones. I. Definition according to profiles of lymphokine activities and secretory proteins. *J Immunol*, **136**, 2348–57.

Musgrove, K. & Morgan, J.K. (1976). Infantile eczema. A long-term follow-up study. *Br J Dermatol*, **95**, 365–72.

Nickoloff, B.J. & Naidu, Y. (1994). Perturbation of epidermal barrier function correlates with initiation of cytokine cascade in human skin. *J Am Acad Dermatol*, **30**, 535–46.

Nishizuka, Y. (1984). The role of protein kinase C in cell surface signal transduction and tumour promotion. *Nature*, **308**, 693–7.

Norris, G., Schofield, O. & Camp, R.D.R. (1988). A study of the role of house dust mite in atopic dermatitis. *Br J Dermatol*, **118**, 435–40.

Ohman, J.D., Hanifin, J.M., Nickoloff, B.J. et al. (1995). Overexpression of IL-10 in atopic dermatitis: contrasting cytokine patterns with delayed-type hypersensitivity reactions. *J Immunol*, **154**, 1956–63.

O'Loughlin, S., Diaz-Perez, J.L., Cleich, G.J., et al. (1977). Serum IgE in dermatitis and dermatosis: an analysis of 497 cases. *Arch Dermatol*, **113**, 309–15.

Oranje, A.P., Aarsen, R.S.R., Mulder, P.G.H. et al. (1992). Food-immediate contact hypersensitivity (FICH) and elimination diet in young children with atopic dermatitis: preliminary results in 107 children. *Acta Derm Venereol (Stockh)*, Suppl. **176**, 41–4.

Parker, C.W., Kennedy, S. & Eisen, A.Z. (1977). Leukocyte and lymphocyte cyclic AMP responses in atopic eczema. *J Invest Dermatol*, **68**, 302–6.

Platts-Mills, T.A.E., Chapman, M.D., Michell, B., Heymann, P.W. & Deuell, B. (1991). Role of inhalant allergens in atopic eczema. In: Ruzicka, T., Ring, J. & Przybilla, B. (eds.) *Handbook of Allergens* in *Atopic Eczema*, pp. 192–203. Heidelberg: Springer-Verlag.

Pochet, R., Delespesse, G. & Demaubeuge, J. (1980). Characterization of beta-adrenoceptors on intact circulating lymphocytes from patients with atopic dermatitis. *Acta Derm Venereol (Stockh)*, **92**, 26–9.

Quinti, I., Brozek, C., Geha, R.S. & Leung, D.Y.M. (1986). Circulating IgG antibodies to IgE in atopic syndromes. *J Allergy Clin Immunol*, 77, 586–94.

Rajka, G. (1975). The clinical aspects of atopic dermatitis. In: *Atopic Dermatitis*, pp. 4–35. London: Saunders.

Rassmussen, H. & Goodman, D.B.P. (1977). Relationship between calcium and cyclic nucleotides in cell activation. *Physiol Rev*, 57, 421–509.

Reed, C.E., Busse, W.W. & Lee, T.P. (1976). Adrenergic mechanisms and the adenyl cyclase system in atopic dermatitis. *J Invest Dermatol*, 67, 333–8.

Reinhold, U., Pawelec, G., Wehrmann, W., Herold, M., Wernet, P. & Kreysel, H.W. (1988). Immunoglobulin E and immunoglobulin G subclass distribution *in vivo* and relationship to *in vitro* generation of interferon-gamma and neopterin in patients with severe atopic dermatitis. *Int Arch Allergy Appl Immunol*, 87, 120–6.

Renz, H., Jujo, K., Bradley, K.L., Domenico, J., Gelfand, E.W. & Leung, D.Y.M. (1992). Enhanced IL-4 production and IL-4 receptor expression in atopic dermatitis and IL-4 receptor expression in atopic dermatitis and their modulation by interferon-gamma. *J Invest Dermatol*, 99, 403–8.

Ring, J., Senter, T., Cornell, R.C., Arroyave, C.M. & Tan, E.M. (1979). Plasma complement and histamine changes in atopic dermatitis. *Br J Dermatol*, 100, 521–30.

Roth, H.L. & Kierland, R.R. (1964). The natural history of atopic dermatitis. *Arch Dermatol*, 89, 209–14.

Rousset, F., Robert, J., Andary, M. et al. (1991). Shifts in interleukin-4 and interferon-γ production by T-cells of patients with elevated serum IgE levels and the modulatory effects of these lymphokines on spontaneous IgE synthesis. *J Allergy Clin Immunol*, 87, 58–69.

Rudzkia, E., Samochocki, Z., Rebandel, P. et al. (1994). Frequency and significance of the major and minor features of Hanifin and Rajka among patients with atopic dermatitis. *Dermatology*, 189, 41–6.

Ruoho, A.E., DeClerque, J.L. & Busse, W.W. (1980). Characterization of granulocyte beta-adrenergic receptors in atopic eczema. *J Allergy Clin Immunol*, 66, 46–51.

Saarinen, U.M. (1984). Transfer of latent atopy by bone marrow transplantation? A case report. *J Allergy Clin Immunol*, 74, 196–200.

Safko, M.J., Chan, S.C., Cooper, K.D. & Hanifin, J.M. (1981). Heterologous desensitization of leukocytes: a possible mechanism of beta-adrenergic blockade in atopic dermatitis. *J Allergy Clin Immunol*, 68, 218–25.

Sampson, H.A. & Jolie, P.L. (1984). Increased plasma histamine concentrations after food challenges in children with atopic dermatitis. *N Engl J Med*, 311, 372–6.

Sampson, H.A. & Albergo, R. (1984). Comparison of results of prick skin tests, RAST, and double-blind placebo-controlled food challenges in children with atopic dermatitis. *J Allergy Clin Immunol*, 74, 26–33.

Sampson, H.A., Broadbent, K.R. & Bernhisel-Broadbent, J. (1989). Spontaneous release factor in patients with atopic dermatitis and food hypersensitivity. *N Engl J Med*, 321, 228–32.

Saurat, J.H. (1985). Eczema in primary immune deficiencies. Clue to the pathogenesis of atopic dermatitis with special reference to the Wiskott–Aldrich syndrome. *Acta Derm Venereol (Stockh)*, Suppl. 114, 125–8.

Schultz Larsen, F. (1993). Atopic dermatitis: a genetic–epidemiologic study in a population-based twin sample. *J Am Acad Dermatol*, 28, 719–23.

Sigurs, N., Hattevig, G. & Kjellman, B. (1992). Maternal avoidance of eggs, cow's milk, and fish during lactation: effect on allergic manifestations, skin-prick tests, and specific IgE antibodies in children at age 4 years. *Pediatrics*, 89, 735–9.

Sladden, M.J., Dure-Smith, B., Berth-Jones, J. et al. (1991). Ethnic differences in the pattern of skin disease seen in a dermatology department – atopic dermatitis is more common among Asian referrals in Leicestershire. *Clin Exp Dermatol*, 16, 348–9.

Stone, S.P., Muller, S.A. & Gleich, G.J. (1973). IgE levels in atopic dermatitis. *Arch Dermatol*, 108, 806–11.

Szentivanyi, A. (1968). The beta adrenergic theory of the atopic abnormality in bronchial asthma. *J Allergy*, 42, 203–32.

Szentivanyi, A., Heim, O., Schultze, P. & Szentivanyi, J. (1980). Adrenoceptor binding studies with 3H (dihydroalprenolol) and 3H (dihydroergocryptine) on membranes of lymphocytes from patients with atopic disease. *Acta Derm Venereol (Stockh)*, 92, 19–21.

Tada, J., Toi, Y., Akyama, J. et al. (1994). Infra-auricular fissures in atopic dermatitis. *Acta Derm Venereol (Stockh)*, 74, 129–31.

Tomlinson, S., MacNeil, S., Walker, S.W., Ouis, C.A., Merritt, L.E. & Brown, B.L. (1984). Calmodulin and cell function. *Clin Science*, 66, 497–508.

Trask, D.M., Chan, S.C., Hirshman, C.A. & Hanifin, J.M. (1985). Effect of histamine on phosphorylation by protein kinases A and C in normal and atopic leukocytes. *J Invest Dermatol*, 84, 330.

Tsicopoulous, A., Hamid, Q., Varney, V. et al. (1992). Preferential messenger RNA expression of Th-1-type cells (IFN-γ+, IL-2 +) in classical delayed-type (tuberculin) hypersensitivity reactions in human skin. *J Immunol*, 148, 2058–61.

Tucker, J., Barnetson, R. & Eden, O.B. (1985). Atopy after bone marrow transplantation. *Br Med J*, 290, 116–7.

Uehara, M. (1985). Clinical and histological features of dry skin in atopic dermatitis. *Acta Derm Venereol (Stockh)*, Suppl. **114**, 82–6.

Uehara, M. & Kimura, C. (1993). Descendant family history of atopic dermatitis. *Acta Derm Venereol (Stockh)*, **73**, 62–3.

Ven der Heijden, F., Wierenga, E.A., Bos, J.D. & Kapsenberg, J.L. (1991). High frequency of IL-4 producing CD4$^+$ allergen-specific T lymphocytes in atopic dermatitis lesional skin. *J Invest Dermatol*, **97**, 389–94.

Van Reijsen, F.C., Bruijnzeel-Koomen, C.A., Kalthoff, F.S. et al. (1992). Skin-derived aeroallergen-specific T-cell clones of the T_{H2} phenotype in patients with atopic dermatitis. *J Allergy Clin Immunol*, **90**, 184–93.

Vercelli, D., Jabara, H.H., Lee, B., Woodland, N., Geha, R.S. & Leung, D.Y.M. (1988). Human recombinant interleukin-4 induces FceR$_2$/CD23 on normal human monocytes. *J. Exp Med*, **167**, 1406–16.

Vercelli, D., Jabara, H.H., Lauener, R.P. & Geha, R.S. (1990). IL-4 inhibits the synthesis of IFN-γ and induces the synthesis of IgE in human mixed lymphocyte cultures. *J Immunol*, **144**, 570–3.

Vickers, C.F.H. (1980). The natural history of atopic eczema. *Acta Derm Venereol (Stockh)*, Suppl. **92**, 113–5.

Walker, R.B. & Warin, R.P. (1956). Incidence of eczema in early childhood. *J Dermatol*, **68**, 182–3.

White, M.I. & Noble, W.C. (1986). Consequences of colonisation and infection by *Staphylococcus aureus* in atopic dermatitis. *Clin Exp Dermatol*, **11**, 34–40.

Wierenga, E.A., Snoek, M., Bos, J.D., Jansen, H.M. & Kapsenberg, M.L. (1990). Comparison of diversity and function of house dust mite-specific T-lymphocyte clones from atopic and non-atopic donors. *J Immunol*, 4651–6.

Williams, H.C. & Pembroke, A.C. (1996). Infraorbital crease, ethnic group, and atopic dermatitis. *Arch Dermatol*, **132**, 51–4.

Williams, H.C., Strachan, D.P. & Hay, R.J. (1994). Childhood eczema: disease of the advantaged? *Br Med J*, **308**, 1132–5.

Williams, H.C., Burney, P.G.J., Hay, R.J., Archer, C.B., Shipley, M.J. et al. (1994a). The UK Working Party's diagnostic criteria for atopic dermatitis: I. Derivation of a minimum set of discriminators for atopic dermatitis. *Br J Dermatol* **131**, 383–96.

Williams, H.C., Burney, P.G.J., Strachan, D., Hay, R.J., Archer, C.B. et al. (1994b). The UK Working Party's diagnostic criteria for atopic dermatitis. II. Observer variation of clinical diagnosis and signs of atopic dermatitis. *Br J Dermatol*, **131**, 397–405.

Williams, H.C., Burney, P.G.J., Pembroke, A.C., Hay, R.J., Archer, C.B. et al. (1994c). The UK Working Party's diagnostic criteria for atopic dermatitis: III. independent hospital validation. *Br J Dermatol*, **131**, 406–16.

Williams, H.C., Pembroke, A.C., Forsdyke, H. et al. (1995). London-born black Caribbean children are at increased risk of atopic dermatitis. *J Am Acad Dermatol*, **32**, 212–7.

Wüthrich, B. (1991). Minimal forms of atopic eczema. In: Ruzicka, T., Ring, J. & Przybilla, B. (eds.) *Handbook of Atopic Eczema*, pp. 46–53. Berlin: Springer-Verlag.

Yates, V.M., Kerr, R.E. & MacKie, R.M. (1983). Early diagnosis of infantile seborrhoeic dermatitis and atopic dermatitis – clinical features. *Br J Dermatol*, **108**, 633–8.

Yates, V.M., Kerr, R.E., Frier, K. et al. (1983). Early diagnosis of infantile seborrhoeic dermatitis and atopic dermatitis – total and specific IgE levels. *Br J Dermatol*, **108**, 639–45.

3

The natural history of atopic dermatitis

Hywel C. Williams and Brunello Wüthrich

Introduction

In a chapter such as this, it is tempting to simply repeat the same list of studies on the natural history of atopic dermatitis (AD) which have been quoted in other texts with little reservation. This would lead to a perpetuation of many of the myths surrounding this area. Instead, we will focus on highlighting the potentially serious flaws in previous studies which have examined the natural history of AD, and draw attention to major gaps in our current knowledge in order for future researchers to move forward in this important area. Before we do this, we should remind ourselves why studying the natural history of AD is important.

First, in the absence of any treatments which influence the natural history of AD, knowledge of disease prognosis is an important item of clinical information for AD sufferers and their families. As two physicians with an interest in AD, parents of children with AD invariably ask us 'will my child grow out of it?' Some ask more probing questions such as '*when* will my child grow out of it?' or 'why did my boy grow out of his eczema when he was aged 5, yet his sister continues to have it at the age of 10?' or 'will my child go on to develop asthma?' These are difficult questions to answer, and explaining prognosis in probabilistic terms to parents requires knowledge (which is scanty), special terms which convey the language of risk to the public (which we are generally poor at), and time (which is often in short supply). Adolescence is a particularly difficult time for AD cases which become persistent. Some adolescents understandably feel angry with previous doctors who had glibly informed them at a younger age that they would 'grow out' of AD (Williams, 1997).

Secondly, the phenomenon of clearance of AD in late childhood is a scientifically fascinating one. If, as many believe, AD is a mainly genetic disease, why should it clear at all? Is this because some genes have become inactive, other inflammatory suppressor genes have become active, or do we need to look for other explanations such as the development of immune tolerance or improved barrier function?

Thirdly, the identification of subgroups of AD sufferers with different prognosis and disease associations may shed light on shared genetic or environmental risk factors. Thus, children with severe AD in infancy who go on to develop asthma and hay fever are often said to represent a different phenotype from the more common mild case of AD in early childhood which clears after a few years (Roth, 1987). The identification of disease subgroups, if confirmed independently in further studies, could be useful in highlighting high-risk patients for public health interventions. However, great care has to be taken in making such *post hoc* assumptions of different disease subgroups on patients who present themselves to hospital, where apparent subsets related to referral patterns may occur (disease severity and concurrence of two or more diseases are both determinants of hospital referral). Only when one examines *all* AD cases in well defined populations can one begin to hypothesize about the possible existence of severe or persistent subgroups, or whether such individuals are simply part of a spectrum within the normal distribution of AD associations and prognosis.

Some past dermatological texts have had a tendency to be overoptimistic about the prognosis of AD. Whilst it is natural for physicians to want to comfort parents of children with this sometimes depressing disease, misleading them with an overoptimistic prognosis is a disservice in the long run. We would like to begin this chapter with the provocative statement that we do not think that one ever 'grows out of' AD. We believe that the increased propensity to react specifically to allergenic and nonspecifically to environmental irritants, along with decreased barrier function, might always be present in the constitutional background of an individual formally affected by AD. Some individuals may apparently be completely free of disease during adolescence, only for the disease to re-emerge in adulthood in a minor and often unreported form following exposure to irritants and other factors (Rystedt, 1986).

We will now examine critically the evidence surrounding the natural history of this common and important disease.

Age of onset

Why measure it?

Although age of onset of AD is usually mentioned in most texts, this information is of little use to parents of children with AD, since their child already has it. The main reason for wishing to know more about age of onset of AD is that it may point to possible causes. If, in fact, around 70% of AD cases are expressed below the age of two years, then it is unlikely that exposures which occur at around the age of 13 years are playing a major part in the incidence of this disease. The early onset of AD is thus a strong pointer to the possible role that factors occurring during the perinatal period and early infancy might have in the expression of AD (Williams, 1995). As Godfrey points out in Chapter 9, there are a number of critical growth periods in early development which might be susceptible to influences from a host of nutritional or metabolic factors, resulting in permanent 'programming' of adult disease. In this

sense, AD is an ideal disease to study using the cohort design. Unlike conditions such as cutaneous melanoma, where one has to wait for around 30 years to accrue sufficient cases, one can assemble a reasonable number of cases from a birth cohort study of AD within a few years.

Knowledge of age of onset is also of some use in separating AD from other inflammatory dermatoses. Indeed, in the multicentre study which developed diagnostic criteria for AD, age of onset below the age of two years was one of the most powerful discriminators for separating AD from other skin diseases (Williams et al., 1994). Thus, although it is possible to develop flexural AD for the first time at the age of 46 years, one is suspicious of such a diagnosis, and one would want to consider other possibilities, such as flexural psoriasis or contact dermatitis, with more vigour than one would at the age of two years.

Problem areas

A number of problems exist with the interpretation of studies which summarize the age of onset of atopic dermatitis. The first is rather obvious – that age of onset will depend on the age of the population of AD subjects examined. Thus, if one examines age of onset in 600 children aged 10 years, then one will miss cases with age of onset at age 12 years. If one looks at 600 adults with AD, this will increase the likelihood of including cases with later disease onset, which will in turn decrease the proportion of cases with onset in the first two years of life. Most AD studies refer to children: this will inevitably tend to bias estimates of age of onset towards early life.

The second problem in interpreting age of onset in AD is that most studies are based on hospital-ascertained cases. By definition, referral to hospital is related to disease severity. If, as other studies consistently suggest (Rystedt, 1986), early disease onset is a predictor of disease severity, then studies of disease onset in hospital cases will again tend to overestimate the true population proportion of early onset cases. Studies which look at entire populations of AD cases in the community are needed to overcome this bias.

Table 3.1. Studies which have recorded some data on age of onset of atopic dermatitis

Author and date	Study design and sample size	Source of cases	Case definition	Age at follow-up	Age of onset	Comments
Nexmand (1948)	Retrospective $n = 100$	Hospital	Dermatologist diagnosis	1 to 40 years	42% by age 1 year and 80% by 5 years	Methods unclear
Helleström & Lidman (1956)	Retrospective $n = 311$	Hospital	Dermatologist diagnosis	Up to 40 years	63% by age 1, 87% by age 5	Methods unclear
Oddoze (1959)	Retrospective $n = 206$	Hospital	Dermatologist diagnosis	Mean age 17 years	75% by age 1, 86% by age 5	Methods unclear
Wagner & Pürschel (1962)	Retrospective $n = 1059$	Three hospital skin clinics	Dermatologist	Up to 30 years	60% by age 1 in males, 67% by age 1 in females	Methods unclear
Wüthrich (1975)	Retrospective $n = 132$	Specialist outpatient clinic	Dermatologist diagnosis	95% up to 15 years	72% by age 1 year	Additional data on asthma and hay fever onset
Wüthrich & Schudel (1983)	Retrospective $n = 121$	Children referred to specialist clinic	Dermatologist	Mean age 15 years	88% by age 1 year (average 5.5 months)	Additional data on asthma and hay fever onset
Rajka (1989)	Retrospective $n = 1200$	Hospital	Dermatologist diagnosis	Up to 50 years	60% by age 1 in males, 55% by age 1 in females	Methods unclear
Quille-Roussel et al. (1985)	Prospective $n = 500$	Hospital	Dermatologist diagnosis	5.7 years	81.5% by age 1, 91% by age 2 years	No association with age of onset and disease severity and sex of child
Åberg & Engstrom (1990)	Retrospective questionnaire 694 eczema cases	Community	Partly validated symptom-based questionnaire	14 years	63% by 7 years	Additional data on asthma and hay fever onset
Williams & Strachan (1988)	Historical cohort study $n = 6877$	Community	Parental report and physician diagnosis	Up to 16 years	66% by age 7	National birth cohort study

The studies

These (Nexmand, 1948; Helleström & Lidman, 1956; Oddoze, 1959; Wagner & Pürschel, 1962; Wüthrich, 1975; Wüthrich & Schudel, 1983; Quille-Roussel, Raynaud & Saurat, 1985; Rajka, 1989; Åberg & Engstrom, 1990; Williams & Strachan, 1998) are summarized in Table 3.1. As predicted in the preceding paragraph, age of onset in the two studies where cases were ascertained from the community (Åberg & Engstrom, 1990; Williams & Strachan, 1998) is later when compared with hospital-based studies. The distribution for age of onset also shifts towards a later onset for studies which include older subjects. No marked sex differences in the age of onset was noted, with the exception of Åberg and Engstrom's study where a female:male ratio 2:1 occurred for AD onset after the age of two years. In the 1958 British birth cohort study (Williams & Strachan, 1998), age of onset was significantly earlier for eczema cases defined during a point examination of the children by medical officers when compared with cases of eczema defined by parental report of symptoms by parents over the last 12 months. One possible explanation of this is that early onset is a predictor of disease chronicity and that there is likely to be an overrepresentation of chronic or severe in prevalence surveys conducted at one point in time.

Conclusions

Most studies based on hospital-ascertained cases have probably overestimated the proportion of cases of AD with early onset because early onset may be a predictor of disease severity. Studies which examine age of onset in case series of younger age groups will also overestimate the proportion of cases with early onset by excluding those who might have disease onset at a later age. Despite these limitations, studies of well defined cases suggest that most (70%) AD cases become manifest within the first five years of life. The early onset of AD suggests that factors operating in early life may be critical for disease expression.

Studies of disease fluctuation over weeks or months

Whilst recording the persistence of disease over many years provides useful clinical and scientific information, there is also a need to understand more about the anatomical site and fluctuation of AD over shorter intervals. If it is true that the distribution of AD changes from cheeks and hands in infants to flexures in older children (Aoki et al., 1992), then this may give us a clue about likely factors which exacerbate disease, such as irritants or aeroallergens. If, as some physicians observe, AD is present one day and is apparently gone within a space of two or three days, then this may tell us something about the type of cells or inflammatory mediators which are likely to be responsible for the visible changes of AD.

Furthermore, if long-term studies suggest that AD tends to recur in the same sites within individuals over long periods, this suggests that such lesions may be associated with collections of abnormal cells, such as tissue specific T-lymphocytes which become 'fixed' at these tissue sites and retain their ability to express surface receptors which can react to circulating antigen or other signals which induce nonspecific inflammation (Boguniewicz, 1998).

Despite the scientific need to gain such information, this area represents a major gap in our knowledge. This is difficult to understand as such information would seem to be readily available by studying cases in hospital settings. Apart from a few isolated studies, our understanding of the short- to medium-term fluctuations in site and activity of AD is scanty and deserves further investigation.

Clinical trials

Inspection of the time course of AD symptoms and signs in control groups which have been used as outcome measures in clinical trials of treatments for AD, suggest large variations in disease activity scores over the course of a few days (Harper et al., 1991). Such data are limited as most control groups exhibit significant placebo effects in atopic eczema.

However, one of the most striking anomalies in clinical trials of treatments for AD over the last 30 years is the obsession with short-term outcome measures. As this chapter demonstrates, AD is a fluctuating disease with relapses and remissions over many months and years, yet almost every clinical trial of treatments for AD to date has examined short-term outcome measures such as erythema, degree of papulation, lichenification, scaling, etc., at periods of usually no longer than six weeks. Whilst it is important to demonstrate that treatment with topical corticosteroids can help to control an isolated exacerbation quite quickly, it is also vital to demonstrate the effects of such treatment on disease chronicity (Van der Meer et al., 1999). Some of our patients who are wary of topical corticosteroid preparations sometimes fear that their use 'makes the condition come back more often' or 'drives the disease into the body only to emerge at a later time as asthma or hay fever'. Such notions may appear simplistic and not in accord with our 'clinical experience', but until evidence is produced in the form of clinical trials which record longer-term end-points for AD, such as number and median duration of 'disease-free periods', we should not dismiss such concerns too readily.

Despite the time course similarities of AD to other chronic relapsing and remitting conditions such as rheumatoid arthritis or multiple sclerosis, nobody to our knowledge has yet attempted to define what is a disease 'remission' for AD. This major methodological obstacle needs to be overcome. Work is currently in progress at Nottingham to try to develop such a scale which is sensitive to patients' views, where techniques such as time series analysis (Bahmer, 1992) could be used to examine repeated events.

Other studies

Some authors have demonstrated that the face and hands are the most common sites of involvement for babies, with flexural involvement predominating in older children (de Graciansky, 1966; Quille-Roussel, Raynaud & Saurat, 1985; Lammintausta et al., 1991). Undoubtedly the most detailed study of the distribution of AD lesions with time in children is that of Aoki et al. (1992). They studied 1012 patients aged under ten years attending a dermatology outpatient clinic in Japan. These children were divided into five age groups (3–5 months, 6–11 months, 1 year, 2–4 years and 5–9 years) and the presence or absence of visible eczema was recorded in 52 specified regions of the body. Findings were compared between different age groups and between those who had a personal or family history of atopy (80%) and those who did not. The study suggested that there was a change in distribution from the head, scalp and around the ears to the neck and flexures between one and two years of age. The trunk was the most common area to be affected, whereas the nose, upper chest, palms and feet were the least commonly involved areas. Only upper arms were affected more frequently on the external side than

the internal side in all age groups. Personal or family history of other atopic disease did not affect these findings. Although it is true that this study did not follow the *same* individual children prospectively in time, the inference of change in distribution of lesions is likely to hold unless there were specific cohort events occurring at that time which could have explained the particular distribution in certain age groups. Because this was a cross-sectional study, it is not possible to comment on the fluctuation of disease activity over time.

In addition to direct clinical observation of patients, other studies which hint at the fluctuating course of AD are epidemiological surveys which have recorded both point and period prevalences of AD. Such studies have suggested a ratio of point to period prevalence of AD of around 1:1.5 (Dotterud et al., 1995; Saval et al., 1993), suggesting that visible or symptomatic disease is present only two thirds of the time in an 'average' case of mild AD. This ratio is likely to change towards a more continuous course when more severe cases are studied, although the exact relationship between disease severity and chronicity is unknown.

Longer term 'clearance' rates

Problem areas

Most studies examining the natural history of AD to date have been retrospective case series, i.e. they have identified previous cases from hospital notes or registers and requested up-to-date information on subsequent clearance or recurrences. The main problems associated with such an approach are difficulties in ensuring a large enough sample, biases which might occur by selecting only the more accessible individuals and difficulty in tracing such individuals over a long period. Case definition is unlikely to be uniform unless a special study was designed at the outset. Hospital cases are likely to exclude those with milder disease, limiting the generalizability of the study. Cases in such retrospective studies are likely to have been assembled at different ages, rendering it difficult to make

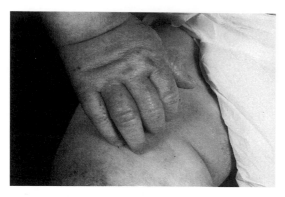

Fig. 3.1. How does one define a true disease remission in atopic dermatitis: when symptoms cease, when there is no visible erythema, or when normal barrier function is restored?

summary statements about prognosis according to age of onset unless very large samples (i.e. 1000+) are employed. Prospective studies are ideally required to examine issues of disease persistence, and recommendations for a 'good' study are given at the end of this chapter (Sackett et al., 1997).

Another challenge facing those who wish to conduct studies of the natural history of AD is defining terms such as 'remission' (Figure 3.1) or real and apparent clearance rates. Most physicians can recall cases of AD who were apparently clear during teenage years only to present with a disease recurrence in early adulthood. The classical example is the case of irritant hand dermatitis superimposed on a background of atopic dermatitis in those taking up wet-work occupations or mothers nursing young children. This begs the question, therefore, of how long a person should be clear of AD before he or she can be declared 'clear'. Defining 'a remission' may also prove difficult – should this refer to cessation of symptoms or the complete restoration of the skin to a normal appearance as judged by the patient or a dermatologist, or should it be defined by tests of barrier function? Many clinicians have anecdotally suggested that the dry or 'sensitive' skin characteristic of atopic dermatitis may persist for life, even in the absence of clinical eczema (Thune, 1989). It is difficult to study this notion further until the debate on whether such dry skin simply represents low-grade eczematous inflammation is clearer (Al-Jabin

& Marks, 1984). Although the methodologies for tackling the above problems are still in their infancy researchers need to record, as a minimum requirement, exactly how they have defined a remission. Attempts should also be made at adjusting 'apparent' clearance rates at one point in time by subsequent recurrences.

Most follow-up studies have relied upon following cohorts of patients at fixed narrow time intervals, recording prevalent disease. Such a strategy will miss some children with transient mild disease. Because of the intermittent nature of AD, it is also clear that the recurrence rate in any study could be directly proportional to the *frequency* of follow-up – thus an AD cohort study which requests information about disease symptoms in its subjects on a weekly basis is likely to report a poorer prognosis for AD than a study which requests information at a point five or ten years later.

As highlighted in Chapter 1, another major problem in AD research in relation to cohort studies is defining a truly incident case. Most definitions of AD utilize elements of disease chronicity. How, therefore, can one define a truly incident case? How can we be sure that those mild transient eczematous rashes which occur just once in infancy are not in fact part of the spectrum of the AD syndrome? Thus, studies which include only well defined AD cases may exclude milder transient cases with a better prognosis. There seems to be no way around this problem until better gold standards are available for defining incident cases.

Studies which have examined real and apparent atopic dermatitis clearance

These (Boddin, 1930; Edgren, 1943; Osborne & Murray, 1953; Vowles, Warin & Apley, 1955; Finn, 1955; Kesten, 1954; Purdy, 1953; Heite, 1961; Burrows & Penman, 1960; Meenan, 1959; Berlinghoff, 1961; Roth & Kierland, 1964; Stifler, 1966; Musgrove & Morgan, 1976; Vickers, 1980; van Hecke & Leys, 1981; Wüthrich & Schudel, 1983; Rystedt, 1986; Quille-Roussel et al., 1985; Businco et al., 1989; Åberg & Engstrom, 1990; Linna et al., 1992; Kissling & Wüthrich, 1993; Lammintausta, Mäkelä & Kalimo,

1995; Williams & Strachan, 1998) are summarized in Table 3.2. Many of the earlier studies are very small, have selected a severe subset of children who were hospitalized, and have poor response rates. The usefulness of such studies, therefore, is severely limited by possible selection and response bias.

Given the limitation in comparing studies which have been performed in different countries with different sources and definitions of subjects, most studies suggest that AD is a chronic disease with ten-year clearance rates of around 50 to 70% for most cases with onset in childhood. The only exception is the Vickers study which reports ten-year clearance rates in excess of 90%. It is difficult to explain the unusually good prognosis reported in Vickers' study (Vickers, 1980). This was a large prospective study with good follow-up rates, and some attempt at adjustment for subsequent recurrences was made. However, disease prognosis according to age of onset cannot be discerned from the data shown in the paper, and the person recording disease status was fully aware of the study's aims. It is also possible that the favourable outcomes could have been the result of enthusiastic treatment by the one investigator who was also responsible for the patients' management. We are not told how often the children were examined or interviewed, or how clearance was defined. Cases of seborrhoeic dermatitis of infancy, which may have a more favourable prognosis, were also included in the inception cohort of Vickers' study.

Studies which have long follow-up periods suggest that many individuals who are apparently clear at one period in their life, subsequently relapse at a later point (Vickers, 1980; Williams & Strachan, 1998). It is possible that if cohorts of AD individuals were followed up frequently enough and for long enough, most individuals would exhibit some form of recurrence at some stage in their life, although many such recurrences will be asymptomatic and clinically unimportant. Some studies suggest that, in the absence of disease clearance, disease severity is also likely to decrease with time, emphasizing the importance of recording severity in relation to morbidity or disability in future natural history studies. Perhaps an appropriate question when considering end-points for future follow-up studies is therefore 'what proportion of people who still have eczema are no longer *bothered* by it?' in addition to recording disease clearance as defined by a doctor.

Determinants of disease prognosis

Not surprisingly, studies which have examined determinants of disease prognosis are largely the same as those which have examined natural history. Such historical cohort studies have been constrained into examining only those features which have been recorded in the inception cohort.

Studies which have examined possible determinants of AD persistence (Wüthrich, 1996; Williams & Strachan, 1993; Lammintausta et al., 1991; Åberg & Engstrom, 1990; Vickers, 1980; Rystedt, 1986; Roth & Kierland, 1964; Vowles, Warin & Apley, 1955; Musgrove & Morgan, 1976; van Hecke & Leys, 1981; Quille-Roussel, Raynaud & Saurat, 1985) are summarized in Table 3.3. Given the limitation that different studies have looked at different risk factors for persistence, there appears to be reasonably consistent evidence that early disease onset, severe early disease, concomitant asthma and family history of atopic dermatitis appear to be the strongest predictors for a poor outlook for childhood AD. Even less is known about the long-term prognosis and determinants of prognosis of adult atopic eczema. One study of 1008 adults with atopic skin disease since their teenage years in Finland (Lammintausta & Kalimo, 1993) suggested that persistence of disease was independent of type of occupation (e.g. nursing work versus office work). Inevitably, there could be a 'healthy worker effect' which could partly bias such studies, i.e. a person with more severe eczema or previous problems with hand eczema as a teenager might be less likely to take up a job such as hairdressing with high exposure to irritants.

Conclusions

Generalizing prognostic studies across time and space is a limited exercise – accessibility, effectiveness and use of health services and treatments is likely to be different within and between

Table 3.2. Studies which have recorded data on the long-term prognosis of atopic dermatitis

Author and date	Sample size	Source of sample	Way disease was defined at follow-up	Age of inception cohort	Length of follow-up in years	Losses to follow-up	Adjusted for recurrent disease?	Clearance rate	Comments
Boddin (1930)	33	Children in hospital	Examination	3–6 months to 9 years	2 years	Not stated	No	43%	Time period of follow-up unclear
Edgren (1943)	311	Hospital inpatients and outpatients	Examination at home (nurse) and questionnaire	Onset before 2 years	17–38 years	Unclear	No	37%	Time period of follow-up unclear
Osborne & Murray (1953)	98	Hospital clinic	Examination	Under 2 years	3–5 years	Not stated	Not stated	20%	Scanty details
Vowles et al. (1955)	84	Hospital inpatients	Questionnaire and examination	Infantile	13–22	26%	No	45%	Severe subset of cases
Finn (1955)	37	Hospital	Questionnaire	Infants	15–22	73%	No	59%	V. poor response rate
Kesten (1954)	200	Hospital clinic	Questionnaire	Unclear	7 years	Not stated	No	35%	Methods unclear
Purdy (1953)	93	Hospital inpatients	Questionnaire	Onset before 1 year	16–22	72%	No	72%	V. poor response rate
Heite (1961)	166	Hospital inpatients	Questionnaire and examination	Onset before 1 year	Unclear	62%	No	66%	V. poor response rate
Burrows & Penman (1960)	43	Hospital inpatients	Questionnaire and examination	Infants	8–11	12%	No	17–37%	Severe subset
Meenan (1959)	42	Hospital inpatients	Questionnaire	Infants	14–27	31%	No	70%	
Berlinghoff (1961)	234	Hospital inpatients	Questionnaire	Infants	8–22	45%	No	56%	
Roth & Kierland (1964)	221	Hospital in- and outpatients	Questionnaire	Children and young adults	20	55%	No	29% for severe cases 40% for mild cases	Poor response rate

Study	N	Setting	Method	Age	Age	%	Follow-up	%	Comments
Stifler (1966)	40	Hospital	Questionnaire	Onset before 1 year	22–25	20%	No	65%	Severe cases
Musgrove & Morgan (1976)	99	Hospital	Examination	Aged under 5 years	15–17	32%	No	42%	Poor response rate
Vickers (1980)	1897	Hospital outpatients	Examination	5–20		5%	Yes	84–92%	Large prospective review by one individual. High response rate. Unclear methods
van Hecke & Leys (1981)	50	Hospital in- and outpatients		Aged less than 5 years	20	37%	No	38%	Poor response rate
Wüthrich & Schudel (1983)	227	Hospital	Questionnaires and examination	Infancy	15 and 23.5	Unclear	Yes	11.3%. Detailed description of different course of disease in different possible subtypes	Other data on asthma and atopy recorded
Rystedt (1986)	955	Inpatients (549) + outpatients (406)	Questionnaire and examination	0–14 years	24–44	Less than 3%	Unclear	38% inpatients 60% outpatients	Careful study with some validation of diagnosis and very low loss to follow-up
Quille-Roussel et al. (1985)	200	Hospital in- and outpatients	Questionnaire and examination	Unclear – up to 5.7 years	Up to 6 years	60%	No	26%	Prospective study of children at different ages with very short follow-up period
Businco et al. (1989)	68	Hospital clinics	Examination by paediatrician	4 months to 10.5 years	5	18%	No	57%	Children selected on the basis of AD and food hypersensitivity

Table 3.2 (*cont.*)

Author and date	Sample size	Source of sample	Way disease was defined at follow-up	Age of inception cohort	Length of follow-up in years	Losses to follow-up	Adjusted for recurrent disease?	Clearance rate	Comments
Aberg & Engstrom (1990)	694	Community	Questionnaire	Unclear	Unclear	Not applicable	Yes	34%	Cross-sectional study of Swedish 14-year-olds with past 'eczema' who were asked when symptoms ceased
Linna et al. (1992)	40	Hospital in-patients	Examination	Under 2 years	11–13	Unclear	No	18%. Less severe in 65%	Additional data on atopy
Kissling & Wüthrich (1993)	106	Hospital clinic	Questionnaire and examination	<2 years	20	12%	Yes	39%	Additional data on atopy
Lammintausta et al. (1995)	801	Hospital outpatients	Questionnaire and examination	12–16 years	Around 20	19%	Unclear	30% for severe cases. 45% for moderate, 70% with minor AD	Large study with low losses to follow-up and additional data on asthma, hay fever and atopy
Williams (1997)	571	Community	Questionnaire and examination	7 years	9	Less than 10%	Yes	53% after 4 years and 65% after 9 years	National birth cohort study. Some additional data at age 23 years

Table 3.3. Studies which have examined possible determinants of a poor prognosis in atopic dermatitis

Author and date	Determinants of poor prognosis	Comment
Wüthrich & Schudel (1983)	Early disease onset Severe disease Small family size Association with respiratory allergy High serum IgE levels	Follow-up study of 121 out of 271 patients with AD in infancy interviewed at ages 15 and 23 years
Williams & Strachan (1998)	Onset of AD in first year of life History of hay fever or asthma History of whooping cough	Birth cohort study of 6877 children. Crude and adjusted analysis given. Many other 'negative' findings
Lammintausta et al. (1995)	Severe AD	Mixture of risk factor analysis and follow-up data in 801 clinic patients with AD in teenage years
Åberg & Engstrom (1990)	Concomitant asthma or hay fever	Retrospective study of 1335 14-year-old children with allergic disease
Vickers (1980)	Early age of onset Extensor distribution in infancy Only child Associated allergic disease Female sex	1897 hospital cases followed up over a long period. Cases of seborrhoeic dermatitis included in inception cohort
Rystedt (1986)	Early onset Severe widespread dermatitis in childhood Family history of atopic dermatitis Associated hay fever or asthma Female sex	Crude and adjusted analyses presented for 955 hospital-ascertained individuals
Roth & Kierland (1964)	Severe disease in childhood	Retrospective survey of 211 out of 492 Mayo Clinic patients
Vowles et al. (1955)	Severe disease in childhood	
Musgrove & Morgan (1976)	Severe disease in childhood Concomitant asthma/hay fever Family history of AD	
van Hecke & Leys (1981)	Severe disease in childhood Concomitant asthma/hay fever	
Quille-Roussel et al. (1985)	Severe disease at onset Flexural site at disease onset Concomitant asthma Family history of atopy	Refers to 2/3 of original sample followed up to age of 5.6 years

countries and it is also likely to have changed with time. It is true that most long-term large studies of representative AD cases suggest that AD is a more chronic disease than earlier reports suggest, with a ten-year prognosis of around 50 to 70% for cases developing in childhood. We know a little about predictors of prognosis, but it is disappointing that those which have been identified so far are not amenable to public health manipulation.

Atopic dermatitis and the development of asthma and hay fever

How many and why?

Studies which have estimated the risk of children with AD developing asthma or hay fever (Lammintausta et al., 1991; Linna et al., 1992; Luoma, Koivikko & Viander, 1983; Kissling & Wüthrich, 1993; Kayahara et al., 1994; Åberg & Engstrom, 1990; Rystedt, 1986) are summarized in Table 3.4. These studies are limited as none has set out to examine issues of allergic disease association and the possible predictors of such associations. Few of the studies have used clear disease definitions for asthma or allergic rhinitis, hay fever or perennial rhinitis. Because knowledge of the association between AD, asthma and hay fever is so widespread, it is likely that subsequent asthma or hay fever is overreported or overdiagnosed in AD subjects, leading to an overestimate of disease co-occurrence. The high rates of concurrent or subsequent asthma in Table 3.4 (20 to 50%) are also likely to reflect the fact that most studies have 'ascertained' their eczema cases from hospital clinics, the implication being that severe AD is a predictor for increased subsequent or concurrent asthma. This is clearly shown in Rystedt's study (1986) where 39% of AD former hospital inpatients developed asthma compared with 22% of former outpatients. One study has suggested that many patients with 'pure' AD are more likely than noneczema sufferers to exhibit bronchoconstriction after bronchial provocation testing (Salob, Laverty & Atherton, 1993).

Other studies suggest that the dry skin of AD may be common to other atopic diseases, even in the absence of AD (Gollhausen, 1991).

A number of studies have suggested that childhood AD is a strong predictor of subsequent asthma (Meijer, 1976), but this is a slightly different question from 'what factors predict the development of asthma in children who already have AD?' Other studies have suggested that concomitant or previous AD are strong predictors of asthma persistence in older children and adults (Rieger, 1983; Terada et al., 1991). It is difficult to say whether the AD is a truly 'independent' predictor of asthma in such studies, or whether it is simply a surrogate measure of the amount of atopic disease burden per se. Such issues will be resolved only when the genetic basis for such allergic diseases becomes elucidated.

The time course of the three main 'atopic' diseases is also interesting in that it may inform us about possible environmental exposures and possible 'time windows' for subsequent allergic disease prevention. Åberg & Engstom's study (1990) of 1335 14-year-old children in the community with a past history of asthma, allergic rhinitis or atopic eczema, suggested that eczema was the first disease to become manifest, followed closely by asthma (41% within a two-year interval). Of those with both atopic eczema and allergic rhinitis, 83% of children developed allergic rhinitis after the atopic eczema, and 33% developed the allergic rhinitis within a two-year interval. Kissling and Wüthrich's (1993) follow-up study of 106 children with AD in infancy suggested that the mean ages at which the associated allergic diseases became manifest were 9.7 years for hay fever, 8.1 years for perennial rhinitis and 6.3 years for asthma. They also showed that the course of AD worsened when the asthma improved or vice versa in 15 of 34 cases, with a parallel course in 5 cases and an apparently independent course in 14 children. Currently, there is no good explanation of why AD should precede asthma and hay fever in such a consistent pattern in atopic individuals. It is unlikely that the quantity and type of allergen exposure is that different in a two-year-old when

Table 3.4. Studies which have documented development of subsequent asthma or hay fever in children who had atopic dermatitis

Author and date	Sample size	Source and ages of inception cohort	Follow-up rate and duration	% developing asthma	% developing hay fever	Comment
Lammintausta et al. (1991)	801	Hospital clinic 12 to 16 years	81% Duration unclear – 10 to 18 years?	10 to 19% (lower in less severe cases)	59 to 69%	A study of teenagers who had been seen in a dermatology unit in the past. Difficult to discern risk of asthma over time from the data.
Linna et al. (1992)	40	Children who had been previously hospitalized because of AD	10 years	53%	78%	Probably a severe subset of AD children.
Luoma et al. (1983)	543	Maternity unit from atopic families ($n = 395$) and non-atopic families ($n = 148$)	5 years	29%	35%	Unclear how data relates to atopic vs. non-atopic families
Kissling & Wüthrich (1993)	121	Hospital clinic	Up to 15 years	28%	33% hay fever 12% perennial allergic rhinitis	Follow-up study of children with AD in infancy.
Kayahara et al. (1994)	48	Hospital clinic	Up to 6 years	48%	Unclear	
Åberg & Engstrom (1990)	694	14-year-old children in the community	Birth to 14 years	16% had a history of concurrent or past asthma	28% had a history of concurrent or past allergic rhinitis	Retrospective large study which suggested that allergic disease co-occurrence is commoner in early onset disease
Rystedt (1986)	955	549 former inpatients with AE and 406 former outpatients	24 to 44 years	39% among former AE inpatients, 22% among outpatients	66% among former inpatients, 53% among outpatients	Large follow-up study with response rates above 90%.

compared with a nine-year-old child, so it is possible that time-related host factors such as differences in tissue-specific T-helper lymphocyte populations or antigen-presenting cells are occurring. Whether such an end-organ imbalance or maturation is under predominantly genetic programming or whether environmental stimuli are needed, is unknown.

Very little is known about what factors increase the risk of a child with AD developing asthma or hay fever. This is a pity since it is a commonly asked question by parents of children with AD, and identification of high-risk children could be the subject of intervention studies which aim to reduce the risk of developing subsequent asthma. Such is the rationale for the ETAC (early treatment of the atopic child) study, a randomized double-blind placebo-controlled clinical trial of cetirizine, antihistamine with some in vitro activity on inhibiting eosinophil migration, which is being sponsored by the manufacturers of cetirizine (ETAC Study Group, 1998). An earlier randomized double-blind placebo-controlled trial of ketotifen in 91 infants with only AD and followed up for 52 weeks suggested that children in the active group developed less asthma and less severe eczema (Ikura et al., 1991). The ETAC study set about comparing the incidence of symptoms of asthma in 817 AD infants aged one to two years with a history of atopic disease in parents or siblings, who took daily cetirizine or placebo for 18 months. No difference was noticed for the intention-to-treat population initially randomized. However, a subgroup analysis suggested a protective effect of cetirizine in those children (approximately 20% of the study population) who were sensitized to grass pollen or house dust mite. Caution has to be exercised in interpreting such post hoc subgroup analyses, but the magnitude of the benefit (relative risk for developing asthma when cetirizine treated of 0.6, 95% confidence intervals 0.4 to 0.9) for those infants sensitized to house dust mite or grass was impressive, and certainly warrants further testing in future trials. It is also crucial to know what happens to the children who have now stopped the cetirizine, i.e. whether the treatment simply suppressed hista-mine-induced asthma symptoms triggered by house dust mite and pollen, whether the treatment has simply delayed the onset of asthma, or whether there is a long-lasting benefit. Interestingly, in the ETAC study, 34% of the children with clinical AD in that study were not atopic in terms of raised total IgE of >30 kU/l, reinforcing concerns raised in Chapter 1 that AD is not necessarily atopic. One advantage of the ETAC study is that observation of the control group alone should provide us with a good opportunity of observing the natural history of AD according to disease severity and sensitization status. Other studies such as the PREVASC study (prevention of asthma in children), conducted in a general practice setting in Maastricht, will also provide pointers to the effectiveness and compliance with prevention programmes for the development of asthma (Schönberger, H., personal written communication, September 1998).

Other long-term disease consequences and associations

Sensitization

The link between the time course of AD and sensitization is unclear, but the few studies which exist suggest that sensitization may be the preceding event. Guillett & Guillett (1992) have followed up sensitization rates in 29 children with severe AD in early infancy. They claimed that food allergy was causal in all cases and that this was still clinically significant at the age of three years. It is unclear how the natural history of sensitization relates to the development of AD in well-defined cohorts of cases ascertained in the community, but studies such as the German multicentre allergy study (MAS) should be helpful in this area as the cohort progresses (Wahn et al., 1997). Some studies suggest that sensitization may occur at a very early age and that such sensitization as determined by analysis of cord blood may predict the later development of AD in affected children.

The relationship between sensitization, atopy and AD has been discussed more fully in Chapter 1.

Bring back the parasites?

In addition to the other 'allergic' diseases discussed in this chapter, other associations with AD have been suggested, some of which may even be advantageous. For instance, it has been suggested that the mast cell–IgE and eosinophil tissue system has been retained in phylogeny because it appears to confer biological advantage in adaptive immunity against a number of helminthic parasites (Moqbel & Prichard, 1990). The notion of an inverse relationship between parasites and manifest allergic disease carries some weight in that atopic subjects have been shown to have a decreased parasite load when compared with nonatopics, and helminth infections have been shown to improve established atopic disease (Grove & Forbes, 1975; Turton, 1976).

Cancer

It has also been suggested that atopic subjects may be at decreased risk of developing subsequent cancer (Sanchez-Borges et al., 1986; Kölmel & Compagnone, 1988), but longitudinal studies with clear case definitions are needed.

Other associations

Other studies of AD subjects have suggested a range of unusual associations, such as increased susceptibility to mosquito bites (Harford-Cross, 1993), increased urinary tract infections (Oggero et al., 1994), genital bleeding (Sumitsuji et al., 1996), recurrent ear infections (Luoma, 1984), decreased numbers of naevi (Broberg, 1996) and an increased tendency to headaches (Mortimer et al., 1993), findings which require further confirmation. Some localized viral infection such as herpes simplex recurrences might be increased in AD (Rystedt, Stannegard & Stannegard, 1986). One small clinical report suggested that viral warts are generally increased in AD children (Currie, Wright & Miller, 1971), a finding which some have interpreted as evidence to support a systemic defect in T-cell mediated immunity, despite the fact that such children do not suffer from more viral infections in general. A

large population study has shown that viral warts are not more common in children with examined eczema (Williams, Pottier & Strachan, 1993), suggesting that earlier observations could have been due to localized defective immunity or epiphenomena of disease severity. One study of cases of fungal infections referred to a university hospital has suggested that atopics were at increased risk of dermatophyte infections (Svejgaard, 1996), but further population studies with well-defined criteria are needed. The association between atopic eczema and allergic or irritant contact dermatitis is discussed by Coenraads and Diepgen in Chapter 4.

Growth

Children with severe AD are significantly shorter than control even after adjusting for concurrent asthma and parental height, for reasons which are still unclear (Pike et al., 1989). In another study of 68 AD children, height was significantly correlated with the surface area of skin affected by AD after adjusting for parental height for those children with over 50% skin involvement, which could not be explained by dietary treatment and topical steroids (Massarano et al., 1993).

Recommendations for future studies which examine the natural history of atopic dermatitis

This chapter has demonstrated the major gaps and methodological obstacles in relation to our current understanding of the natural history of atopic dermatitis. It is difficult to understand why our knowledge is so poor, given that AD is a common disease and that its manifestations are visible and amenable to recording. The early onset of the disease also makes it a very suitable condition for investigation by means of the cohort study, yet few such studies exist to date.

Given this lack of knowledge, there is a strong case for setting up further cohort studies relating to the natural history of AD. Such studies need to consider the following design issues.

Issues relating to assembling the cohort

It has already been shown that the natural history of AD in hospital subjects is not necessarily the same as that of milder cases ascertained through the community. If studies are to be generalized to all AD sufferers, it is essential that the inception cohort selects a representative sample from the community. Given the difficulties and continued debate on what constitutes a case of definite AD in very early infancy, there is a strong argument for beginning the inception cohort at the age of one year.

In order to explore possible predictors of prognosis, features such as disease severity, disease pattern, disease associations and family history, as well as potential gestational and perinatal risk factors that might be amenable to change, should be collected at the onset of the study. An open mind should be kept when selecting possible predictors of disease persistence since they may be different from the more established risk factors for disease occurrence.

Issues relating to definitions

It is important that studies use a valid and repeatable definition of AD in order to allow comparison with other studies. These are discussed more fully in Chapter 1. Similarly, there should be clear definitions of disease remission (which are not yet fully developed) and disease clearance. Equal rigour needs to be given to defining other associated diseases such as asthma and hay fever.

Issues relating to follow-up

Every effort should be made to ensure a high follow-up rate (i.e. around 90%) and the characteristics of those lost to follow-up should be recorded. Disease severity and other disease associations should be recorded in addition to presence or absence of disease at specific time points. It is important that every possible attempt is made to reduce information bias in such a study by ensuring that those requesting information on disease recurrences are unaware of the initial characteristics of the children by following a standardized protocol. Information on recurrences should be sought frequently (at least every three years) in order to capture the intermittent nature of the disease. Consideration should also be given to recording possible consequences of such effects on occupation, morbidity, school performance, marriage, cancer rates and mortality. Information should also be gathered on the frequency and predictors of associated asthma and hay fever.

Issues relating to analysis and interpretation

Sensitivity analyses which include and exclude those lost to follow-up should be performed in order to explore the possible consequences of loss to follow-up. Care should be taken in the interpretation of post hoc findings, e.g. of disease subgroups which could have arisen by chance in small samples. Constraint should also be demonstrated in attributing poor prognosis to certain factors when many variables have been recorded, especially if they have not been declared at the study onset or suggested by previous studies. Appropriate statistical techniques such as survival curves or time series analysis should be used for investigating events which are connected in time.

We conclude this chapter by providing some recommendations for future studies (Laupacis et al., 1994). These are summarized in Box 3.1.

Box 3.1. Recommendations for future studies of the natural history of atopic dermatitis

Is the disease definition clear and valid?

Is the sample representative of all persons with the condition?

Has the inception cohort been assembled at a uniform and early point of the disease?

Was the follow-up sufficiently long and complete?

Were a range of clinically relevant and objective outcome measures examined?

Were outcome measures recorded in a blind fashion?

Were prognostic subgroups identified a priori?

Summary of key points

- Most studies based on hospital-ascertained cases have probably overestimated the proportion of cases of atopic dermatatis (AD) with early onset because early onset may be a predictor of disease severity.

- Studies which examine age of onset in case series of younger age groups will also overestimate the proportion of cases with early onset by excluding those who might have disease onset at a later age.

- Despite these limitations, studies of well defined cases suggest that most (70%) AD cases become manifest within the first five years of life.

- The early onset of AD suggests that factors operating in early life may be critical for disease expression.

- The change in distribution of AD lesions with time might be a pointer to understanding the factors which exacerbate the disease and to recognize different subtypes of disease.

- Little is known about short- to medium-term fluctuations in AD disease activity.

- Research is urgently needed to develop ways of defining a 'remission' of AD so that the effects of treatments on the chronicity of the disease can be explored.

- Previous texts have tended to give the erroneous impression that the prognosis of AD is very good.

- Most large studies of well defined and representative studies suggest that around 60% of childhood AD cases are clear or free of symptoms in early adolescence.

- Many such apparently clear cases are likely to recur in adulthood.

- The strongest and most consistent factors which appear to predict more persistent AD are early disease onset, severe widespread disease in early life, concomitant asthma or hay fever and a family history of AD.

- There is a strong case for more studies which investigate the natural history of AD.

- Such studies should try to avoid the pitfalls of previous studies by ensuring high follow-up rates, long follow-up periods and the use of clear disease definitions in representative populations.

References

Åberg, N. & Engstrom, I. (1990). Natural history of allergic disease in children. *Acta Paediat Scand*, **79**, 206–11.

Al-Jabin, H. & Marks, R. (1984). Studies of the clinically uninvolved skin in patients with dermatitis. *Br J Dermatol*, **11**, 437–43.

Aoki, T., Fukuzumi, J., Adachi, K. et al. (1992). Re-evaluation of skin lesion distribution in atopic dermatitis. *Acta Dermatol Venereol (Stockh.)*, Suppl. 176, 19–23.

Bahmer, F. A. (1992). ADASI score: atopic dermatitis area and severity index. *Acta Dermatol Venereol (Stockh)*, Suppl. 176, 32–3.

Berlinghoff, W. (1961). Die Prognosis des Säuglingsekzems. *Dtsch Gesundheitswes*, **16**, 110–13.

Boddin, M. (1930). Beitrag zur Klinik des neurogenen Ekzems im Kindesalter. *Med Klin*, **26**, 270–2.

Boguniewicz, M. (1998). Progress in understanding and treatment of atopic dermatitis. In: *Conversations from the American Academy of Allergy, Asthma and Immunology 54th Annual Meeting*, Washington, UCB Institute of Allergy, pp. 1–4.

Broberg, A. (1996). Atopic dermatitis and melanocytic naevi. In: *Proceedings of the 6th International Symposium on Atopic Dermatitis*, Åarhus, June 7th to 9th 1996.

Burrows, D. & Penman, R.W.B. (1960). Prognosis of the eczema–asthma syndrome. *Br Med J*, **ii**, 825–8.

Businco, L., Ziruolo, M.G., Ferrara, M. et al. (1989). Natural history of atopic dermatitis in childhood. *Allergy*, **44** (Suppl. 9), 70–8.

Currie, J.M., Wright, R.C. & Miller, O.G. (1971). The frequency of warts in atopic patients. *Cutis*, **8**, 243–5.

de Graciansky, P. (1966). Eczéma constitutionnel. *Bull Mem Soc Med Hop (Paris)*, **117**, 765–88.

Dotterud, L.K., Kvammen, B., Lund, E. & Falk, E.S. (1995). Prevalence and some clinical aspects of atopic dermatitis in the community of Sør-Varanger. *Acta Dermatol Venereol*, **75**, 50–3.

Edgren, G. (1943). Prognose und Erblichkeitsmomente bei Ekzema Infantum. *Acta Paediat*, **30** (Suppl. II), 30–6.

ETAC Study Group (1998). Allergic factors associated with the development of asthma and the influence of cetirizine in a double-blind, randomised, placebo-controlled trial: first results of ETAC®. *Pediat Allergy Immunol*, **9**, 116–24.

Finn, O.A. (1955). Long-term prognosis in infantile eczema. *Br Med J*, **i**, 772.

Gollhausen, R. (1991). Irritable skin in atopic eczema. In: Ring, J. & Przybilla, B. (eds.) *New Trends in Allergy III*, pp. 207–21. Berlin: Springer-Verlag.

Grove, D.I. & Forbes, I.J. (1975). Increased resistance to helminth infestation in an atopic population. *Med J Aust*, **1**, 336–8.

Guillett, G. & Guillett, M-H. (1992). Natural history of sensitizations in atopic dermatitis. *Arch Dermatol*, **128**, 187–92.

Harford-Cross, M. (1993). Tendency to being bitten by insects among patients with eczema and with other dermatoses. *Br J Gen Pract*, **43**, 339–40.

Harper, J.I., Mason, U.A., White, T.R. et al. (1991). A double-blind placebo-controlled study of thymostimulin (TP-1) for the treatment of atopic eczema. *Br J Dermatol*, **125**, 368–72.

Heite, H-J. (1961). Katamnestische Erhebungen, Klinische Untersuchungen und Testungen zur Spätprognose des Eczema infantum. *Arch Klin Exp Dermatol*, **213**, 460–70.

Helleström, S. & Lidman, H. (1956). Studies of Besnier's prurigo. *Acta Dermatol Venereol (Stockh.)*, **36**, 11–22.

Ikura, Y., Baba, M., Mikawa, H., Nishima, S. et al. (1991). [A double blind study of the effectiveness of ketotifen in preventing the development of asthma in atopic dermatitis patients] (Japanese). *Arerugi – Japanese Journal of Allergology*, **40**, 132–40.

Kayahara, M., Murakami, G., Adachi, Y. et al. (1994). [Bronchial hypersensitivity and development of bronchial asthma in children with atopic dermatitis] (Japanese). *Arerugi – Japanese Journal of Allergology*, **43**, 759–65.

Kesten, B.M. (1954). Allergic eczema. *N Y J Med*, **54**, 2441–7.

Kissling, S. & Wüthrich, B. (1993). Verlauf der atopischen Dermatitis nach derm Kleinkindatter. *Hautarzt*, **44**, 569–73.

Kölmel, K.F. & Compagnone, D. (1988). Melanoma and atopy. *Dtsch Med Wochenschr*, **113**, 169–71.

Lammintausta, K. & Kalimo, K. (1993). Does a patient's occupation influence the course of atopic dermatitis? *Acta Dermatol Venereol (Stockh.)*, **73**, 119–22.

Lammintausta, K., Kalimo, K., Raitala, R. & Forsten, Y. (1991). Prognosis of atopic dermatitis. *Int J Dermatol*, **30**, 563–8.

Lammintausta, K., Mäkelä, L. & Kalimo, K. (1995). Long-term course of atopic dermatitis. *Allergologie*, **18**, S460 (abstract).

Laupacis, A., Wells, G., Richardson, W.S. & Tugwell, P. (1994). How to use an article about prognosis. *J Am Med Ass*, **272**, 234–7.

Linna, O., Kokkonen, J., Lahtela, P. & Tammela, O. (1992). Ten-year prognosis for generalised infantile eczema. *Acta Paediat*, **81**, 1013–16.

Luoma, R. (1984). Environmental allergens and morbidity in atopic and non-atopic families. *Acta Paediat Scand*, **73**, 448–53.

Luoma, R., Koivikko, A. & Viander, M. (1983). Development of asthma, allergic rhinitis and atopic dermatitis by the age of five years. *Allergy*, **38**, 339–46.

Massarano, A.A., Hollis, S., Devlin, J. & David, T.J. (1993). Growth in atopic eczema. *Arch Dis Childh*, **68**, 677–9.

Meenan, F.O.C. (1959). Prognosis in infantile eczema. *Irish J Med Sci*, **398**, 79–83.

Meijer, A. (1976). High risk factors for childhood asthma. *Ann Allergy*, **37**, 119–22.

Moqbel, R. & Prichard, D.I. (1990). Parasites and allergy; evidence for a 'cause and effect' relationship. *Clin Exp Allergy*, **20**, 611–18.

Mortimer, M.J., Kay, J., Gawkrodger, D.J. et al. (1993). The prevalence of migraine in atopic children: an epidemiological study in general practice. *Headache*, **33**, 427–31.

Musgrove, K. & Morgan, J.K. (1976). Infantile eczema. A long-term follow-up study. *Br J Dermatol*, **95**, 365–72.

Nexmand, P-H. (1948). *Clinical Studies of Besnier's Prurigo*, pp. 20–30. Copenhagen: Rosenkilde and Bagger.

Oddoze, L (1959). Notre statistique sur l'étiologie du prurigo de Besnier en France. *Acta Allergol*, **13**, 410–4.

Oggero, R., Monti, G., Fiz, A. et al. (1994). Atopic dermatitis of infancy and urinary tract infections. *Dermatology*, **189**, 139–41.

Osborne, E.D. & Murray, P.F. (1953). Atopic dermatitis: a study of its natural course and of wool as a dominant allergenic factor. *Arch Dermatol*, **68**, 619–26.

Pike, M.G., Chang, C.L., Atherton, D.J., Carpenter, R.G. et al. (1989). Growth in atopic eczema: a controlled study by questionnaire. *Arch Dis Childh*, **64**, 1566–9.

Purdy, M.J. (1953). The long-term prognosis in infantile eczema. *Br Med J*, **i**, 1366–9.

Quille-Roussel, C., Raynaud, F. & Saurat, J-H. (1985). A prospective computerized study of 500 cases of atopic dermatitis in childhood. *Acta Dermatol Venereol (Stockh.)*, Suppl. 114, 87–92.

Rajka, G. (1989). *Essential Aspects of Atopic Dermatitis*, pp. 7–16. Berlin: Springer-Verlag.

Rieger, C.H. (1983). Asthma bronchiale. Langzeittherapie und Prognose. *Monatsschrift Kinderheilkunde*, **131**, 128–31.

Roth, H.L. (1987). Atopic dermatitis revisisted. *Int J Dermatol*, **26**, 139–49.

Roth, H.L. & Kierland, R.R. (1964). The natural history of atopic dermatitis. *Arch Dermatol*, **89**, 209–14.

Rystedt, I. (1986). Long term follow-up in atopic dermatitis. *Acta Dermatol Venereol (Stockh.)*, Suppl. 114, 117–20.

Rystedt, I., Strannegard, I.L. & Strannegard, O. (1986). Recurrent viral infections in patients with past or present atopic dermatitis. *Acta Dermatol Venereol (Stockh.)*, **114**, 575–82.

Sackett, D.L., Richardson, W.S., Rosenberg, W. & Haynes, R.B. (1997). *Evidence-based Medicine*, pp. 129–32. London: Churchill Livingstone.

Salob, S.P., Laverty, A. & Atherton, D.J. (1993). Bronchial hyper-responsiveness in children with atopic dermatitis. *Pediatrics*, **91**, 13–16.

Sanchez-Borges, M., de Orozco, A., Arellano, S. et al. (1986). Preventive role of atopy in lung cancer. *Clin Immunol Immunopathol*, **41**, 314–19.

Saval, P., Fuglsang, G., Madsen, C. & Østerballe, O. (1993). Prevalence of atopic disease among Danish school children. *Pediat Allergy Immunol*, **4**, 117–22.

Stifler, W.C. (1996). A 21-year follow-up of infantile eczema. *J Pediat*, **66**, 166–7.

Sumitsuji, H., Endo, K., Fukuzumi, T. et al. (1996). Atopic dermatitis and dysfunctional genital bleeding. In: *Proceedings of the 6th International Symposium on Atopic Dermatitis*, Åarhus, June 7th to 9th 1996.

Svejgaard, E. (1986). Epidemiology and clinical features of dermatomycoses and dermatophytoses. *Acta Dermatol Venereol (Stockh.)*, Suppl. 121, 19–26.

Terada, M., Ishioka, S., Hozawa, S., Yasumatsu, Y. et al. (1991). [A statistical investigation of the importance of the influence of allergic factors on intractable asthma by multiple factor analysis] (Japanese). *Arerugi – Japanese Journal of Allergology*, **40**, 1289–96.

Thune, P. (1989). Evaluation of the hydration and the water-holding capacity in atopic skin and so-called dry skin. *Acta Dermatol Venereol (Stockh.)*, Suppl. 144, 133–5.

Turton, J.A. (1976). IgE, parasites and allergy. *Lancet*, **2**, 686.

Van der Meer, J.B., Glazenburg, E.J., Mulder, P.G.H., Eggink, H.F. & Coenraads, P-J. (1999). The management of moderate to severe atopic dermatitis in adults with topical fluticasone propionate. *Br J Dermatol*, **140**, 1114–21.

van Hecke, E. & Leys, G. (1981). Evolution of atopic dermatitis. *Dermatologica*, **163**, 370–5.

Vickers, C.F.H. (1980). The natural history of atopic eczema. *Acta Dermatol Venereol (Stockh.)*, Suppl. 92, 113–5.

Vowles, M., Warin, R.P. & Apley, J. (1955). Infantile eczema: observation on natural history and prognosis. *Br J Dermatol*, **67**, 53–9.

Wagner, G. & Pürschel, W. (1962). Klinisch-analytische Studie zum Neurodermitis-Problem. *Dermatologica*, **125**, 1–32.

Wahn, U., Lau, S., Bergmann, R. et al. (1997). Indoor allergen exposure is a risk factor for sensitization during the first three years of life. *Clin Immunol*, **99**, 763–9.

Williams, H.C. (1995). Atopic eczema – why we should look to the environment. *Br Med J*, **311**, 1241–2.

Williams, H.C. (1997). Diagnosis and management of teenage eczema. *Prescriber*, **8**, 69–73.

Williams, H.C. & Strachan, D. (1993). The natural history of childhood eczema. *Br J Dermatol*, **129**, 26.

Williams, H.C. & Strachan, D.P. (1998). The natural history of childhood eczema: observations from the 1958 British cohort study. *Br J Dermatol*, **139**, 834–9.

Williams, H.C., Pottier, A. & Strachan, D. (1993). Are viral warts seen more commonly in children with eczema? *Arch Dermatol*, **129**, 717–21.

Williams, H.C., Burney, P.G.J., Hay, R.J. et al. (1994). The UK working party's diagnostic criteria for atopic dermatitis. I: Derivation of a minimum set of discriminators for atopic dermatitis. *Br J Dermatol*, **131**, 383–96.

Wüthrich, B. (1975). In: Wüthrich, B. (ed.) *Zur Immunpathologie der Neurodermitis constitutionalis*, pp. 53–5. Bern: Verlag Hans Huber.

Wüthrich, B. (1996). Epidemiology and natural history of atopic dermatitis. *Allergy Clin Immunol Int*, **8**, 77–82.

Wüthrich, B. & Schudel, P. (1983). Die Neurodermitis atopica nach dem Kleinkindesalter. Eine katamnestische Untersuchung anhand von 121 Fällen. *Z Hautkr*, **58**, 1013–23.

4

Occupational aspects of atopic dermatitis

Pieter-Jan Coenraads and Thomas L. Diepgen

Introduction

Children with atopic dermatitis (AD) often struggle at school (Saval et al., 1993), and adults with AD do their best to keep their job (Lammintausta & Kalimo, 1993). Looking at AD as a disease with many predisposing, precipitating and perpetuating factors (Williams, 1997) it is obvious that occupational factors can precipitate and perpetuate. While it is unlikely that occupational factors are predisposing (although a role of occupational factors operating on the fetus in utero cannot be ruled out), there is a vast body of literature pointing towards certain jobs causing more skin trouble for people with AD. A preliminary reading of this literature generates a few questions, which one would like to have answered before one is convinced that there is really a problematic association between AD and occupation. One question, for example, is whether the patients with whom the publication deal really have AD. In other words, was AD correctly assessed, without observer bias? Another question is how the patients came to be in their present jobs? In other words, to what extent may AD have influenced the fact that patients selected or avoided a particular occupation? One would also like to know more about those with AD who do not seem to have a (skin) problem within their occupation; maybe they use adequate protection measures at work or avoid domestic exposure, or maybe they have a milder or different type of AD. Some issues, such as a discussion on diagnostic criteria

for AD, are dealt with elsewhere in this book. For the time being, a variability in the assessment of AD, which affects the interpretation of most studies, must be accepted. The following paragraphs will show that a certain degree of selection and observation bias is inevitable in most published studies dealing with occupation and AD. A review of the available literature on occupational aspects guides us towards the following domains as components of this chapter:

1 The triangle: occupational skin disease, hand eczema and AD.
2 Sick leave and change of work due to AD.
3 Risk factors for hand eczema: AD as an effect modifier.
4 On the quantification of risk.
5 Occupational guidelines for people with AD.

The triangle of occupational skin disease, hand eczema and atopic dermatitis

Occupational skin diseases are mostly (about 90%) a subtype of contact dermatitis (Coenraads, Diepgen & Smit, 1999; Rycroft, 1995). Rarely is there exclusive involvement of the trunk: almost always (in about 90% of all cases) are the hands affected. Thus, occupational skin disease is mostly a matter of hand eczema. When occupational factors are the subject of a published study, hand eczema appears. This does not rule out the fact that occupation-related flare-ups of AD, not located on the hands, are well documented in persons handling animals to which

Table 4.1. Type IV contact allergy and skin atopy among hairdressers 1990–1993 in the North Bavaria district of Germany (Tacke et al., 1995)

	Skin atopics ($n = 215$)	Nonatopics ($n = 312$)
Occupational allergens		
glycerylmonothioglycolate	48%	54%
p-phenylenediamine	28%	30%
ammonia persulphate	22%	26%
Nonoccupational allergens		
nickel sulphate	49%	45%
balsam of Peru	2%	4%

they are allergic: examples are veterinarians and farmers.

Major studies on the role of atopy in occupational hand eczema appear in the 1980s (Bäurle et al., 1985; Rystedt, 1985a, 1985b; Lammintausta & Kalimo, 1981; Meding & Swanbeck, 1990). There are no systematic studies on occupational factors and AD not restricted to the hands, except for a study from Finland (Lammintausta & Kalimo, 1993), and this study confirms, for AD of the hands, a correlation between eczema and occupational exposure to irritants. There has been much debate on the issue of whether patients with AD are more (or less) prone to (occupational) contact allergy. While some argue that there may be a slightly decreased risk, at least a 'classical' type IV contact allergy to common sensitizers does not seem to be more prevalent among atopics (Rystedt, 1985b). This is supported by data from a study among hairdressers (Table 4.1): even in this group, which is heavily exposed to occupational allergens, there are no significant differences in sensitization rates between those with atopic manifestations on the skin and nonatopics (Diepgen et al., 1999). With type I (IgE-mediated) contact urticarial reactions, which can develop into hand eczema, the situation is different. Immediate type contact reactions to latex (gloves used by health-care personnel), to alpha-amylase (yeast used by bakers) or to food

proteins are more common among atopics (Rycroft, 1995; Lahti, 1995).

Among persons with AD exposed to irritants, it is difficult to distinguish between hand eczema based on atopy and hand eczema as a manifestation of irritant contact dermatitis. There is a consensus that exposure to irritants precipitates or aggravates hand eczema in individuals with a history of AD (Rystedt, 1985b; Meding & Swanbeck, 1990). Most of this consensus is derived from a perceived overrepresentation of skin atopy among those with irritant contact dermatitis of the hands. This overrepresentation stems mainly from studies with a kind of cross-sectional design, with a posterior assessment of skin atopy. A few studies look at hand eczema and occupational factors in atopics (instead of atopy in persons with hand eczema), and even fewer have any kind of follow-up design. Rystedt's study has elements of a cohort study: work-related hand eczema was assessed in persons diagnosed with or without AD more than 24 years earlier (Rystedt, 1985a). Although details about the inclusion and exclusion critertia are lacking, Lammintausta's study also consists of a cohort of teenage AD patients, re-examined in adulthood (Lammintausta & Kalimo, 1993). In both studies, however, the (historical) 'cohorts' were assembled retrospectively, mostly based on hospital records.

A follow-up study on hand eczema by Nilsson is based on a cohort of newly employed workers in whom a pre-employment questionnaire identifies atopics (Nilsson, 1986). The above-mentioned studies are discussed further later in this chapter.

Other methodological problems emerge: for example, do we deal with irritant contact dermatitis or with AD as a manifestation of hand eczema. Several studies mentioned in Table 4.2 show that a considerable number of individuals with a personal history of AD manage to work with irritant exposure without developing hand eczema. Therefore, a discussion on the role of AD as an effect modifier (i.e. whether AD makes a person more likely to develop hand eczema from occupational exposure) or on the role of AD of the hands independent of occupational

Table 4.2. The relationship between hand eczema (HE) and atopy

HE among atopics			
Cronin et al. (1970)	AD	$n = 233$	68% HE
Breit et al. (1972)	AD	$n = 130$	69%
Rystedt (1985b)	Severe AD	$n = 549$	60%
	Moderate AD	$n = 406$	48%
	Respiratory	$n = 222$	14%
	Nonatopics	$n = 199$	11%
Diepgen & Fartasch (1994)	AD	$n = 428$	72%
Atopics among HE			
Lammintausta & Kalimo (1981)	HE in hospital wet work	$n = 259$	54% atopics
Cronin (1985)	HE in women	$n = 263$	34% personal history of atopy
Meding & Swanbeck (1990)	HE in population-based sample	$n = 1238$	27% childhood eczema
			28% asthma/hay fever
Lodi et al. (1992)	Pompholyx	$n = 104$	50% personal or family history of atopy
Tacke et al. (1995)	HE in bakers	$n = 107$	50% aetiological fraction

factors, seems appropriate. Some older studies on the role of occupational skin exposure mention 'atopy' without distinction between mucosal atopy (asthma, hay fever) and atopic dermatitis. In the meantime, there is sufficient evidence that mucosal atopy, without skin manifestations, is not associated with increased risk of irritant contact dermatitis (Rystedt, 1985b; Diepgen & Fartasch, 1994). An association between skin risk and 'atopy' is probably based on the inclusion of patients who have mucosal atopy and AD.

Sick leave and change of work due to atopic dermatitis

Sick leave or absence from work due to AD has never been studied from reviewing employment records or other registries. One of the main reasons is that most records are not detailed enough to distinguish between AD and other (skin) dieases. In a Finnish cohort, patients with AD did not take sick leave any more often than others (Lammintausta & Kalimo, 1993), but among those with moderate or severe AD their sick leave was more often due to the problems with their skin. Also, the duration of a period of absence from work due to AD was longer than

average, but the total number of compensated days in this study was no different from the number of days due to other diseases.

An analysis of cost, including days of work lost, is presented in a study based on an occupational disease registry (Shmunes & Keil, 1983). Unfortunately the conclusions, indicating more days of work lost among the atopics, are based on a subset of responders which comprises only 13% of all registered cases, and are therefore likely to be affected by selection bias.

Not only is sick leave multifactorial, but also the decision to change work. Studying the role of AD in changing occupation is fraught with difficulties, and is virtually impossible by a cross-sectional design. In the above-mentioned Finnish study, the majority of patients with AD had learned to work and live with their skin symptoms (Lammintausta & Kalimo, 1993). A low level of education was associated with occupational changes, and it is possible that educated patients tend to avoid occupations which may be harmful to their skin. A cross-sectional study, comparing AD patients with and without hand eczema, showed a higher rate of occupational change among those with hand involvement and whose first job was wet and dirty (Forsbeck et al.,

1983). A questionnaire-based study among patients who had in the past been hospitalized for AD and psoriasis showed no differences in the frequency of occupational change, but those with AD more often gave their skin problem as a reason for change (Odia et al., 1994). However, due to its design, that study was unable to detect a possible impact of AD on work history. No adjustment was made for the age difference between the groups: age, for example, may have been a confounder because it undoubtedly reflects differences in occupational environment, education and employment prospects.

In a follow-up of newly employed female hospital workers, sick leave and change of work occurred more often in those with AD and among those with a history of hand eczema (Nilsson, 1986). However, all assessments, including the assessment of the occurrence of hand eczema, were made by questionnaire; the absence of any clinical verification may have led to responder bias. Sick leave and medical consultations due to hand eczema were uncommon and had occurred in only 8% of those with AD who were employed in wet work. Among the reasons given for not consulting a doctor were a mild dermatitis and self-medication. Nurses especially may avoid medical consultation deliberately and have easy access to topical self-medication.

Risk factors for hand eczema: atopic dermatitis as an effect modifier

Exposure to irritants may cause irritant contact dermatitis of the hands. Patients with moderate to severe AD often have hand dermatitis. Assessing the contribution of eczema caused by irritant exposure to the hand is very difficult when the study is restricted to such patients. Many studies have resorted to hand eczema, assessed whether or not there is AD, and have tried to associate the findings with occupational exposure. Usually, atopy or AD is studied as a 'risk factor' for hand eczema. In the context of this chapter, it is more logical to look at AD as an effect modifier, i.e. the question as to what extent the presence of AD will elicit more skin reac-

tions (hand eczema) from occupational exposure. As shown in this paragraph, most papers give summaries of relative risks of exposure on hand eczema, and do not give clear estimates of effect modification of this exposure by AD. No study has ever attempted to estimate the aetiological fraction (attributable risk) of occupational exposure in AD and/or AD-related hand eczema.

In the context of a larger study, two cohorts of 549 and 406 individuals who had been diagnosed with AD during the period 1952–1956 were identified and contacted by questionnaire more than 25 years later (Rystedt, 1985a). There was a high (97%) response rate. A subsample was examined clinically and hand eczema was present in 34–48% of the patients in that sample. Hand eczema was significantly more prevalent in those with exposure to irritants. Rystedt concentrates on the role of irritants in patients with AD, and does not give an estimate of the effect of AD on the relationship between occupational exposure and hand eczema. Although the material was heavily biased towards hospital cases, the severity of childhood AD appeared to be a decisive factor for the development of hand eczema, and irritant contact dermatitis seemed to be the subordinate diagnosis after 'endogenous' (mostly atopic) hand eczema. The bias towards hospital cases may reflect the severe end of the spectrum of AD. It was a cross-sectional assessment of exposure, and patients may well have adapted their occupational exposure to their skin problems. In a separate analysis, domestic exposure to irritants was more clearly associated with hand eczema in this group of patients (Rystedt, 1985c). The study demonstrates that a careful assessment of exposure (occupational as well as domestic) is needed for further conclusions about the role of AD in any occupation. In a study on the occurrence of hand eczema in Finnish workers exposed to wet work, the concept of atopic skin diathesis as a minor variant of overt AD was introduced (Lammintausta & Kalimo, 1981). The definition of this atopic diathesis includes a low threshold of pruritus to nonspecific irritants. Because of this definition, it is likely that a clear association was found between hand eczema and AD.

In a large cross-sectional sample of the general population Meding studied the relative importance of various risk factors for hand eczema by regression analysis (Meding & Swanbeck, 1990). As with findings in other studies, it showed that childhood eczema, which is more or less equivalent to childhood AD, was the most important 'predictive' factor for hand eczema. It also showed that, among those with a history of childhood AD, there was a tendency to avoid occupations with irritant exposure. Occupational exposure seemed to raise the predicted probability of having hand eczema by about a third. The significantly raised rates among women arouses the suspicion that domestic exposure to household irritants plays a major role.

Nilsson studied a large cohort of about 2600 newly employed hospital workers (Nilsson, 1986). The history of AD and/or visible AD was assessed during the pre-employment examination, and all workers were followed-up for 20 months. It should be borne in mind that all data were gathered by questionnaire only. About half the subjects identified with AD had hand eczema before they began their present work. It was not clear whether relevant occupational factors were present in their previous jobs, but bias should be suspected: of the office workers (no occupational exposure) 23% had hand eczema prior to their current job, in contrast to 8% among craftsmen. A history of AD increased the odds ratio of developing hand eczema about three times in wet and in dry work. This points towards AD as a constant multiplicative effect modifier for any kind of exposure. In general, the predicted probability of developing hand eczema during the observation time (20 months) was 38% for office workers with AD and 72% for nurses with AD. It should be borne in mind that AD meant a combination of firm AD with atopic mucosal symptoms when interpreting these figures.

The study leads to the question of how those individuals with mild skin atopy would perform in these occupations. A grading of skin atopy seems, therefore, an important variable to be included in such studies. Such a severity grading system could be based on, for example, mucosal symptoms only, history of childhood AD, recent active AD, or on a scoring of points (Diepgen et al., 1989, 1996).

An interesting analysis on the contribution of skin atopy to the total number of cases of occupational skin disease was performed in the food and catering sector, especially bakers and cooks (Tacke et al., 1995). It was a population-based study, meaning that the total number of employees in the study region was known, and all cases of occupational skin disease (mainly hand eczema) were well documented with respect to atopy. An assumption had to be made about the prevalence of AD in the general population. Assuming this background prevalence is 10%, the risk of an employee with AD developing occupational skin disease (mainly hand eczema) was on average eight times greater. The aetiological fraction of AD (attributable risk) in all cases of occupational skin diseases among bakers was about 50%.

In an ongoing follow-up study among 2100 new employees in a car factory, skin atopy was assessed and graded during the pre-employment examination (Funke et al., 1996). Thus far, for hand eczema the relative risk was about three for workers who had a history of AD. The study divides the cohort into four groups with different (assumed) risk levels for the development of hand eczema: it distinguishes between those with overt AD with signs of hand eczema, AD without hand eczema and those with minor AD criteria versus no signs of skin atopy. Preliminary results point towards a doubling of the hand eczema risk when there is exposure to wet work for more than three hours per day.

On the quantification of risk

Public health authorities, especially occupational health services, and also individual patients are interested in having an answer to the broad question: how employable is a person with AD? In other words, what is the magnitude of risk for somebody with AD that his or her skin problems will get worse or develop hand involvement for the first time

Table 4.3. Some estimates of 'predicted' risk for hand eczema in adults with and without atopic dermatitis (AD). Selection bias may be in operation

	Follow-up period	No AD, no exposure	AD, no exposure	AD, with irritant exposure
Meding & Swanbeck (1990)	12 months	5–9%	14–23%	34–48%
Nilsson (1986)	20 months	16%	38%	62–72%
Rystedt (1985b)	24 years	5%	37–50%	60–81%

because of occupational exposure, and will eventually interfere with work? Obviously, the question has the hidden fear that someone with AD will be handicapped, irrespective of occupational exposure.

Summarizing the studies that are discussed in the preceding paragraphs, it is clear that a precise overall estimate is meaningless. It would disregard the importance of the level of skin exposure to irritants, including domestic exposure, and the importance of the degree of severity of skin atopy. As explained earlier, consequences of occupational exposure are usually described as hand eczema.

Estimates expressed as relative risk (with or without confidence limits) may be elegant from a statistical point of view, but are difficult to interpret intuitively when there is no notion about the 'normal' background risk. From the literature it is clear that the risk of hand eczema, irrespective of exposure, is considerable in subgroups of individuals with AD or a history of AD. In view of this, a relative risk due to exposure of the order of two affects a considerable additional number of employees.

The probability of having hand eczema in a 12-month period, without any supposed risk factor in operation (i.e. no atopy, no occupational exposure), was calculated in Gotenburg (Meding & Swanbeck, 1990). Within the limitations of a cross-sectional design, this probability was estimated at 5% for males and 9% for females. With a history of childhood eczema, irrespective of occupational exposure, the calculated probability of hand eczema was 14% (males) and 23% (females). Occupational exposure in general raises this probability by a third, and occupational exposure in service work doubles the probability to 34% (males) and 48% (females) among those with a history of AD.

The questionnaire-based study by Nilsson among hospital employees, where AD was defined as past or present signs of AD, calculates much higher absolute risks: the predicted probability of hand eczema in nonatopic craftsmen was 16% (Nilsson, 1986). AD increased the risk about three times, and this tripled risk is present in high and low levels of exposure. This seems to be in agreement with Meding's observed triplication of risk among patients with a history of AD (Meding & Swanbeck, 1990). For office workers with AD a predicted probability of 38% was calculated, and for nurses 62–72% (Nilsson, 1986). In this material exposure to irritants seems to increase the risk by a factor of two.

In Rystedt's follow-up study of childhood AD cases, occupational exposure to irritants did not seem to increase the risk of hand eczema by very much. But in a separate analysis among women there were about twice as many cases among those who were exposed to domestic work (Rystedt, 1985a, 1985c). Pooling of domestic and occupational exposure to irritants seemed to indicate a rise of hand eczema prevalence by less than a third. The selection of cases which were at the moderate-to-severe end of the spectrum is reflected in a 'background' risk of hand eczema of 40–50% in AD patients without exposure, versus 5–11% among nonAD individuals. Table 4.3 summarizes the abovementioned studies which have attempted to calculate absolute risks in terms of predicted probabilities. As explained in the previous paragraph, these absolute figures should be interpreted with caution, since they are highly dependent on the chosen study design, and may suffer from selection bias. In terms of relative risk, the data from the different studies show a rather consistent pattern: a history of AD without exposure

Table 4.4. Relative risks (estimated by odds ratios) for hand eczema in different studies among hairdressers, demonstrating similarity in the factors AD and exposure to wet work (Diepgen et al., 1997)

	Prospective cohort study hairdressers: $n = 574$						Case-control study hairdressers: 103 cases; 156 controls		
	Crude odds ratios			Logistic regression model[†]			Logistic regression model[†]		
	OR	95% Cl	p value	OR	95% Cl	p value	OR	95% Cl	p value
AD (10 pts.)	2.6	1.7–3.9	***	2.1	1.4–3.2	***	2.1	1.2–3.7	**
Resp. atopy	1.0	0.7–1.7	n.s.	0.8	0.4–1.4	n.s.	0.5	0.2–1.1	n.s.
Wet work (4 h)	2.3	1.6–3.3	***	2.1	1.4–3.0	***	2.3	1.3–3.9	***
Permanent wave (1 h)	1.9	1.3–2.7	***	1.7	1.1–2.4	**	1.4	0.7–2.6	n.s.
Nickel sensitivity	1.5	1.1–2.2	*	1.3	0.9–1.9	n.s.	1.7	1.0–2.9	n.s.

Notes:

***$p<0.001$ **$p<0.01$ *$p<0.05$; n.s. = not significant

[†] ORs adjusted for all other variables mentioned in this table.

at least doubles the risk for hand eczema, and occupational exposure doubles this risk again. This is a multiplicative effect, which means that the risk of hand eczema in patients with AD who perform work that is unfriendly to their hands is four times increased. This is supported by data from two different studies among hairdressers (Diepgen et al., 1999). As shown in Table 4.4, the relative risks (calculated as odds ratios) are almost identical in a prospective study and a case-control study. The model defines AD cases as those with at least ten points on a scale of criteria (Diepgen et al., 1989, 1996). Again, a doubling of risk is shown for patients with AD, multiplied by two by exposure to wet work, with a possible additional increase of risk due to exposure to special high-risk tasks such as permanent waving. The data do not present a possible (statistical) interaction of AD on the relationship between wet work and hand eczema.

Occupational guidelines for patients with atopic dermatitis

Summarizing the evidence thus far, it is clear that AD patients run a certain risk of developing hand eczema, and that this risk is dependent on the severity of their AD. In this severity, a history of hand involvement or a present involvement of the hands plays a central role. Proper advice at a pre-employment examination is essential, and regular follow-up and counselling of patients with an increased risk will help them to keep functioning in their jobs. Recently, the German occupational organizations (which also administer the occupational insurance funds) have reached consensus on a series of guidelines for pre-employment advice (G-24) to employees opting for occupations which carry increased skin risk (G-24, 1996). As an analogy, this chapter can be concluded with Table 4.5, presenting guidelines if one is confronted with a request for preventive advice to individuals with AD. As a first step, the risk category is defined, and as a second step the corresponding advice is formulated.

Although the guidelines are restricted to occupational aspects, it is clear that domestic exposure, such as household wet work or handicraft work, should not be neglected and that this should be an important component of occupational counselling. In an ongoing study in an automobile factory the above-mentioned risk categories are being validated (Funke et al., 1996). Preliminary results pointed towards increased risk due to domestic handicraft work, car repair and house building.

Table 4.5. A practical guide for occupational pre-employment counselling in persons with (possible) atopic dermatitis

Step 1: Defining the occupational risk category	Step 2: Occupational counselling for each risk category

First risk category
   moderate to severe AD with hand involvement
   chronic hand eczema
   change of work due to irritant contact dermatitis
	For the first risk category:
	   occupations with wet work or other exposure to irritants not advisable.
	   pre-employment medical–occupational counselling and medical advice is required.

Second risk category
   AD without involvement of the hands
   dyshidrosis (history of pompholyx)
   allergic rhinitis or asthma in occupations with increased risk for type I allergies (e.g. bakers)
	For the second risk category:
	   technical and organizational protection measures.
	   personal protection measures.
	   repeated follow-up examinations every three months in the first year, and every six months in the second year.

Third risk category
   evidence for low threshold to nonspecific irritants:
      wool intolerance
      itch due to sweating
      unusually dry skin
	For the third risk category:
	   technical and organizational protection measures.
	   follow-up examinations after 6, 12 and 24 months.

Summary of key points

- Occupational irritants precipitate atopic dermatitis (AD).
- Occupational contact urticaria is more common in atopics.
- Patients with AD are at risk of developing hand eczema.
- A history of (childhood) involvement of the hands is a major risk factor.
- AD is probably an effect modifier for occupational exposure.
- A history of AD doubles the risk of hand eczema.
- In severe AD this increase in relative risk is probably higher.
- Exposure to occupational irritants multiplies this risk by at least a factor of two, and in some professions it is greater than this.
- Severity grading of skin atopy is recommended for future studies.
- It is unclear how many patients avoid certain occupations, adapt to their jobs, or change occupation.
- Occupational counselling must take a history of AD into account.

References

Bäurle, G., Hornstein, O.P. & Diepgen, T.L. (1985). Professionelle Handekzeme und Atopie. Eine klinische Prospektivstudie zur Frage des Zusammenhangs. *Dermatosen*, **33**, 161–5.

Breit, R., Leutgeb, C. & Bandmann, H.J. (1972). Zum neurodermitischen Handekzem. *Arch Dermatol Res*, **244**, 353–4.

Coenraads, P.J., Diepgen, T.L. & Smit, H.A. (2000). Epidemiology. In: Rycroft, R.J.G., Menné, T. Frosch, P.J. & Lepoittevin, J.P. (eds.) *Textbook of Contact Dermatitis*, 3rd edn. Berlin: Springer-Verlag. In Press.

Cronin, E., Bandmann, H.G., Calnan, T.D. et al. (1970). Contact dermatitis in the atopic. *Acta Dermatol Venereol (Scand.)*, **50**, 183–9.

Diepgen, T.L. & Fartasch, M. (1994). General aspects of risk factors in hand eczema. In: Menné, T. & Maiback, H.I. (eds.) *Hand Eczema*, pp. 141–56. Boca Raton: CRC Press.

Diepgen, T.L., Fartasch, M. & Hornstein, O.P. (1989). Evaluation and relevance of atopic basic and minor features in patients with atopic dermatitis and in the general population. *Acta Dermatol Venereol (Stockh.)*, Suppl. 144, 50–54.

Diepgen, T.L., Fartasch, M. & Schmidt, A. (1999). Hand eczema in hairdressers. (Submitted)

Diepgen, T.L., Sauerbrei, W. & Fartasch, M. (1996). Development and validation of diagnostic scores for atopic dermatitis incorporating criteria of data quality and practical usefulness. *J Clin Epidemiol*, **49**, 1031–8.

Forsbeck, M., Skog, E. & Asbrink, E. (1983). Atopic hand dermatitis: a comparison with atopic dermatitis without hand involvement, especially with respect to influence of work and development of contact sensitization. *Acta Dermatol Venereol, (Stockh.)*, **63**, 9–13.

Funke, U., Diepgen, T.L. & Fartasch, M. (1996). Risk-group related prevention of hand eczema at the workplace. *Curr Prob Dermatol*, **25**, 123–32.

G-24 (1996). Berufsgenossenschaftlicher Grundsatz für arbeitsmedizinische Vorsorgeuntersuchungen. G-24: Hauterkrankungen (mit Ausnahme von Hautkrebs). In: *Arbeitsmedizin Sozialmedizin Umweltmedizin*, Heft 6, Stuttgart: Gentner Verlag.

Lahti, A. (1995). Immediate contact reactions. In: Rycroft, R.J.G., Menne, T., Frosch, P.J. & Benezra, C. (eds.) *Textbook of Contact Dermatitis*, 2nd edn, pp. 62–74. Berlin: Springer-Verlag.

Lammintausta, K. & Kalimo, K. (1981). Atopy and hand dermatitis in hospital wet work. *Contact Dermatitis*, **7**, 301–8.

Lammintausta, K. & Kalimo, K. (1993). Does a patient's occupation influence the course of atopic dermatitis? *Acta Dermatol Venereol (Stockh.)*, **73**, 119–22.

Lodi, A., Betti, R., Chiarelli, G., Urbani, C.E. & Crosti, C. (1992). Epidemiological, clinical and allergological observations on pompholyx. *Contact Dermatitis*, **26**, 17–21.

Meding, B. & Swanbeck, G. (1990). Predictive factors for hand eczema. *Contact Dermatitis*, **23**, 154–61.

Nilsson, E. (1986). Individual and environmental risk factors for hand eczema in hospital workers. *Acta Dermatol Venereol*, Suppl. 128, 1–63.

Odia, S.G., Pürschel, W.C., Vocks, E. & Rakoski, J. (1994). Noxen und irritantien im beruf. Berufsrelevante Fragestellung bei 1156 Patienten mit Neurodermitis constitutionalis atopica und psoriasis vulgaris. *Dermatosen*, **42**, 179–83.

Rycroft, R.J.G. (1995). Occupational contact dermatitis. In: Rycroft, R.J.G., Menné, T., Frosch, P.J. & Benezra, C. (eds.) *Textbook of Contact Dermatitis*, 2nd edn, pp. 343–400. Berlin: Springer-Verlag.

Rystedt, I. (1985a). Factors influencing the occurrence of hand eczema in adults with a history of atopic dermatitis in childhood. *Contact Dermatitis*, **12**, 185–91.

Rystedt, I. (1985b). Hand eczema and long term prognosis in atopic dermatitis (thesis). *Acta Dermatol Venereol (Stockh.)*, **117** (Suppl), 1–59.

Rystedt, I. (1985c). Work-related hand eczema in atopics. *Contact Dermatitis*, **12**, 164–71.

Saval, P., Fuglsang, G., Madsen, C. & Osterballe, O. (1993). Prevalance of atopic disease among Danish school children. *Pediat Allergy Immunol*, **4**, 117–22.

Shmunes, E. & Keil, J.E. (1983). Occupational dermatosis in South Carolina: a descriptive analysis of cost variables. *J Am Acad Dermatol*, **9**, 861–8.

Tacke, J., Schmidt, A., Fartasch, M. & Diepgen, T.L. (1995). Occupational contact dermatitis in bakers, confectioners and cooks. A population-based study. *Contact Dermatitis*, **33**, 112–17.

Williams, H.C. (ed.) (1997). Inflammatory skin diseases. I: Atopic dermatitis. In: *The Challenge of Dermatoepidemiology*. Boca Raton: CRC Press.

PART II

Descriptive studies which indicate the size of the problem

5

Geographical studies of atopic dermatitis

Nicholas McNally and David Phillips

The range and potential of spatial health research

Medical geography and the geography of health care have an established place in the study of disease occurrence and the concomitant need for health care. This chapter focuses on the role of spatial (geographical) approaches in the understanding of atopic dermatitis (AD). The main traditional areas of spatial health research have been identified as disease mapping and medical cartography, associative analyses and spatio-temporal diffusion studies (Phillips, 1981; Joseph & Phillips, 1984; Douven & Scholten, 1995). In epidemiological terms, these correspond with descriptive studies, ecological studies, and those subdivided by time and place (Parry, 1979; Beaglehole et al., 1993). At a more exploratory level, disease mapping and associative analyses have generally been undertaken and, for diseases such as AD, detailed spatio-temporal analyses have, to date, rarely been performed as their modelling techniques often require considerable and refined data. Douven & Scholten (1995) summarize the stages which can be identified in a chain linking aggregate spatial health studies to the identification of possible causal factors. These stages are useful in considering the spatial epidemiology of AD and are shown in Box 5.1.

The need for a geographical epidemiology approach in atopic dermatitis

Atopic dermatitis is the most common inflammatory skin disease in children, affecting 10–15% of children in the developed world (Williams et al.,

Box 5.1. Key stages in associative spatial research

(1) The *collection* and *preparation* of disease data.
(2) The *mapping* of data to identify spatial disease patterns at a variety of scales.
(3) Applying objective *statistical tests* in order to consider whether the variation is significant and, if so, at what spatial scales.
(4) *Measuring* the *association* between disease and other spatially varying factors.
(5) *Interpretation* of the results of the previous stages, the indication of areas interesting for further research and, eventually, the generation of hypotheses.
(6) *Searching* for *possible causal relationships*.

1995; Kay et al., 1994) and, increasingly, those in the developing world. It can be a distressing condition, influencing children's well-being, personal and educational development and family life. It can continue into adulthood. There is also reasonably strong evidence to suggest that the prevalence of AD has increased substantially over the last three decades (Williams, 1992). Explanations for the increase remain largely unknown although there is a growing body of work which suggests that environmental agents are important in the aetiology of the disease (Williams, 1995).

Temporal trends in the occurrence of AD feature in many of the recent epidemiological studies but consideration of geographical aspects of the disease is far less common. However, comparison of disease prevalence and incidence rates between different places can serve as the descriptive starting points for further, more detailed investigations which utilize the methods of analytical epidemiology (Hutt & Burkitt, 1986; English, 1992). For example, if the prevalence of AD was found to vary spatially, it could suggest that studying genetic, ethnic or environmental factors might yield more insights into the aetiology and assist in the management of the disease (Neame et al., 1995). Ecological approaches have achieved great success throughout epidemiology, most notably in studies of cancer and cardiovascular disease where they have helped throw light on many possible associated factors (Mayer, 1983, 1986). For example, in an ecological study of primary acute pancreatitis in Nottingham, Giggs et al. (1980) have shown the total number of cases of the disease to be significantly greater than could have occurred by chance in one of Nottingham's six water supply areas. Moreover, the association between overcrowding and tuberculosis mortality in England and Wales has been highlighted using an ecological approach (Elender & Bentham, 1996).

The problem of unreliable data over time and space

One of the most significant problems encountered when trying to describe the geography of any disease, and perhaps the principal reason for a lack of spatial work with regard to AD, is the varied reliability of disease data over both space and time (Cliff & Haggett, 1988). Even relatively 'hard' mortality data and diagnoses are often incomplete, but this is of far greater concern when considering morbidity data which are frequently unavailable or inappropriate (Olumide, 1986). While prevalence data for AD have for some time become more widely available from European nations, knowledge at a global scale remains severely limited (Rajka, 1986). To date, there has been a virtual absence of data from African and Latin American countries (Kottenhahn & Heck, 1994), although the International Study of Asthma and Allergies in Children (ISAAC) will provide wider comparable standardized data with numerous reporting points in the developing world (see below). Again, to date, even when prevalence estimates have been available in different countries, the lack of standardized data renders the comparison of

studies difficult. As a result, any observed differences in the prevalence of disease between studies may reflect differences in disease definition, population sampling and evaluation criteria as well as any real spatial differences (Neame et al., 1995).

International variation in the prevalence of atopic dermatitis

An appreciation of different disease definitions, time period for reporting symptoms, size of the study group and age range and representativeness of the sample are imperative in any review of prevalence studies. Burkholter & Schiffer (1995) have provided a selective review of prevalence studies of atopic disease during the 1980s, which includes some consideration of the criteria and methods of each study. Table 5.1 provides a summary of some of the more recent prevalence studies from around the world. Only studies from the 1990s have been systematically recorded since earlier data are often more difficult to interpret because many have not been collected on comparable bases.

There is a strong indication that the prevalence of AD varies considerably from one country to another although, in the absence of a standardized definition and methodology, it is impossible to make any firm quantitative comparisons from this review. The lowest prevalence estimates are found in parts of the developing world (Henderson, 1995; Leung & Ho, 1994). Multi-centre studies from south-east Asia (Leung & Ho, 1994) and northern Europe (Schultz Larsen et al., 1996), which use common protocols and standardized procedures, have also shown large variations in AD.

Preliminary findings from the International Study of Asthma and Allergies in childhood (ISAAC), which uses standardized definitions of AD, have confirmed that marked variations in the prevalence of the disease exist on an international scale (Williams et al., 1999). The study used cross-sectional questionnaire surveys conducted on random samples of schoolchildren aged 6–7 years and 13–14 years from centres in 56 countries throughout the world. A history of an itchy relapsing skin rash in the last 12 months which had affected the skin creases at some

Table 5.1. Summary of prevalence estimates published in the 1990s.

Location (author and year)	Prevalence	Definitions and data	Age group	Comments and findings
London, England (Williams et al., 1995)	11.7% ($n = 693$)	Point prevalence (dermatologist's examination)	3–11 years	Prevalence found to be significantly higher in Black Caribbean children (16.3%) than in White children (8.7%)
Birmingham, England (Kay et al., 1994)	11.5% ($n = 1104$)	One-year period prevalence (questionnaire)	3–11 years	No protective effect of breast feeding was found
Leicester, England (Neame et al., 1995)	14% ($n = 446$)	Point prevalence (trained observer's examination)	1–4 years	No ethnic difference in prevalence was observed
Livingston, Scotland (Herd et al., 1996b)	8.1% ($n = 9786$)	One-year period prevalence (dermatologist's examination)	2–11 years	Prevalence of AD showed a continuous reduction with increasing age
Aberdeen, Scotland (Ninan & Russell, 1992)	12% ($n = 409$)	Lifetime prevalence (questionnaire)	Primary school	Prevalence of all manifestations of eczema, wheezing and hay fever was shown to have increased over a 25-year period
Hanover, Germany (Buser et al., 1993)	11.8% ($n = 4651$)	Point prevalence (questionnaire)	Primary school	Forms part of a validation study
Bavaria, Germany (Schäfer et al., 1993)	22.1% ($n = 1066$)	Lifetime prevalence (questionnaire)	5–6 years	The manifestation of all forms of atopy was not related to the patient's month of birth
West and east Germany (Behrendt et al., 1993)	12.9% 15.7% ($n = 1154$)	Current symptoms (questionnaire)	6 years	A tendency to higher total serum IgE levels in cities with higher levels of air pollution was found
Bavaria, Germany (Dold et al., 1992)	19.5% ($n = 6665$)	Lifetime prevalence (questionnaire)	9–11 years	Children of parents with AD were found to be at higher risk of development of AD
Denmark, Germany, Sweden (Schultz Larsen et al., 1996)	22.9% 13.1% 15.5% ($n = 2655$)	Lifetime prevalence (questionnaire)	7 years	Comparative survey of three northern European populations
Karlskoga, Sweden (Gustafsson et al., 1992)	5.3% ($n = 736$)	Point prevalence (medical records)	7 years	Cow's milk-based formula was not found to be related to the prevalence of AD
Viborg, Denmark (Saval et al., 1993)	7% ($n = 4952$)	One-year period prevalence (questionnaire)	5–16 years	Prevalence of AD in girls found to be significantly higher (10.7%) than in boys (5.7%)

Table 5.1 (*cont.*)

Location (author and year)	Prevalence	Definitions and data	Age group	Comments and findings
Hordaland county, Norway (Bakke et al., 1990)	25% ($n = 4992$)	Lifetime prevalence (questionnaire)	15–70 years	No differences in prevalence of AD were found between urban and rural areas. Prevalence of AD was found to be associated with occupational dust or gas exposure
Sør Varanger, Norway (Dotterud et al., 1995)	26% ($n = 424$)	Point prevalence (questionnaire)	7–12 years	Detailed study of an isolated rural community, close to the Russian border
Turku, Finland (Varjonen et al., 1992)	9.7% ($n = 416$)	Lifetime symptoms (history and examination)	15–16 years	The prevalence estimates of this study compare favourably with those found in similar studies 10 years earlier
Finland (Pöysä et al., 1991)	4.3% ($n = 3649$)	Lifetime prevalence (questionnaire)	3–18 years	The prevalence of atopy was found to be highest in southern, urbanized areas of Finland
Switzerland (Wüthrich, 1996)	13% ($n = 4465$)	Lifetime prevalence (questionnaire)	Schoolchildren	Part of the Swiss Scarpol study on childhood allergy. Also found a significant social class gradient with the highest prevalence in social class I
Poland (Breborowicz et al., 1995)	12.9%	Questionnaire	Schoolchildren	Family history of allergy was shown to increase the risk of allergic diseases
Western Siberia (Toropova et al., 1996)	11.2% ($n = 4117$)	Point prevalence (doctor's examination)	4–7 years	Prevalence of AD found to have increased since 1970
Ankara, Turkey (Kalyoncu et al., 1994)	6.1% ($n = 1036$)	One-year period prevalence (questionnaire)	6–12 years	The first epidemiological survey of atopic disease in Turkey
Czech Republic (Bobák et al., 1995)	3.9% boys 6.3% girls ($n = 2060$)	One-year period prevalence (questionnaire)	3–5 years	No apparent relationship between atopy and atmospheric pollution was found
Okinawa, Japan (Okuma, 1994)	9.5% ($n = 10\,137$)	Point prevalence (questionnaire)	Elementary schools	Large survey of atopic diseases in Okinawa
Japan (Sugiura et al., 1997)	20%	Point prevalence (dermatologist's examination)	3 years	A declining prevalence with age was observed. The prevalence estimates were found to be similar to those of a similar study 20 years before
Korea (Park et al., 1996)	10% (6–8 years) 5.4% (10–12 years) 2.5% (16–18 years)	Lifetime prevalence (questionnaire)	6–18 years	Breast feeding was shown to have a significant positive effect on AD

Table 5.1 (*cont.*)

Location (author and year)	Prevalence	Definitions and data	Age group	Comments and findings
Hong Kong, Malaysia, China (Leung & Ho, 1994)	20.1% 7.6% 7.2% (n = 2208)	Lifetime prevalence (questionnaire)	Secondary schools	Large questionnaire survey of atopic disease in three South-east Asian populations. Extensive discussion of possible aetiology
Tanzania (Henderson, 1995)	0.7% (n = 548)	Point prevalence (doctor's examination)	7–18 years	A significant difference in prevalence of AD was observed between two villages in rural Tanzania
New South Wales, Australia (Peat et al., 1994)	28.0% (n = 1668)	Cumulative incidence (questionnaire)	8–10 years	Survey of atopic diseases in school children in Belmont and Wagga Wagga, New South Wales
Victoria, Australia (Kilkenny et al., 1997)	11.8% (primary) 7.8% (secondary) (n = 2500)	Point prevalence (dermatologist's examination)	4–18 years	Part of the School Skin Survey which aims to determine the prevalence and severity of common skin diseases
New Zealand (Barry et al., 1991)	15.9% (n = 873)	Cumulative incidence (questionnaire)	12 years	Survey of atopic diseases in school children

time was used as the main outcome measure. Figure 5.1 illustrates the global distribution of the prevalence of symptoms of AD in the last 12 months based on 458 623 individuals aged 13–14 years. Figure 5.2 suggests the presence of a band of low disease prevalence extending from China through Asia and the eastern Mediterranean to eastern Europe. With the exception of some African centres, higher values in northern Europe and Australasia suggest a possible latitude gradient. Similar patterns were observed for 6–7-year-olds based on 256 410 children. These findings are suggestive of a critical role of environmental factors in determining disease expression (Williams et al., 1999).

Atopic dermatitis and westernization

Atopic dermatitis therefore appears to be a common problem in developed nations but relatively unusual in the developing world (Paajanen, 1994; Failmezger, 1992). However, there are some indications that the prevalence of atopic diseases in developing countries is not static but is subject to dramatic increases which could reach epidemic proportions as traditional lifestyles are eroded by increasing adaptation to the living patterns exhibited by industrialized societies (Turner, 1987). This appears to be particularly the case in urban areas where economic development is often polarized. For example, a consistent rise in the incidence of AD since the 1960s has been observed using numerator data from the Nigerian city of Ibadan (George, 1989).

Migrant studies inherently have a strong geographical component. Several studies have shown the disease experience of migrant groups to differ from that of genetically similar populations in their country of origin and are discussed in detail in Chapter 13. For example, a study of children who migrated from Tokelau to New Zealand has shown a large increase in the prevalence of AD in the migrant children compared with similar genetic groups in their country of origin (Waite et al., 1980). Atopic dermatitis has also been found to occur far more frequently in Chinese than in Caucasian children living

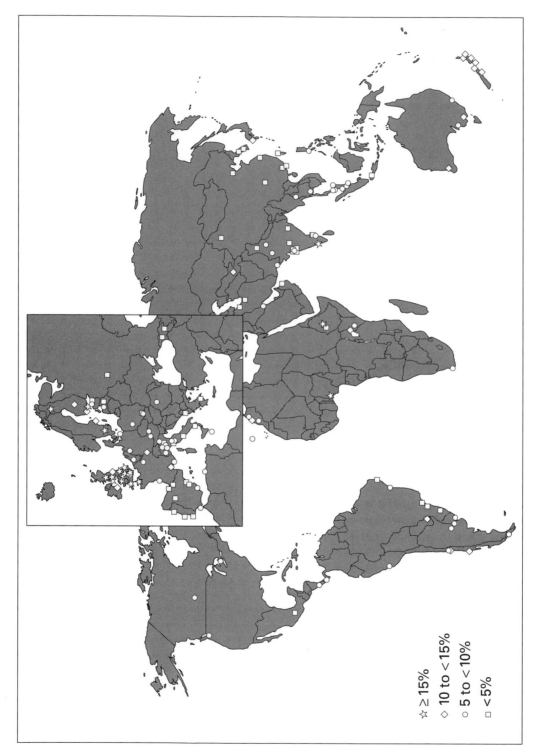

Fig. 5.1. The global distribution of eczema symptoms in the last 12 months based on 458623 individuals aged 13–14 years who took part in the International Study of Asthma and Allergies in Childhood (ISAAC)

☆ ≥ 15%
◇ 10 to <15%
○ 5 to <10%
□ <5%

in San Francisco and Hawaii (Worth, 1962). Asian children born in Australia have been shown to be at a higher risk of AD than those who have recently immigrated (Leung, 1994). Black Afro-Caribbean children residing in London have been shown to be at twice the risk of AD than Whites (Williams et al., 1995). Another study indicates the prevalence of atopic disease to be significantly higher in a Turkish population residing in Sweden than among Swedes (Kalyoncu & Stålenheim, 1993).

A number of potential causes are suggested by such studies which are more likely to be environmental than genetic given the similarity between the migrant and indigenous population. The increased atopic disease observed in the migrant populations could result from exposure to new or increased levels of allergens brought about by the migration. Factors such as urbanization and overcrowding, exposure to industrial pollution, different housing design, central heating, smoking, a diet poor in free radical scavengers and the eradication of parasites, may all contribute to the observed differences in disease frequency, either by enhancing sensitization or by directly influencing allergen levels (Williams, 1992). However, it is unlikely that factors such as pollution and loss of parasites alone explain the increase in prevalence of AD over the last 20 years in Britain where, for example, peak air pollution has generally fallen.

Epidemiological transition

Certain exogenous factors associated with modernization appear to help to explain the disease experiences of migrant groups. Therefore, future trends to increased prevalence of AD in the developing world may lead to a growing burden of the disease in many of these countries as the processes of economic development gather pace. A greater knowledge of the exogenous factors which are involved in the aetiology of AD is needed in order to prevent or reduce the impact of the increasing problem of AD in developing nations.

The earlier review of prevalence studies suggest that the increased prevalence of AD is linked to environmental causes and triggers that are associated

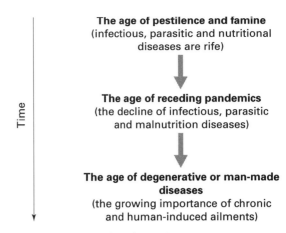

Fig. 5.2. The epidemiological transition

with 'modern' lifestyles. The concept of epidemiological transition and the somewhat broader health transition may be useful in general terms (Frenk et al., 1991). This concept involves changes in the sources of mortality and morbidity with development. In particular, an era of decline in infectious, parasitic and malnutrition diseases, with high levels of morbidity and mortality and low expectation of life, will be superseded by an age of 'receding pandemics'. During this phase, sources of morbidity and mortality move towards chronic and man-made (human-induced) ailments. This then merges into an era in which these diseases come to predominate (see Figure 5.2). The concept is widely accepted although whether epidemiological change is inevitably a linear progression is open to challenge. Many Third World countries and those such as the former Yugoslavia, in which health services have been damaged by war and economic problems, may face a reverse transition. There is also evidence of a dual or delayed transition in many developing countries, in which the better-off residents move rapidly towards a modern 'Western' disease profile and the even poorer suffer from infectious and nutritional disorders; they may also face rises in heart disease and cancers, experiencing the worst of both aspects of epidemiological change. Areas of poor hygiene may also be those with the worst general environmental conditions from household, industrial and vehicular pollution, and also at risk from poor diets (Phillips, 1990; Gribble & Preston, 1993).

This concept, of mortality and morbidity change with modernization, has obvious implications for changing incidence and prevalence of dermatological problems. However, as always, the chief limitation is data availability. As a result, virtually all research on epidemiological transition to date has focused on gross changes in mortality and, even then, data are not widely available over sufficient time-spans in many developing countries. A few exceptions, such as Hong Kong and some other countries in south-east Asia, illustrate very clear changes in mortality (Phillips & Verhasselt, 1994). The challenge for the future is to begin gathering comparable information on morbidity from AD (amongst other skin conditions) to see how epidemiological change is progressing in terms of nonlife-threatening morbidity. This is an important area of work since, if the incidence of AD increases in developing countries at anything like the rate it has in some developed countries, it will provide another huge cost of medication to be met either by public sector health services or (more likely) by individual household budgets (Herd et al., 1996a). The scope for research within and between countries is huge. The suggestion that factors of modernization are involved in the expression of the disease also needs to be explored at more detailed smaller scales, such as between different urban subareas and urban–rural differences. The reasons for a possible levelling-off of prevalence in some countries which have very rapidly modernized, such as Japan (Sugiura et al., 1997), are also very worthy of research. The search for possible associations at such a large geographical scale is necessary as there may be important aetiological factors which are homogeneous within large populations and therefore will not be detected by case-control or cohort methodologies (Rose, 1985).

Regional variation in the prevalence of atopic dermatitis

A common approach in geographical research is to study the distribution of various phenomena at different spatial scales: global, international/continental, national, regional, subregional, local and so on, to gain increasing insight into associations and possible causation (Pyle, 1979). With regard to AD, there are some studies at the subnational or regional scale. In Finland, for example, the disease has been shown to be most common in the southern, more urbanized region of the country (Pöysä et al., 1991). The lowest prevalence of the disease was found in the eastern region of the country, an area dominated by agricultural land use. While the observed variation may represent the greater availability of health services in the south of the country, and hence perhaps higher rates of reporting, at least part of the difference may reflect a real increased risk of AD in large towns and southern parts of the country. Some support for these findings was provided by another Finnish study which found the occurrence of AD in urban areas to be significantly higher than that for rural areas, although this difference did not exist for other manifestations of atopy (Luoma & Koivikko, 1982).

In contrast to the Finnish studies, analyses of both the 1970 British Cohort Study (BCS70) (Golding & Peters, 1987) and the National Child Development Study (NCDS) (McNally et al., 1998a) are suggestive of a higher prevalence of AD in rural areas than in urban areas (Golding & Peters, 1987; McNally, 1998). Region of residence emerged as a significant predictor of atopic disease in the British birth cohort studies. The common distributional feature from both major cohort studies was a low prevalence in Scotland and higher prevalence in southern regions of Britain. Further analysis of these data found a fairly consistent pattern of dermatitis and hay fever. The geographical pattern of wheezing in childhood was found to differ from that observed for the other manifestations of atopy. The observed regional variations in the prevalence of asthma at age 5–7 in both of these cohorts appear to be related to region of current residence rather than region at birth (Strachan et al., 1990).

Existing research therefore suggests that there is a reasonably marked regional variation in the risk of AD in Britain. However, because of the use of large administrative units in the studies, more detailed interpretation of the findings is a difficult and troublesome task. Analysis of the cohort data using finer divisions of region would help to verify or refute the findings. However, the relatively low number of individuals in the study means that mapping the data at scales lower than the county level would be of questionable value, as the resulting prevalence estimates will be inherently variable or unstable, fluctuating considerably with the addition or deletion of even a single case (Gatrell & Bailey, 1996).

The following diagrams illustrate the results of mapping AD in Britain using the pre-1975 county configuration. Due to the low population of a number of counties, particularly those in Scotland and Wales, some counties have been amalgamated to make larger regional units. Figure 5.3 shows the crude prevalence of parentally-reported dermatitis by the age of seven years. All nonmigrants by seven years have been excluded from the analysis because of the complicated exposure history of this group. Figure 5.4 shows the lifetime prevalence of AD among nonmigrants at the age of 16 years, calculated by amalgamating the data from the three cohort sweeps. Figure 5.5 maps standardized data for AD at seven years, taking into account the effect that social class could have on the spatial distribution as a confounding variable.

A fairly consistent spatial patterning of AD is found in all of the maps and supports the earlier findings using these data which suggest markedly different prevalence between regions of Britain. The disease appears to be most common in southern and central counties stretching in a 'belt' of high prevalence from the south-west through central areas to central eastern areas. Lower prevalence is found in northern areas and Scotland, although some eastern counties of Scotland also have higher prevalence. The consistencies between the crude data and the standardized data are suggestive of a residual regional effect on the disease.

Geographical clues to environmental associations

Most analysis to date on the geography of AD has been largely descriptive, analogous to descriptive

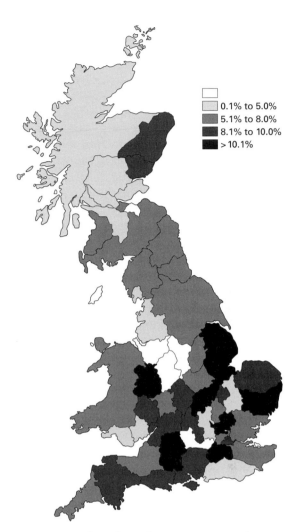

Fig. 5.3. Reported prevalence of eczema among nonmigrants by seven years of age

epidemiological studies. More refined research is emerging and a growing number of studies have begun to address possible links between atopic disease and broad environmental factors, most notably air quality due to its plausibility as an important factor in the expression of respiratory diseases. The studies are at a fairly basic level and have commonly sought to compare prevalence estimates between urban areas. One such study of atopic disease in five Czech towns, for example, found no apparent relationship between any manifestation of

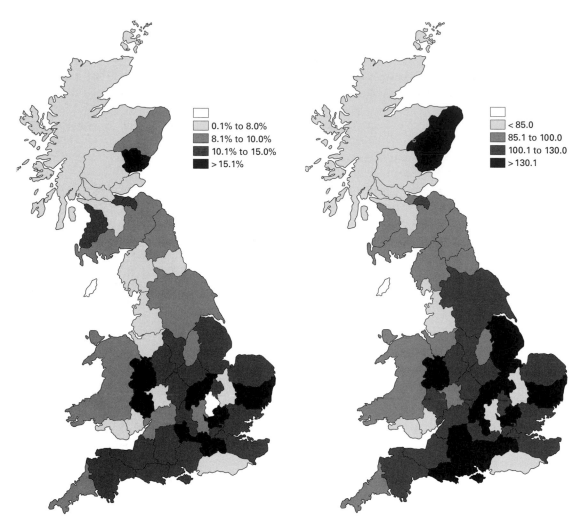

Fig. 5.4. Lifetime reported prevalence of eczema by 16 years

Fig. 5.5. Standardized morbidity ratios (SMRs) for eczema at seven years

atopy – including reported symptoms of AD – and levels of air pollution (Bobák et al., 1995).

The occurrence of atopic diseases in the former East Germany, with its purported poor environmental record, provides an interesting comparison with western Germany where environmental exposures are likely to have differed over the last half a century. One study found a significantly higher prevalence of AD in several urban areas of eastern Germany than in three cities in western Germany (Behrendt et al., 1993). However, conflicting findings emerged in a

study which compared the prevalence of atopic disease in Munich and Leipzig. A slightly lower prevalence was actually observed in Leipzig in former East Germany, than its western counterpart (von Mutius et al., 1992). The higher concentrations of nitrogen dioxide and automobile exhaust in Munich perhaps suggest that it is more important to consider the effects of specific air pollutants on atopic disease expression than merely to treat air pollution as a single factor. Indeed, residence closer than 50 metres from a high traffic road has been identified as an independent risk factor for AD in a subsequent Bavarian study (Behrendt et al., 1996). These studies are discussed further in Chapter 12.

The findings of these largely descriptive, regional studies are somewhat inconclusive, but serve as an introduction to further analyses which seek to determine whether spatial differences in the occurrence of AD are related to broad environmental factors such as industrial and automobile pollutants, water supply constituents and pesticide residues (such as organophosphorous which is secreted in breast milk). For example, one recent study investigated the potential association between AD and water hardness (McNally et al., 1998b). The study used Geographical Information Systems (GIS) to link the geographical distribution of a school survey with underlying exposure data relating to the characteristics of the local water supply. Strong trends in the prevalence of AD were found with increasing water hardness. The strongest trends were found for one-year period prevalence, implying that hard water may be more a determinant of disease chronicity rather than just incidence. Clearly, more refined studies are needed in order to test hypotheses such as these and particularly to identify the influence of specific factors or constituents in these media.

A more explanatory geographical approach?

The problems incurred when reviewing the geography of AD relate primarily to the inadequacies of the data available for geographical analysis. Geographically-encoded data, or data which can be spatially referenced, are needed which compare the occurrence of the disease between localities using standardized disease definitions. Spatial associations can become possible when recorded data are gathered at specific geographical locations and at particular points in time. Repeated recording of disease characteristics at each given spatial location would add a temporal dimension to the already spatially-referenced data, so that in effect changes over time can be identified. If such prospective studies are carried out on a sufficiently large population basis then the effects of purported environmental

risk factors can be traced through time and space (Cliff & Haggett, 1988). Geographical Information Systems (GIS) also have a great potential for future associative work, particularly for the exploration of the risk associated with proximity to certain factors (de Lepper et al., 1995). In this respect, GIS would be useful for further investigations of the already suggested risks associated with proximity to major roads (Behrendt et al., 1996) and a wide range of other environmental phenomena.

The key to developing geographical research which can provide aetiological clues and evidence in AD, as Williams emphasizes in Chapter 1, is the use of consistent disease definition and diagnosis and also consistency with regard to spatial and temporal referencing. If such data can be derived, geographical studies have a huge potential for clarifying associations between a puzzling condition such as AD and environmental factors, as well as for generating new hypotheses for investigation in further studies at an individual level.

Summary of key points

- Medical geography and the geography of health care have an established place in the study of disease occurrence and the concomitant need for health care.
- Temporal trends in occurrence of AD feature in many of the recent epidemiological studies but consideration of geographical aspects of the disease is far less common.
- The principal reason for a lack of spatial work with regard to AD is the varied reliability and the traditional lack of standardization of disease data over space and time.
- There is a strong indication that the prevalence of AD varies considerably from one country to another.
- The International Study of Asthma and Allergies in Childhood (ISAAC), which uses standardized definitions of AD, has confirmed that marked variations of the disease exist on an international scale.
- The findings of ISAAC suggest that a band of low

prevalence exists in low latitudes and that the disease is more common at higher latitudes.

- Migrant studies have shown large differences in the prevalence of AD between migrant groups and similar genetic groups in their own country, suggesting that factors associated with the transition to developed lifestyles are important in the expression of the disease.
- The concept of the epidemiological transition has important implications for the changing incidence and prevalence of AD.
- A regional variation in the prevalence of AD has been illustrated in Finland and the United Kingdom.
- There are consistencies between the regional distribution of AD and the county level distribution in the UK – the disease is seemingly more common in southern and eastern areas.
- Geographical mapping techniques have been used to identify strong trends in the prevalence of AD with increasing water hardness.
- Further studies which use geographically-encoded data are needed which compare the occurrence of AD between different localities using standardized disease definitions.

References

Bakke, P., Gulsvik, A. & Eide, G.E. (1990). Hay fever, eczema and urticaria in southwest Norway. *Allergy*, **45**, 515–22.

Barry, D., Burr, M. & Limb, E. (1991). Prevalence of asthma among 12 year old children in New Zealand and South Wales: a comparative survey. *Thorax*, **46**, 405–9.

Beaglehole, R., Bonita, R. & Kjellstrom, T. (1993). *Basic Epidemiology*. Geneva: WHO.

Behrendt, H., Krämer, U., Dolgner, R., Hinrichs, J., Willer, H., Hagenbeck, H. & Schlipköter, H.W. (1993). Elevated levels of total serum IgE in East German children: atopy, parasites, or pollutants? *Allergy J*, **2**, 31–40.

Behrendt, H., Krämer, U., Ring, J. & Schäfer, T. (1996). The role of environmental pollutants in atopic eczema. *Conference Abstract*.

Bobák, M., Koupilová, I., Williams, H.C., Leon, D.A., Dnov, J. & Kriz, B. (1995). Prevalence of asthma, atopic eczema and hay fever in five Czech towns with different levels of air pollution. *Epidemiology*, **6** S35 (abstract).

Breborowicz, A., Burchardt, B. & Pieklik, H. (1995). Asthma, allergic rhinitis and atopic dermatitis in schoolchildren. *Pneumonolgia I Alergologia Polska*, **63**, 157–61.

Burkholter, D. & Schiffer, P. (1995). The epidemiology of atopic diseases in Europe – a review. *All Clin Immunol Int*, **7**, 113–25.

Buser, K., von Bohlen, F., Werner, P., Gernhuber, E. & Robra, B-P. (1993). Neurodermitis-Pravalenz bei schulkindern in landkreis Hannover. *Dtsch Med Wschr*, **118**, 1141–5.

Cliff, A.D. & Haggett, P. (1988). *Atlas of Disease Distributions*. Oxford: Blackwell Scientific.

Dold, S., Wjst, M., von Mutius, E., Reitmeir, P. & Stiepel, E. (1992). Genetic risk for asthma, allergic rhinitis, and atopic dermatitis. *Arch Dis Childh*, **67**, 1018–22.

Dotterud, L.K., Kvammen, B., Lund, E. & Falk, E.S. (1995). Prevalence and some clinical aspects of atopic eczema in the community of Sør-Varanger. *Acta Dermatol Venereol (Stockh.)*, **75**, 50–53.

Douven, W. & Scholten, H.J. (1995). Spatial analysis in health research. In: de Lepper, M.J.C., Scholten, H.J. & Stern, R.M., *The Added Value of Geographical Information Systems in Public and Environmental Health*, pp. 117–33. Dordrecht: Kluwer Academic Publishers for WHO.

Elender, F. & Bentham, G. (1996). Tuberculosis mortality in England and Wales during 1982–92: its association with overcrowding, poverty, ethnicity and AIDS. *Proceedings of the VIIth International Symposium in Medical Geography*, pp. 377–80.

English, D. (1992). Geographical epidemiology and ecological studies. In: Elliot, P., Cuzick, J., English, D. & Stern, R. (eds.) *Geographical and Environmental Epidemiology: Methods for Small-Area Studies*, pp. 3–13. Oxford University Press.

Failmezger, C. (1992). Incidence of skin disease in Cuzco, Peru. *Int J Dermatol*, **31**, 560–61.

Frenk, J., Bobadilla, J.L., Stern, C., Frejka, T. & Lozano, R. (1991). Elements for a theory of health transition. *Hlth Transit Rev*, **1**, 21–38.

Gatrell, A.C. & Bailey, T.C. (1996). Interactive spatial data analysis in medical geography. *Soc Sci Med*, **42**, 843–55.

George, A.O. (1989). Atopic eczema in Nigeria. *Int J Dermatol*, **28**, 237–9.

Giggs, J.A., Ebdon, D.S. & Bourke, J.B. (1980). The epidemiology of primary acute pancreatitis in the Nottingham defined population area. *Trans Inst Br Geography*, **NS5**, 229–42.

Golding, J. & Peters, T.J. (1987). The epidemiology of childhood eczema. *Paediat Perinat Epidemiol*, **1**, 67–79.

Gribble, J.N. & Preston, S.H. (eds.) (1993). *The Epidemiological Transition: Policy and Planning Implications for Developing Countries*. Washington, DC: National Academy Press.

Gustafsson, D., Löwhagen, T. & Andersson, K. (1992). Risk of developing atopic disease after early feeding with cows' milk formula. *Arch Dis Childh*, **67**, 1008–10.

Henderson, C.A. (1995). The prevalence of atopic eczema in two different villages in rural Tanzania. *Br J Dermatol*, **133**, Suppl. 45, 50.

Herd, R.M., Tidman, M.J., Prescott, R.J. & Hunter, J.A.A. (1996a). The cost of atopic eczema. *Br J Dermatol*, **135**, 20–23.

Herd, R.M., Tidman, M.J., Prescott, R.J. & Hunter, J.A.A. (1996b). Prevalence of atopic eczema in the community: the Lothian atopic dermatitis study. *Br J Dermatol*, **135**, 18–19.

Hutt, M.S.R. & Burkitt, D.P. (1986). *The Geography of Non-infectious Disease*. Oxford University Press.

Joseph, A.E. & Phillips, D.R. (1984). *Accessibility and Utilization: Geographical Perspectives on Health and Health Care*. London: Harper and Row.

Kalyoncu, A.F. & Stålenheim, G. (1993). Survey on the allergic status in a Turkish population in Sweden. *Allergol Immunopathol*, **21**, 11–14.

Kalyoncu, A.F., Selçuk, Z.T., Karakoca, Y., Emri, A.S., Çöplü, L., Sahin, A.A. & Baris, Y.I. (1994). Prevalence of childhood asthma and allergic diseases in Ankara, Turkey. *Allergy*, **49**, 485–8.

Kay, J., Gawkrodger, D.J., Mortimer, M.J. & Jaron, A.G. (1994). The prevalence of childhood atopic eczema in a general population. *J Am Acad Dermatol*, **30**, 35–9.

Kilkenny, M., Marks, R., Jolley, D. & Merlin, K. (1997). Prevalence of common skin diseases in children and adolescents in Victoria, Australia. *J Invest Dermatol*, **108**, 366 (abstracts).

Kottenhahn, R.K. & Heck, J.E. (1994). Prevalence of paediatric skin diseases in rural Honduras. *Trop Doctor*, **24**, 87–8.

de Lepper, M.J.C., Scholten, H.J. & Stern, R.M. (eds.) (1995). *The Added Value of Geographical Information Systems in Public and Environmental Health*. Dordrecht: Kluwer Academic Publishers for WHO.

Leung, R. (1994). Asthma, allergy and atopy in South-East Asian immigrants in Australia. *Aust N Z J Med*, **24**, 255–7.

Leung, R. & Ho, P. (1994). Asthma, allergy, and atopy in three south-east Asian populations. *Thorax*, **49**, 1205–10.

Luoma, R. & Koivikko, A. (1982). Occurrence of atopic diseases in three generations. *Scand J Soc Med*, **10**, 49–56.

Mayer, J.C. (1983). The role of spatial analysis and geographic data in the detection of disease causation. *Soc Sci Med*, **17**, 1213–21.

Mayer, J.D. (1986). Ecological associative analysis. In: Pacione, M. (ed.) *Medical Geography: Progress and Prospect*, pp. 64–83.

McNally, N.J. (1998). The environment, lifestyle and atopic eczema: a geographical perspective. *Unpublished PhD Thesis, University of Nottingham*.

McNally, N.J., Phillips, D.R. & Williams, H.C. (1998a). The problem of atopic eczema: aetiological clues from the environment and lifestyles. *Soc Sci Med*, **46**, 729–41.

McNally, N.J., Williams, H.C., Phillips, D.R., Smallman-Raynor, M.R., Lewis, S., Venn, A. & Britton, J. (1998b). Atopic eczema and domestic water hardness. *Lancet*, **352**, 527–31.

von Mutius, E., Fritzsch, C., Weiland, S.K., Roll, G. & Magnussen, H. (1992). Prevalence of asthma and allergic disorders among children in united Germany: a descriptive comparison. *Br Med J*, **305**, 1395–9.

Neame, R.L., Berth-Jones, J., Kurinczuk, J.J. & Graham-Brown, R.A.C. (1995). Prevalence of atopic eczema in Leicester: a study of methodology and examination of possible ethnic variation. *Br J Dermatol*, **132**, 772–7.

Ninan, T.K. & Russell, G. (1992). Respiratory symptoms in Aberdeen schoolchildren: evidence from two surveys 25 years apart. *Br Med J*, **304**, 873–5.

Okuma, M. (1994). Prevalence rate of allergic diseases among schoolchildren in Okinawa. *Jap J Allergol (Arergui)*, **43**, 492–500.

Olumide, Y.M. (1986). The incidence of atopic eczema in Nigeria. *Int J Dermatol*, **25**, 367–8.

Paajanen, H. (1994). Common skin diseases. In: Lankinen, K.S., Bergstrom, S., Makela, P.H. & Peltomaa, M. (eds.) *Health and Disease in Developing Countries*, pp. 271–80. London: Macmillan.

Park, C.J., Kim, T.Y., Kim, J.W. & Kim, C.W. (1996). Atopic dermatitis in Korea: the prevalence, the cumulative incidence, and environmental factors. *J Invest Dermatol*, **106**, 893 (abstract).

Parry, W.H. (1979). *Communicable Diseases*, 3rd edn. London: Hodder and Stoughton.

Peat, J.K., van den Berg, R., Green, W., Mellis, C.M., Leeder, S.R. & Woolcock, A.J. (1994). Changing prevalence of asthma in Australian children. *Br Med J*, **308**, 1591–6.

Phillips, D.R. (1981). *Contemporary Issues in the Geography of Health Care*. Norwich: GeoBooks.

Phillips, D.R. (1990). *Health and Health Care in the Third World*. London: Longman.

Phillips, D.R. & Verhasselt, Y. (eds.) (1994). *Health and Development*. London: Routledge.

Pöysä, L., Korppi, M., Pietiäinen, M., Remes, K. & Juntunen-Backman, K. (1991). Asthma, allergic rhinitis and atopic eczema in Finnish children and adolescents, *Allergy*, **46**, 161–5.

Pyle, G.F. (1979). *Applied Medical Geography*. London: John Wiley.

Rajka, G. (1986). Atopic eczema: correlation of environmental factors with frequency. *Int J Dermatol*, **25**, 301–4.

Rose, G. (1985). Sick individuals and sick populations. *Int J Dermatol*, **14**, 32–8.

Schäfer, T., Przybilla, B., Ring, J., Kunz, B., Greif, A. & Überla, K. (1993). Manifestation of atopy is not related to patients' month of birth. *Allergy*, **48**, 291–4.

Schultz Larsen, F., Holm, N.V. & Henningsen, K. (1986). Atopic eczema: a genetic–epidemiologic study in a population-based twin sample. *J Am Acad Dermatol*, **15**, 487–94.

Schultz Larsen, F., Diepgen, T. & Svensson, A. (1996). The occurrence of atopic eczema in North Europe: an international questionnaire study. *J Acad Deratol*, **34**, 760–4.

Strachan, D.P., Golding, J. & Anderson, H.R. (1990). Regional variations in wheezing illness in British children: effect of migration during early childhood. *J Epidemiol Commun Hlth*, **44**, 231–6.

Sugiura, H., Uchiyama, M., Omoto, M., Sasaki, K. & Uehara, M. (1997). Prevalence of infantile and early childhood eczema in a Japanese population: comparison with the disease frequency examined 20 years ago. *Acta Dermatol Venereol (Stockh.)*, **77**, 52–3.

Toropova, N.P., Sinyavskaya, O.A., Kashirskaya, E.N. & Anashkina, T.I. (1996). Epidemiology of atopic eczema (AD) in the Urals and Western Siberia. *Abstract from the 6th International Symposium on Atopic Eczema.*

Turner, K.J. (1987). Epidemiology of atopic disease. In: Lessof, M.H., Lee, T.H. & Kemeny, D.M. (eds.) *Atopy: An International Textbook*, pp. 337–45. London: John Wiley.

Varjonen, E., Kalimo, K., Lammintausta, K. & Terho, P. (1992). Prevalence of atopic disorders among adolescents in Turku, Finland. *Allergy*, **47**, 243–8.

Waite, D.A., Eyles, E.F., Tonkin, S.L. & O'Donnell, T.V. (1980). Asthma prevalence in Tokelauan children in two environments. *Clin Allergy*, **10**, 71–5.

Williams, H.C. (1992). Is the prevalence of atopic eczema increasing? *Clin Exp Dermatol*, **17**, 385–91.

Williams, H.C. (1995). Atopic eczema: we should look to the environment. *Br Med J*, **311**, 1241–2 (Editorial).

Williams, H.C., Pembroke, A.C., Forsdyke, H., Boodoo, G., Hay, R.J. & Burney, G.J. (1995). London-born black Caribbean children are at increased risk of atopic eczema. *J Am Acad Dermatol*, **32**, 212–7.

Williams, H.C., Robertson, C.F., Stewart, A.W., Aït-Khaled, N., Anabwani, G., Anderson, H.R., Asher, M.I., Beasley, R., Björkstén, B., Burr, M., Clayton, T., Crane, J., Ellwood, P., Keil, U., Lai, C.K.W., Mallol, J., Martinez, F., Mitchell, E.A., Montefort, S., Pearce, N., Shah, J.R., Sibbald, B., Strachan, D., von Mutius, E. & Weiland, S.K. (1999). Worldwide variations in the prevalence of symptoms of atopic eczema in the International Study of Asthma and Allergies in Childhood. *J Allergy Clin Immunol*, **103**, 125–38.

Worth, R.M. (1962). Atopic eczema among Chinese infants in Honolulu and San Francisco. *Hawaii Med J*, **22**, 31–4.

Wüthrich, B. (1996). Epidemiology and natural history of atopic eczema. *Allergy Clin Ummunol Int*, **8**, 77–82.

6

The morbidity and cost of atopic dermatitis

Robert M. Herd

Age-specific prevalence

In contrast with other atopic diseases, there are few good population-based epidemiological studies of atopic dermatitis (AD). It is hard to decipher any prevalence trend in published studies because of the various measures of frequency and different age groups. Most have avoided the inherent sampling difficulties of studying entire populations by concentrating on schoolchildren who are accessible and have a high prevalence of AD. The lack of firm diagnostic criteria has usually been glossed over and data have been collected from postal questionnaires, health visitor and general practitioner records and, rarely, by dermatologist examination.

It is acknowledged that the prevalence of AD is rising (Williams, 1992) and that there are regional variations (Golding & Peters, 1987). The true prevalence today must be determined from recent reports from representative populations.

The prevalence of atopic dermatitis in young schoolchildren

The results of prevalence estimates in some recent studies of young schoolchildren are discussed in Chapter 5 and listed in Table 5.1. Those which have included a skin examination are shown in Table 6.1.

Many of the studies listed have estimated lifetime prevalence. But memory becomes less reliable with passing time and lifetime prevalences, based on parental recall, will be subject to variation even if diagnostic accuracy can be assumed. Furthermore, the lifetime prevalence gives no information about age-specific rates: it does not tell us how many had only infantile eczema, and how many were still suffering from active eczema.

This problem can be addressed by using a point prevalence or one-year age-specific prevalence which have been quoted in three recent British studies. In an English general practice, the one-year period prevalence varied from 14.3% in the age group 3–5, to 10.2% in the age group 9–11 (Kay et al., 1994). These data were collected retrospectively from medical records and there was no clear definition of AD. Children aged 3–11 in three London primary schools were the subject of another UK study (Williams et al., 1995). This well executed survey found a point prevalence of 11.7%. A further community study from Lothian in Scotland estimated the one-year age-specific prevalence at age 2–11 to be 8.1% (Herd et al., 1996a).

It is difficult to draw firm conclusions about the prevalence of AD in the UK. Geographical differences reported in the 1970 national birth cohort study demonstrate a prevalence in Scotland lower than that in the rest of the UK (Golding & Peters, 1987). From available evidence, the lifetime prevalence at age 12 appears to be about 12–16% and the one-year period prevalence age 3–11 is in the region of 8–14%.

Prevalence estimates worldwide appear to be high in industrialized countries and low in poorly developed communities (Chapter 5).

Table 6.1. Prevalence of atopic dermatitis quoted in recent studies which included a skin examination

City/area	Publication	Age groups	Frequency	Comments
Italy	Astarita et al. (1988)	9–15	1.1% Point prevalence	Survey of six Italian towns
Denmark	Schultz Larsen (1993)	7	11.5% Lifetime prevalence	Twin study
Germany	Schäfer et al. (1993)	5–6	22.2% Lifetime prevalence	Community survey
Birmingham	Kay et al. (1994)	3–11	11.5% One-year period prevalence	GP interview
London	Williams et al. (1995)	3–11	11.7% Point prevalence	Survey of schoolchildren
Norway	Dotterud et al. (1995)	7–12	26% One-year prevalence	Rural community survey
Leicester	Neame et al. (1995)	1–4	14% Point prevalence	Community survey
Lothian	Herd et al. (1996a)	2–11	9% Point prevalence	Community survey

The prevalence of atopic dermatitis in other age groups

Preschoolchildren

Recent data on preschoolchildren are few although the prevalence seems to be high. One infant study from New Zealand estimated a lifetime prevalence of 20.3% at three years of age (Fergusson et al., 1981), and there have been two reports of the lifetime prevalence in 0–4-year-olds: one estimate in Norwegian Lapps was 15% and another in Leicester was 14% (Falk, 1993; Neame et al., 1995). The one-year period prevalence in Lothian at age 0–1 was 9.8% and this would be equivalent to a lifetime prevalence close to the other estimates in this age group (Herd et al., 1996a).

Teenagers and adults

Teenagers and adults have been as neglected as infants but appear to be affected less. The prevalence in 12–16-year-olds was 3% in 1980 (Larsson & Liden, 1980). The 20-year-old Lambeth study gives prevalences for adults, but these estimates are so high as to suggest the inclusion of diagnoses other than AD under the banner of 'eczema' (Rea et al., 1976). AD in Danish 'Royal Life Guard' recruits aged 17–24 was estimated to be 3.3% (Svejgaard et al., 1986). The source of information for a more recent US survey was government health statistics (Johnson & Roberts, 1978). They covered all ages from 1 to 74, but their low prevalence of AD for age 6–11 of 1.0% is inconsistent with European studies. The prevalence at age 35–44 was 0.06% but rose to 0.18% at age 55–64. Most recently one-year period prevalences were reported in Scotland: 2.2% at age 12–15, 2.1% age 16–24, 2.0% age 25–40 and 0.2% age over 40 (Herd et al., 1996a).

There are gaps in our knowledge of the prevalence of AD. Over one third of AD patients are aged over 16 and yet this group has been largely ignored in prevalence studies (Herd et al., 1996a). The study of AD in different age groups is necessary to examine possible cohort effects of rising prevalence over time which might show effects due to shared early harmful exposures. Without rigorous research, using consistent methodology, any reports of a rising prevalence are open to question. Good community data, covering all age groups, and not just those presumed to have a high prevalence, are needed.

Burden in absolute terms

The prevalence of AD tells us the rate in the population. It can illustrate how populations and subpopulations differ, but without a measure of severity the disease burden is uncertain: the greater the severity, the larger the burden on primary and secondary health services. For example, in a recent community survey (Herd et al., 1996a) it was found that the majority of children defined as having AD were mildly affected. It is possible that these children and their parents were not particularly troubled by their condition or that they coped well within their family resources and knowledge, and consequently seldom used community services.

Regarding severity, AD presents certain unique problems. A severity scoring system must take account of atypical presentations, differences between age groups and stage of treatment. It must be simple and quick to complete in a clinical and epidemiological setting and should be suitable for monitoring disease activity. If comparisons between individuals and populations are to be made there must be low inter-observer variation.

Should symptoms form part of a severity score? Symptoms are subjective, affected by influences unrelated to severity and are more appropriately included in measures of health status. For instance, an individual with severe AD whose treatment has improved but not cleared his skin, may experience relief from pruritus and consequently be untroubled by symptoms, even though his skin remains affected profoundly. The impact of symptoms may be altered by mood as well as extent of inflammation. On the other hand, disease severity should be assessed objectively, on the basis of clinical appearance and not on the effect of the disease on the individual.

The inclusion of disease extent is also questionable. The estimate of the surface area affected in psoriasis has not been reproducible (Ramsay & Lawrence, 1991; Tiling-Grosse & Rees, 1993). The problems are compounded in AD with indistinct margins and widespread areas that are diffusely, rather than confluently, affected which make extent difficult to ascertain. However, the characteristic distribution of AD has been exploited by some authors to avoid the difficulty with estimates of disease extent by limiting severity assessment to certain sites (Stalder et al., 1994).

The assessment of vesiculation and oedema is poorly correlated between observers and perhaps should be excluded (Hanifin, 1989; Berth-Jones, 1996).

Severity indices currently available

The available severity scoring systems range from the short and simple method proposed by Rajka & Langeland (1989) to some long and complex measures described below and recently reviewed (Finlay, 1996).

The PASI score has gained wide acceptance for grading psoriasis severity (Frederiksson & Pettersson, 1978). Attempts to translate this system from psoriasis to AD led to the ADSI (atopic dermatitis severity index) (de Rie et al., 1991) which was refined to the ADASI (atopic dermatitis area severity index) score (Bahmer et al., 1991). The ADASI score was promising in its attempt to simplify the alternative systems. Scoring requires the use of body diagrams superimposed on a 2 cm grid. The affected areas are colour graded: green indicates discrete erythema with or without some scaling and no infiltration; blue indicates erythema with some infiltration and more or less scaling; and red indicates marked erythema with infiltration, with or without scaling; or lichenification with or without excoriation, and with or without superinfection. The number of points on the grid which fall on affected areas are counted and scored with a weighting towards the severely involved areas. To obtain the final score a 'pruritus intensity' factor of 1–5 is included which gives a score of 1–18. The author reports that he can carry out the scoring very quickly, but the ADASI score has failed to gain widespread acceptance, perhaps because the symptom of itch is included and because the score is dependent on the position in which the grid falls on the diagram; it is possible to have severe eczema but a low score. This anomaly may be unimportant in large clinical trials but could certainly affect the score when monitoring an individual's disease.

Some have used 20 area severity charts (Wahlgren et al., 1990) where 20 body sites are graded 0–3 for severity within each zone, giving a score of 0–60. In a variation on this theme 20 areas have been scored for severity and area, resulting in a maximum score of 180 (Sheehan & Atherton, 1992). However, AD preferentially affects certain sites and concentrating on these leads to a more efficient and elegant system.

The SCORAD is the result of collaborative work by the European Task Force on AD (European Task Force on Atopic Dermatitis, 1993). The extent is assessed using the rule of nines and, in a representative area, a score of 0–3 is given to six items: erythema, oedema/papulation, oozing/crusts, excoriation, lichenification and dryness. The patient grades pruritus, sleep loss and 'overall skin condition' – the last included as a global measurement of quality of life – on a 0–10 visual analogue scale. Various weights are attached to these elements before a combined score is calculated.

Although considerable time was expended developing the SCORAD it does have some shortcomings. First, the inherent problems of measuring severity have been discussed above. Secondly, it is a point severity measure which does not reflect disease fluctuations over the previous weeks or months. Thirdly, much of the information collected may be redundant because of overlap between scaling, erythema, lichenification, etc.: the same information could be extracted from a small group of signs. Fourthly, its validity has never been formally assessed and the interpretation of a score of, for instance, 23.2 is not immediately apparent. It is still quite complicated and time-consuming and, although it has been used in a number of large trials, is unlikely to be incorporated into routine clinical practice.

The most recent contribution is the SASSAD (six area six sign AD) severity score (Berth-Jones, 1996).

It is a refinement of previous systems (Lever et al., 1988; Berth-Jones & Graham-Brown, 1990) in which a grading of 0–3 is given to erythema, exudation, excoriation, dryness, cracking and lichenification at six sites: arms, hands, legs, feet, head and neck, and trunk. The maximum score is 108. This takes account of the usual distribution of AD and does not allow the arbitrary choice of a 'representative area'. It has been tested in clinical trials and is suitable for use in children and adults. It lacks the sophistication of weighted systems, but it is quick and easy to use by untrained practitioners and, of the available schemes, must be considered a good compromise.

Population studies of severity

Having established a means of grading AD, the range of severity in the population can be ascertained. The evolution of severity scores has been driven by the need to measure treatment response in clinical trials, not epidemiological studies. Consequently, detailed population-based studies of severity do not exist but those that have addressed severity are listed in Table 6.2.

There is a published report of the increasing prevalence of atopic diseases in Swedish schoolchildren which classifies eczema severity on empirical grounds (Åberg et al., 1995). It states that 63% had suffered 'severe' eczema over the previous year. One English study, which primarily addressed racial differences, examined severity and found that 13% of 45 children had 'severe' AD (Neame et al., 1995). Lastly, a report from Norway found that severity was distributed as 64% mild, 31% moderate and 3% severe. In each of these reports severity was an incidental part of the investigation.

In a study of ethnic groups in London severity was assessed by a dermatologist on the basis of the strength of treatment (Williams et al., 1995); but anomalies exist where the skin is clear because of strong treatment and, conversely, an individual is severely affected despite using mild treatment. The answer must be more detailed attention to severity in epidemiological studies.

Table 6.2. Recent studies which included assessment of severity

Country	Publication	Year	Comments
England	Williams et al.	1995	Study of ethnic variation. No significant difference in severity found between white and Black Afro-Caribbean children
Sweden	Åberg et al.	1995	63% had severe eczema over previous year
Norway	Dotterud et al.	1995	Community survey found 66% mild, 33% moderate and 3% severe disease
England	Neame et al.	1995	13% had 'severe' atopic dermatitis

Table 6.3. Items of expenditure that were enumerated over a two-month period. Subjects were asked to keep the following records

(1) Keep containers for all treatments whether bought over the counter or prescribed by the family doctor
(2) Record dates of consultations with family doctor and expenses involved
(3) Record dates of visits to hospital and expenses involved
(4) Record all dates off work or school
(5) Record any loss of salary
(6) Record any extra clothing or laundry because of atopic dermatitis
(7) Any other expenses related to skin

Direct and indirect financial costs

Medical practice is becoming increasingly shackled by economic constraints. Some understanding of the financial implications of different diseases is now necessary, particularly for the most common ones such as AD.

The economic aspects of AD have received scant attention. Only one publication in recent years has dealt with the cost of AD (Lapidus et al., 1993). This paper, from the USA, estimated the annual cost of treating children in that country to be $364 million. The analysis was limited for three reasons: it dealt only with children; treatment in the community was not included; and the cost to patients was omitted.

The financial burden in the UK

A community study from Scotland has addressed this issue (Herd et al., 1996b). Over a two-month period patients were asked to record on a proforma (Table 6.3) all expenditure related to their AD. From this information it was possible to separate personal costs, health service costs and society costs. For instance, personal costs to patients and families arise from prescriptions, over-the-counter preparations, travel to and from the general practitioner or hospital, salary loss, and clothing and laundry expenses; health service costs are due to prescribed drugs, and the provision of primary and secondary care; and the cost to society is due to lost working days.

One hundred and forty-six subjects completed the study. Some patients remained in remission over the study period and had no expenditure. However, three patients spent over £150 and ten spent over £100 in two months. The mean annual expenditure in 1994 was £153 per patient. Clothing and laundry led to the highest expense of £70 per annum, followed by over-the-counter preparations and salary loss (Figure 6.1).

The mean annual health service cost was £97 per patient, 68% for drugs, 28% for general practitioner consultations and 6% for hospital consultations. In two months there were 58 lost working days and 17 lost school days.

Any extrapolation to a wider population is subject to error; but if these figures are assumed to be representative, they reveal an annual personal expenditure by patients and families of £297 million, a charge to the health service of £125 million, and cost to society of £43 million for a country such as the United Kingdom in 1994. This adds up to a total of

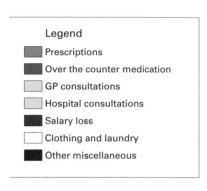

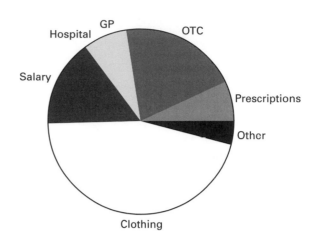

Fig. 6.1. Pie chart illustrating the distribution of expenditure by patients and their families

£465 million per annum, or a per capita cost of £7.38 per annum.

Chronic skin diseases differ from most other medical conditions when their costs are being assessed. A plethora of over-the-counter preparations is available for problems ranging from acne to warts. Remedies for treating dry skin conditions like AD are particularly numerous, and vary greatly in their price. Articles in the media often advertise new, expensive, 'holistic' treatments which claim to cure eczema or psoriasis, but at a price. A further drain on patients' resources comes from the need for new clothing or bedding, and from the laundry costs which accounted for 45% of expense to patients in the whole study, and 63% of the costs to families with children aged under 16. One ten-year-old boy in the above study needed new cotton sheets every two months, partly because of repeated washing, but also because nocturnal scratching led to extra wear and tear.

The continuing rise in the cost of providing health care calls for a more rigorous examination of clinical effectiveness. When treatment outcomes are shown to be similar, cost effectiveness becomes a central variable in drawing conclusions about clinical practice. Costing is important to help clinicians make rational decisions about resource allocation, and it is therefore important that clinicians have an understanding of the significance of costing and the methods involved in calculating these costs.

Morbidity and social costs

The issues of cost and quality of life are closely linked. All clinicians have to play a part in the difficult task of allocating scarce resources within the health service (Lazarus, 1994). To do this properly they need to know which treatments lead to an improved outcome for their patients, and which are cost effective (Detsky & Naglie, 1990; Cunliffe et al., 1991). Reliable measures of quality of life can help here by providing an accurate estimate of the benefits conferred by any individual line of treatment.

Many countries now operate in a purchaser/provider era with an economic approach to setting priorities in their health services. Dermatology services are perhaps at a disadvantage when competing for resources because they deal mainly with illnesses that do not threaten life, and are therefore seen as less serious and of low priority by purchasers of health care. Measures of quality of life impairment should be incorporated into these assessments of priority (Delamothe, 1994).

Where quality of life has been measured it is often added as an afterthought (Bergner, 1989). It is seldom the principal focus and in a survey of 100 publications using the term 'quality of life', it was seldom defined (van Dam et al., 1981). This remains a contentious issue (Siegrist & Junge, 1989).

The concept of quality of life

Quality of life has been defined as 'the extent to which hopes and ambitions are matched by experience' and the key aim of medical care should be to 'narrow the gap between a patient's hopes and aspirations and what actually happens' (Calman, 1984). Quality of life was initially promoted as a measure of outcome in 1986, as an alternative to more traditional end-points such as death or myocardial infarction (Croog et al., 1986). However, this early attempt to measure quality of life included physical, cognitive, emotional and social function which usually form part of health status measures.

Quality of life must be distinguished from health status and functional status, concepts that can be measured in a tangible way (Bergner, 1989). Health status measures were developed to improve the care and health of individuals. They include items relating to physical functioning as well as measures of emotional status and perceptions of health (Patrick & Deyo, 1989). Functional status is the assessment of activities of daily living. Two examples of functional status measurements are the Karnofsky Performance Status and the New York Heart Association Classification, which have been used for assessing eligibility for clinical trials (New York Heart Association, 1979; Karnofsky et al., 1980). They are concise and specific to one disease.

In contrast, quality of life is intangible. It should rely on the statements of patients, should not be restricted to one moment in time, and should be able to compare different periods of time (van Dam et al., 1981).

The measurement of quality of life in atopic dermatitis

Patients with AD find that their sleep, work and relationships are all affected by their disease (Jowett &

Ryan, 1985; Reid & Lewis-Jones, 1995). Good qualitative data, generated by outcome measures which truly capture the impact and relavance of AD to patients, are needed as a gauge to the degree to which individuals' lives are altered.

A survey of 11 500 members of the National Eczema Society examined disease impact (Long et al., 1993). The results may be biased on two accounts: the population may not have been representative of all patients with AD, and the response rate was only 29%. They did, however, confirm the important effect on work, household activities and personal relationships, and a survey of parents of children with AD demonstrated that sleep loss was the most important area.

A follow-up survey one year later, targeting individuals with severe AD, generated some interesting data (Finlay, 1994). Quality of life impairment was severe. There was an average of £5000 lost income and five lost working days per annum. Subjects were given a brief description of bronchitis and asked whether they considered it to be worse than AD: the majority would rather have had bronchitis. Such a comparison can be criticized as being unrealistic in that most subjects had not experienced both, but even the few individuals who had both AD and bronchitis felt that AD was worse. Some 50% were willing to spend two hours per day on treatment to make their skin normal, and 70% would spend one hour. Half would pay £10 000 for a cure and 75% would pay £1000. When these results were corrected for income, patients were prepared to spend up to 75% of their annual income on such a cure.

Specific measures of quality of life used in atopic dermatitis

There has been one attempt to develop a quality of life measure specific to AD (Eun & Finlay, 1990). Fifty-five AD patients over 20 years old completed a questionnaire designed to determine which aspects of their lives were most affected, and a questionnaire was constructed using their responses (see Box 6.1). This may have been the basis for a good quality of life measure but it has not been validated. Construct validity (i.e. the extent to which a new measure relates to established measures of severity) was significant at only $p<0.05$, and reliability (i.e. the extent to which a test or measurement result is reproducible) and criterion validity (i.e. the extent to which a new measure correlates with established measures of quality of life) were not tested.

Box 6.1. Desirable elements of a quality of life measure for AD

(1) Should rely on the statements of patients
(2) The severity of items identified by patients should be rated
(3) There should be a composite score
(4) Should not be restricted to one moment in time
(5) Different periods of time should be compared

Few measures of disability are valid, reliable and responsive to change, or are practicable for everyday use. The Dermatology Life Quality Index (DLQI) is a simple practical measure of quality of life for use in clinical practice (Finlay & Khan, 1994). It was established by studying 120 consecutive dermatology out-patients who were asked to identify how their skin disease affected their lives. From this information, a ten-item questionnaire was constructed, each question scoring 0–3, with high scores representing severely impaired quality of life (Table 6.4). Correlation coefficients, as opposed to chance-corrected agreement measures, were erroneously used to examine reliability using the test–retest method which gave a significant correlation ($p<0.001$). Further work on external validity testing is underway but has not yet been published.

Another measure that has been used in dermatology is the Patient Generated Index (PGI). It was developed for back pain, and shown to be valid, reliable and to correlate with measures of severity (Ruta et al., 1994). The elements of life affected by the condition are chosen by individuals completing the questionnaire. Subjects differ in their living conditions, jobs, hobbies, sports and social activities, and consequently their lives are affected in a variety of ways by the same disease. For instance, patients with

Table 6.4. The dermatology life quality index

(1) Over the last week, how itchy, sore, painful or stinging has your skin been?
(2) Over the last week, how embarrassed or self-conscious have you been because of your skin?
(3) Over the last week, how much has your skin interfered with you going shopping or looking after your home or garden?
(4) Over the last week, how much has your skin influenced the clothes your wear?
(5) Over the last week, how much has your skin affected your social or leisure activities?
(6) Over the last week, how much has your skin made it difficult for you to do any sport?
(7) Over the last week, has your skin prevented you from working or studying? If 'No', over the last week how much has your skin been a problem at work or studying?
(8) Over the last week, how much has your skin created problems with your partner or any of your close friends or relatives?
(9) Over the last week, how much has your skin caused any sexual difficulties?
(10) Over the last week, how much of a problem has the treatment for your skin been, for example by making your home messy, or by taking up time?

Reproduced, with permission, from Finlay & Khan (1994).

AD are more affected if they clean their own house than if they employ a domestic, and a nurse is more likely to have her ability to work impaired than a secretary. The PGI not only encompasses the disability attributable to different lifestyles but can theoretically be used for any condition in which quality of life is important.

It is completed in three stages. These are illustrated in Table 6.5 which demonstrates an example of a 32-year-old woman with AD. First, patients identify the five areas or activities most influenced by their disease: for instance work, socializing, swimming, housework and sleep are nominated in this example. Secondly, each of these areas is given a score of 0–100. The lower the score the greater the impairment of life quality: in the example sleep is given the lowest score of 10 implying that it is most

Table 6.5. An example of the calculation of the Patient Generated Index

Activity	Score	Points	Total score
Work	20×	20 [÷60]	= 6.7
Socializing	20×	10 [÷60]	= 3.3
Swimming	30		
Housework	20×	10 [÷60]	= 3.3
Sleep	10×	20 [÷60]	= 3.3
Other aspects of life	30		
Total			16.7

severely affected. A sixth line is provided for areas or activities other than those already mentioned, which may or may not be related to the subject's skin disease. Finally, patients are given 60 points to 'spend', with most points being allocated to areas they most want to improve: sleep and work were the areas to which the woman in our example attached most importance. From this information an overall score of 0–100 is calculated.

The PGI and DLQI were used to determine quality of life in a community study of AD (Herd et al., 1997). The scores from each measure correlated significantly. The DLQI was not devised as a measure of disability specific to AD, but in skin conditions in general; this may explain why it was found that certain questions in the DLQI were not correlated with life quality as measured by the PGI whereas other items not in the DLQI, such as sleep and contact with animals, did appear to be important to AD patients.

Conclusions from this study must be guarded. First, it was a community study in which the severity of AD was mild compared with that seen in hospital practice. Secondly, the PGI needs further validation to assess its responsiveness to change in perceived health or quality of life over time. The numerous skin conditions cause a wide variety of changes in patients' lives. As an open-ended questionnaire, the PGI may be applicable over a range of dermatological disorders but it must be shown to be reliable and adaptable.

Quality of life should be a uniquely personal perception of the way individuals react to their health status (Gill, 1995). A review of 75 quality of life articles found the majority deficient in several ways: they did not define quality of life; they did not identify the specific areas of life on which they intended to focus; and they did not aggregate their results into a composite score (Gill & Feinstein, 1994). The PGI was given special mention, along with two other articles, for 'showing promise' (Ruta et al., 1994; O'Boyle et al., 1992; Joyce, 1994). Three attributes were mentioned which a quality of life measure should possess, based on the hypothesis that quality of life comprises many different characteristics which are the province of the individual. First, patients should identify the areas that are important to them. Secondly, the severity should be rated. Thirdly, patients should be invited to rate the relative importance of these items to their quality of life.

At present, prevalence studies are generally restricted to children while quality of life studies relate to adults. This may be convenient for research workers but it is illogical. More studies of the whole cross-section of the population are required. Children's quality of life assessment is difficult, but there is now a Children's Dermatology Life Quality Index that allows an entry into the world of disability measurement in children (Lewis-Jones & Finlay, 1995). Further work on the impact of AD on children and their families will be illuminating.

Summary of key points

- Atopic dermatitis (AD) surveys concentrate on children, but one study has suggested that one third of AD sufferers are adults.
- Because adults have severe and chronic disease they may occupy a relatively greater proportion of the social and economic cost.
- There is little information about disease burden in the community.
- Several measures have been developed for AD severity for use in clinical trials but have not been validated in epidemiological studies.

- A knowledge of the proportion of patients in the community with mild, moderate and severe disease would help health services provide appropriate care.
- Direct and indirect financial costs have been estimated for AD and are considerable for those most severely affected, both in terms of personal expense and cost to health services.
- An important area of development is in the evaluation of the social burden.
- New measures of quality of life, such as the Patient Generated Index, are helping to reveal the ways that AD influences lives.

References

Åberg, N., Hesselmar, B., Åberg, B. & Eriksson, B. (1995). Increase of asthma, allergic rhinitis and eczema in Swedish schoolchildren between 1979 and 1991. *Clin Exp Allergy*, **25**, 815–19.

Astarita, C., Harris, R.I., de Fusco, R., Franzese, A., Biscardi, D., Mazzacca, F.R.M. & Altucci, P. (1988). An epidemiological study of atopy in children. *Clin Allergy*, **18**, 341–50.

Bahmer, F.A., Schäfer, J. & Schubert, H.J. (1991). Quantification of the extent and the severity of atopic dermatitis: the ADASI score. *Arch Dermatol*, **127**, 1239–40.

Bergner, M. (1989). Quality of life, health status, and clinical research. *Med Care*, **27**, S148–S156.

Berth-Jones, J. (1996). Six area and six sign AD (SASSAD) severity score: a simple system for monitoring disease activity in atopic dermatitis. *Br J Dermatol*, **135** (Suppl. 48), 25–30.

Berth-Jones, J. & Graham-Brown, R.A.C. (1990). Failure of papaverine to reduce pruritus in atopic dermatitis: a double-blind, placebo-controlled cross-over study. *Br J Dermatol*, **122**, 553–7.

Calman, K.C. (1984). Quality of life in cancer patients – a hypothesis. *J Med Ethics*, **10**, 124–7.

Croog, S.H., Levine, S., Testa, M.A., Brown, B., Bulpitt, C.J., Jenkins, C.D., Klerman, G.L. & Williams, G.H. (1986). The effects of antihypertensive therapy on the quality of life. *New Engl J Med*, **314**, 1657–64.

Cunliffe, W.J., Gray, J.A., Macdonald-Hull, S., Hughes, B.R., Calvert, R.T., Burnside, C.J. & Simpson, N.B. (1991). Cost effectiveness of isotretinoin. *J Dermatol Treat*, **1**, 285–8.

Delamothe, T. (1994). Using outcomes research in clinical practice. *Br Med J*, **308**, 1583–4.

De Rie, M.A., Meinardi, M.M.H.M. & Bos, J.D. (1991). Lack of efficacy of topical cyclosporin A in atopic dermatitis and allergic contact dermatitis. *Acta Dermatol Venereol (Stockh.)*, **71**, 452–4.

Detsky, A.S. & Naglie, I.G. (1990). A clinician's guide to cost-effectiveness analysis. *Ann Int Med*, **113**, 147–54.

Dotterud, L.K., Kvammen, B., Lund, E. & Falk, E.S. (1995). Prevalence and some clinical aspects of atopic dermatitis in the community of Sør-Varanger. *Acta Dermatol Venereol (Stockh.)*, **70**, 50–53.

Eun, H.C. & Finlay, A.Y. (1990). Measurement of atopic dermatitis disability. *Ann Dermatol*, **2**, 9–12.

European Task Force on Atopic Dermatitis (1993). Severity scoring of atopic dermatitis: the SCORAD Index. *Dermatology*, **186**, 23–31.

Falk, E.S. (1993). Atopic diseases in Norwegian Lapps. *Acta Dermatol Venereol*, Suppl. 182, 10–14.

Fergusson, D.M., Horwood, L.J., Beautrais, A.L., Shannon, F.T. & Taylor, B. (1981). Eczema and infant diet. *Clin Allergy*, **11**, 325–31.

Finlay, A.Y. (1994). Quality of life survey. *Exchange*, **73**, 22.

Finlay, A.Y. (1996). Measurement of disease activity and outcome in atopic dermatitis. *Br J Dermatol*, **135**, 509–15.

Finlay, A.Y. & Khan, G.K. (1994). Dermatology life quality index (DLQI) – a simple practical measure for routine clinical use. *Clin Exp Dermatol*, **19**, 210–16.

Frederiksson, T. & Pettersson, U. (1978). Severe psoriasis – oral therapy with a new retinoid. *Dermatologica*, **157**, 238–44.

Gill, T.M. (1995). Quality of life assessment: values and pitfalls. *J R Soc Med*, **88**, 680–2.

Gill, T.M. & Feinstein, A.R. (1994). A critical appraisal of the quality of quality-of-life measurements. *J Am Med Ass*, **272**, 619–26.

Golding, J. & Peters, T.J. (1987). The epidemiology of childhood eczema. I. A population-based study of associations. *Paediat Perinatal Epidemiol*, **1**, 67–79.

Hanifin, J.M. (1989). Standardized grading of subjects for clinical research studies in atopic dermatitis: workshop report. *Acta Dermatol Venereol (Stockh.)*, Suppl. 144, 28–30.

Herd, R.M., Tidman, M.J., Prescott, R.J. & Hunter, J.A.A. (1996a). Prevalence of atopic eczema in the community: the Lothian atopic dermatitis study. *Br J Dermatol*, **135**, 18–19.

Herd, R.M., Tidman, M.J., Prescott, R.J. & Hunter, J.A.A. (1996b). The cost of atopic eczema. *Br J Dermatol*, **135**, 20–23.

Herd, R.M., Tidman, M.J., Ruta, D.A. & Hunter, J.A.A. (1997). Measurement of quality of life in atopic dermatitis: correlation and validation of two different methods. *Br J Dermatol*, **136**, 502–7.

Johnson, M.L. & Roberts, J. (1978). Skin conditions and related needs for medical care among persons 1–74 years, United States 1971–1974, US Department of Health, Education and Welfare, Publ. No (PHS) 79–1660 1978: 1–67.

Jowett, S. & Ryan, T. (1985). Skin disease and handicap: an analysis of the impact of skin conditions. *Soc Sci Med*, **20**, 425–9.

Joyce, C.R. (1994). Health status and quality of life: which matters to the patient? *J Cardiovasc Pharmacol*, **23** (Suppl. 3), S26–S33.

Karnofsky, D.A., Abelmann, W.H. & Craver, L.F. (1980). The use of nitrogen mustards in the palliative treatment of carcinoma. *Cancer*, **1**, 634.

Kay, J., Gawkrodger, D.J., Mortimer, M.J. & Jaron, A.G. (1994). The prevalence of childhood atopic eczema in a general population. *J Am Acad Dermatol*, **30**, 35–9.

Lapidus, C.S., Schwartz, D.F. & Honig, P.J. (1993). Atopic dermatitis in children: who cares? who pays? *J Am Acad Dermatol*, **28**, 699–703.

Larsson, P.A. & Liden, S. (1980). Prevalence of skin diseases among adolescents 12–16 years of age. *Acta Dermatol Venereol (Stockh.)*, **60**, 415–23.

Lazarus, G.S. (1994). Managed care in California. Daunting new realities for dermatology and academic medicine. *Arch Dermatol*, **130**, 1539–42.

Lever, R., Hadley, K., Downey, D. & Mackie, R. (1988). Staphylococcal colonization in atopic dermatitis and the effect of topical mupirocin therapy. *Br J Dermatol*, **119**, 189–98.

Lewis-Jones, M.S. & Finlay, A.Y. (1995). The Children's Dermatology Life Quality Index (CDLQI): initial validation and practical use. *Br J Dermatol*, **132**, 942–9.

Long, C.C., Funnell, C.M., Collard, R. & Finlay, A.Y. (1993). What do members of the National Eczema Society really want? *Clin Exp Dermatol*, **18**, 516–22.

Neame, R.L., Berth-Jones, J., Kurinczuk, J.J. & Graham-Brown, R.A.C. (1995). Prevalence of atopic dermatitis in Leicester: a study of methodology and examination of possible ethnic variation. *Br J Dermatol*, **132**, 772–7.

New York Heart Association (1979). *Nomenclature and Criteria for Diagnosis of Diseases of the Heart and Great Vessels*, 8th edn. Boston: Little, Brown.

O'Boyle, C.A., McGee, H., Hickey, A., O'Malley, K. & Joyce, C.R. (1992). Individual quality of life in patients undergoing hip replacement. *Lancet*, **339**, 1088–91.

Patrick, D. & Deyo, R. (1989). Barriers to the use of health status measures in clinical investigation. *Med Care*, **27**, S217.

Rajka, G. & Langeland, T. (1989). Grading of the severity of atopic dermatitis. *Acta Dermatol Venereol (Stockh.)*, Suppl. 144, 13–14.

Ramsay, B. & Lawrence, C.M. (1991). Measurement of involved surface area in patients with psoriasis. *Br J Dermatol*, **124**, 565–70.

Rea, J.N., Newhouse, M.L. & Halil, T. (1976). Skin disease in Lambeth. A community study of prevalence and use of medical care. *Br J Prevent Soc Med*, **30**, 107–14.

Reid, P. & Lewis-Jones, M.S. (1995). Sleep difficulties and their management in preschoolers with atopic eczema. *Clin Exp Dermatol*, **20**, 38–41.

Ruta, D.A., Garratt, A.M., Leng, M., Russell, I.T. & MacDonald, L.M. (1994). A new approach to the measurement of quality of life. The patient-generated index. *Med Care*, **32**, 1109–26.

Schäfer, T., Przybilla, B., Ring, J., Kunz, B., Greif, A. & Überla, K. (1993). Manifestation of atopy is not related to patient's month of birth. *Allergy*, **48**, 291–4.

Schultz Larsen, F. (1993). Atopic dermatitis: a genetic–epidemiologic study in a population-based twin sample. *J Am Acad Dermatol*, **28**, 719–23.

Sheehan, M.P. & Atherton, D.J. (1992). A controlled trial of traditional Chinese medicinal plants in widespread non-exudative atopic eczema. *Br J Dermatol*, **126**, 179–84.

Siegrist, J. & Junge, A. (1989). Background material for the workshop on QALYs. *Soc Sci Med*, **29**, 463–8.

Stalder, J.F., Fleury, M., Sourisse, M., Rostin, M., Pheline, F. & Litoux, P. (1994). Local steroid therapy and bacterial skin flora in atopic dermatitis. *Br J Dermatol*, **131**, 536–40.

Svejgaard, E., Christophersen, J. & Jelsdorf, H.M. (1986). Tinea pedis and erythrasma in Danish recruits. *J Am Acad Dermatol*, **14**, 993–9.

Tiling-Grosse, S. & Rees, J. (1993). Assessment of area of involvement in skin disease: a study using schematic figure outlines. *Br J Dermatol*, **128**, 69–74.

Van Dam, F.S.A.M., Somers, R. & van Beek-Couzijn, A.L. (1981). Quality of life: some theoretical issues. *J Clin Pharmacol*, **21**, 166S–168S.

Wahlgren, C.F., Scheynius, A. & Hägermark, Ö. (1990). Antipruritic effect of oral cyclosporin A in atopic dermatitis. *Acta Dermatol Venereol (Stockh.)*, **70**, 323–9.

Williams, H.C. (1992). Is the prevalence of atopic dermatitis increasing? *Clin Exp Dermatol*, **17**, 385–91.

Williams, H.C., Pembroke, A.C., Forsdyke, H., Booboo, G., Hay, R.J. & Burney, P.G.J. (1995). London-born black Caribbean children are at increased risk of atopic dermatitis. *J Am Acad Dermatol*, **32**, 212–17.

Is the prevalence of atopic dermatitis increasing?

Thomas L. Diepgen

Introduction

There is a widespread belief that the prevalence of atopic disorders (atopic dermatitis, allergic rhinitis, allergic asthma) has been increasing over recent decades. Most of these trends were reported with asthma and allergic rhinitis according to the results of epidemiological studies. In this chapter published studies on recent secular trends in atopic dermatitis (AD) will be reviewed in the light of potential sources of methodological error, and possible reasons for these trends will be discussed.

Summary of available secular trend studies

On the basis of several cross-sectional studies from northern Europe the cumulative incidence in children (up to seven years) seems to be less than 3% if they were born before 1960, 4 to 8% for those children born between 1960 and 1970, 8 to 12% for those born after 1970, rising to over 15% according to recent studies (Table 7.1). The interpretation of these cross-sectional studies, however, must be drawn very carefully and should not be overinterpreted because of several sources of methodological error. Due to methodological heterogeneities given in Table 7.2, extrapolation of data obtained from separate individual studies to establish secular trends in whole communities is fraught with uncertainty. Changes in diagnostic criteria or labelling and a better understanding of the word *eczema* can easily lead to false interpretation of changes in repeated prevalence studies. Repeated cross-sectional studies that use

Table 7.1. Frequency of atopic dermatitis according to year of birth before 1960, between 1960 and 1979, and after 1970. Selection of cross-sectional studies (modified according to Schultz Larsen & Hanifin, 1992)

Author		Frequency (%)
Year of birth before 1960		
Service	1939	2.9
Eriksson-Lihr	1955	2.5
Walker & Warin	1956	3.1
Brereton et al.	1959	1.6
Freeman & Johnson	1964	1.4
Larsson & Lidén	1980	2.0
Year of birth 1960–70		
Arbeiter	1967	6.8
Turner et al.	1974	8.8
Kjellman	1977	8.3
Larsson & Lidén	1980	6.1
Engbaek	1982	3.8
Year of birth after 1970		
Fergusson et al.	1982	20.4
Engbaek	1982	9.1
Taylor et al.	1984	12.2
Schultz Larsen et al.	1986	10.2
Storm et al.	1986	8.9
Schultz Larsen	1993	11.5

the same methodology (disease definition, questions, sampling frame and method) on samples of children also suggest an increase of AD, but they too tend to suffer from the above-mentioned methodological problems.

Table 7.2. Sources of methodological errors for the interpretation and comparison of cross-sectional studies

Source of errors due to	Reasons for not comparable or biased data
Study design	Prospective versus retrospective data collection result in different quality of data. Cohort studies versus cross-sectional studies differ in strength.
Study population	Hospital versus community based data allow different conclusions. Heterogeneity of groups in terms of age, sex, ethnic origin, socioeconomic standards can cause bias. Sample size often too small and confidence limits not given.
Outcome variable	Differences in disease definition and/or differences in the severity of eczema make study populations not comparable.
Instruments	Questionnaire-based data versus medical examination have different strengths and validation of instruments is often missing.
Standardization	Sensitivity, specificity and predictive value are often small or even unknown.
Measures	Point prevalence, period prevalence and incidence rates are different epidemiological measures.
Systematic errors	Selection, information, recall bias and confounding distort results and interpretation.

Taylor et al. (1984) showed that the prevalence of a history of eczema (determined by parental recall when the children were aged between 5 and 7 years) increased from 5.1% in children born in 1946 to 7.3% in those born in 1958 and to 12.2% in the 1970 cohort. The results of this important study, however, must be interpreted with caution because of the following points. The three birth cohorts were recorded

Table 7.3. Sources of misinterpretation in time trend studies (examples)

- More public awareness of allergy and atopy due to mass media
- Increased acceptability of the word *eczema* in the population
- Ignoring of mild or moderate skin complaints because of more serious illness or severe economic problems to worry about
- More medical use of the term eczema
- Improved diagnostic methods for atopy
- Less misclassification of imitating diseases

at slightly different age groups (five to seven years) and drawn from three separate studies which used slightly different methods of data collection. In only the 1958 cohort the diagnosis according to the reports by health visitors interviewing mothers at home (7.1%) was validated against physicians' records (2.5%). Such validation is difficult to interpret as atopic eczema is a rapidly fluctuating disease. Additionally, possible alternative explanations can be given for this trend, such as changes in the acceptability or medical use of the word 'eczema', improved diagnostic methods or misclassification of similar diseases such as irritant dermatitis from the use of nappies. It must also be assumed that parents and children in the 1940s and 1950s had more serious illnesses or other economic problems to worry about, and mild to moderate childhood eczema has been ignored (Table 7.3).

In two elegant Danish population-based twin studies, Schultz Larsen demonstrated a rising cumulative incidence of atopic eczema in twins (Figure 7.1) (Schultz Larsen, 1993; Schultz Larsen et al., 1986). The cumulative incidence rate, up to seven years of age, increases to 3% in twins born between 1960 and 1964, and to 12% in twins born between 1975 and 1979. The diagnosis was achieved by a questionnaire and case ascertainment was still based on recall of eczema as a child according to the patient and/or parent. In a recent cross-sectional study using the same questionnaires the cumulative

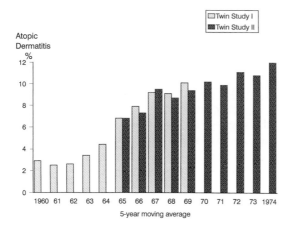

Fig. 7.1. The cumulative incidence rates for atopic dermatitis in Danish twins according to the year of birth between 1960 and 1979 (modified according to Schultz Larsen, 1993; Schultz Larsen et al. 1986)

incidence of AD rises to 15.6% (95% confidence interval 14.2–17.0) in seven-year-old schoolchildren in Denmark, Germany and Sweden (Schultz Larsen et al., 1996).

A Scottish study reported an increase of atopic eczema between 1964 and 1989 from 5.3 to 12% in children aged from 8 to 13 years attending primary schools in Aberdeen (Ninan & Russell, 1992). The main objection against this study is that the first data collection was by interview and the second by questionnaire, and the wording of questions was changed. In another study from Scotland (Austin & Russell, 1997) the prevalence rose from 14% (in 1992) to 18% (in 1994). This time span seems, however, to be too short for studying time trends.

In a recent Japanese study Sugiura et al. (1997) came to the conclusion that the prevalence of infantile and early childhood atopic eczema has not changed over the last 20 years. The authors observed eczema in 30% of four-month-old infants, in 32% of ten-month-old infants, and in 20% of three-year-old children at the time of clinical examination. The majority of cases were mild. The results were compared with a similar study performed 20 years earlier by Uehara et al. (1975), who had observed similar prevalence rates at the same time of the year (spring)

by using the same guidelines for diagnosis during physical examination. The authors conclude that the prevalence of atopic eczema in infants did not increase over the last 20 years in Japan. In their opinion, one reason for the difference from other studies, which have described an increase of the frequency of atopic eczema, might be the possibility that mild cases of eczema have been ignored in the previous studies based on recall bias.

In a questionnaire-based study from Switzerland the authors also found no increase in the prevalence of atopic dermatitis between 1968 (children aged 4–6 years: 2.2%; aged 15 years: 2.3%) and 1981 (children aged 4–6 years: 2.8%; aged 15 years: 1.5%) (Varonier et al., 1984).

An analysis of the prevalence of allergic diseases among Swedish conscripts showed a relatively constant prevalence of flexural dermatitis between 1973 and 1978, i.e. among the males born between 1955 and 1960 (Hedberg, 1994). Since then, there has been a steady increase in the prevalence of flexural dermatitis from 0.8 to 2.6% up to 1993. The same increase was observed for asthma (from 2 to 6%) and hay fever (from 5 to 15%) (Figure 7.2). In Swedish conscripts an increase in allergic diseases was also observed between 1971 and 1981 (Aberg, 1989). The frequency of atopic eczema increased from 4.9 to 8.4% during this period.

Other epidemiological studies performed with 10–20-year intervals in the same region using a similar methodology indicate that there has been an increase in both the prevalence of allergic asthma among children (Burr et al., 1989; Burney, 1993) and the proportion of subjects with at least one positive skin-prick test reaction (Sibbald et al., 1990; Barbee et al., 1987) over the past few decades. After the unification of Germany an increasing prevalence of hay fever and eczema was reported among children (aged 9–11 years) in East Germany. In the first survey (1991–92) the prevalence rates were 2.3% for hay fever and 12.1% for eczema; in the second survey (1995–96) they were 5.1% for hay fever and 14.2% for eczema (von Mutius et al., 1998). Interestingly, the authors could not detect an increase in the prevalence of asthma between these two periods.

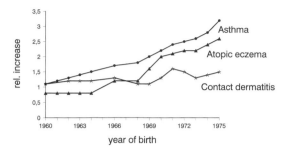

Fig. 7.2. Relative increase in the prevalence of atopic dermatitis, allergic asthma and contact dermatitis among 18-year-old male conscripts in Sweden 1978–1993 in relation to their year of birth (modified according to Björkstén, 1997)

Possible sources of error

Definition of the outcome variable

Although most dermatologists have little difficulty in making a firm diagnosis in most cases of AD, there may be problems in mild cases and in differentiating this condition from other rashes, especially in early infancy. It is crucial for epidemiological studies to have a good disease definition. Atopic dermatitis, however, is a difficult disease to define because of variable distribution and morphology, variable time course, and the lack of a diagnostic test.

Additionally, in every country several synonyms are in common use by physicians and patients for the disease which is here named atopic dermatitis. Given these difficulties it is not surprising that there have been a range of different methods and definitions for AD, ranging from questionnaire recall of 'eczema during childhood' and parental recall, to health visitor and physician recall.

In a study in Brandenburg, Germany, we could show in a sample of 5055 schoolchildren aged between five and six years, that the lifetime prevalence of AD was 10.2% according to physical examination and 7.0% according to physician's diagnosis (Ellsasser & Diepgen, 1998). Clinical signs of atopic disease (atopic dermatitis, allergic rhinitis and asthma) were found in 26.4% but only 12.9% of the children were diagnosed as atopics at former medical consultations.

Clinical diagnostic features of AD were based largely on experience of cases attending hospitals and outpatient clinics (e.g. Hanifin & Rajka, 1980) and these criteria are very helpful in describing the various aspects of the clinical syndrome of AD, but are less useful in epidemiological studies because of their complexity and unknown validity. Various other diagnostic tools have been suggested based on clinical examination (Diepgen & Fartasch, 1992; Diepgen et al., 1989, 1996; Svensson et al., 1985) or questionnaire (Schultz Larsen & Hanifin, 1992). Williams et al. (1994) have proposed and validated a minimum set of diagnostic criteria for AD which are recommended to be used as a one-year period prevalence measure in epidemiological studies. These UK criteria were shown to have a sensitivity and specificity of 80 and 96%, respectively, in children attending hospital dermatology outpatients, when compared to a dermatologist's diagnosis (Williams et al., 1994). In a community survey of London children aged 3–11 years, of mixed ethnic and socioeconomic groups, the sensitivity and specificity for AD prevalence were 80 and 97%, respectively, when using these UK criteria (Williams et al., 1996).

Studies which have examined a defined population over time by using uniform standardized criteria are rare. Therefore, it has to be considered that much, or even all, of the change of reported AD is due to secular trends in diagnosis. Increasing public awareness of rising trends in the prevalence of allergic diseases may have influenced both diagnostic labelling by physicians and parental reports of doctors' diagnoses and children's symptoms of atopic diseases.

Validation of the outcome variable

None of the definitions of the outcome variable for atopic dermatitis is 100% valid. Individuals who carry an atopic disposition are often missed, while others are wrongly designated as cases of AD. In order to ascertain the validity of a used instrument the terms 'sensitivity', 'specificity' and 'predictive value' are used. The sensitivity stands for the chance that cases with AD are correctly diagnosed, the

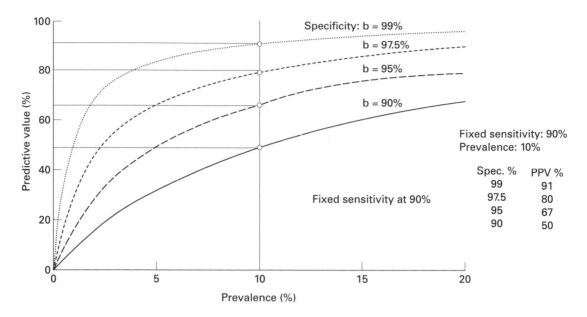

Fig. 7.3. Graphic representation of the positive predictive value (PPV) as a function of the prevalence p for atopic dermatitis for four values of the diagnostic specificity b, given a test sensitivity of 90%

Table 7.4. A hypothetical example of how an increase in the prevalence of AD can be explained by a decrease in specificity

	First study	Second study
True prevalence of AD	10%	10%
Sensitivity	95%	95%
Specificity	95%	90%
Sample size	1000	1000
Estimated number of cases with AD	135	185
Study estimate of AD prevalence	13.5%	18.5%

specificity that the nonAD cases are correctly stated in the investigation. However, it is important not only to know the sensitivity and specificity of the used instruments, it will be more essential to calculate the positive predictive value (PPV), which is the proportion of those individuals diagnosed by the used instrument who actually are atopics. It is important to mention that the PPV is a function of the true prevalence of AD in the population, the sensitivity and the specificity. In Figure 7.3 the PPV is shown as a function of the prevalence p, given a fixed value of 90% for the sensitivity, and four different values for the specificity. If, for example, the prevalence of AD is 10% and the specificity of a questionnaire 90%, then a positive answer result is 50% of cases diagnosed correctly. On the other hand, a specificity of 99% gives a PPV of around 91%. The value of PPV depends strongly on the specificity and only to a limited extent on the sensitivity in the relevant area of 60–100%.

Theoretically, from a statistical point of view an observed increase of the prevalence of AD can be explained by a decrease of specificity over time because of an increased awareness of allergic diseases in the population (resulting in more false positives). Assuming a true prevalence of 10%, a sensitivity of 95% and a specificity of 95%, the percentage of individuals diagnosed as cases of AD would be 13.5%. If the specificity decreases over time to 90%, then 18.5% would be diagnosed as AD cases (Table 7.4). This example also demonstrates that an overestimation of the true prevalence must be

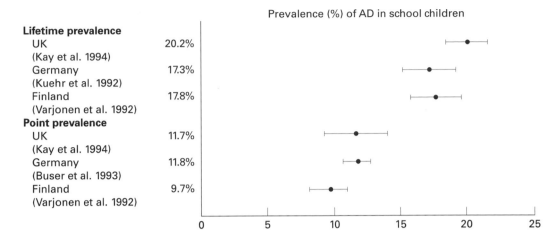

Lifetime prevalence
UK (Kay et al. 1994)	20.2%
Germany (Kuehr et al. 1992)	17.3%
Finland (Varjonen et al. 1992)	17.8%

Point prevalence
UK (Kay et al. 1994)	11.7%
Germany (Buser et al. 1993)	11.8%
Finland (Varjonen et al. 1992)	9.7%

Fig. 7.4. Recent prevalence surveys of atopic dermatitis in schoolchildren in Europe. The point and period prevalence and the corresponding 95% confidence intervals are shown.

assumed in most studies, and comparing studies using different instruments (even with seemingly minor differences regarding sensitivity and specificity) can lead to false conclusions.

Prevalence and incidence

Prevalence of a disease is a cross-section 'snap-shot' of the total number of diseased subjects (new and old) within a defined population at a point of time (point prevalence) or in a defined period (period prevalence), and should not be confused with incidence which gives the number of new cases in a defined period. In Figure 7.4 the results of some recent prevalence studies (point versus period prevalence) are shown for Europe. According to the investigated sample size the 95% confidence intervals were calculated. The point prevalence seems to be half of the period prevalence. Another problem of point prevalence estimates is the fact that AD is a chronically relapsing disease with an age-specific pattern (highest frequencies within the first two years of life) which differs from that of other atopic diseases, such as hay fever or asthma. Thus, the prevalence rate depends on the age of the investigated sample.

Prevalence reflects disease determinants of disease duration as well as incidence. Without knowing whether disease chronicity has changed over time, the interpretation of prevalence data is hazardous and incidence data are preferable for examining the changes in the biology of a disease.

If it is increasing, why?

The above mentioned deficiencies, problems and limitations of the available data and studies need to be borne in mind when discussing the question whether AD and other atopic manifestations have been increasing over recent years. Which plausible reasons can support a real increase in the prevalence of atopic diseases over recent decades?

Genetic susceptibility

There is no doubt that the general propensity of atopy is genetically determined. The likelihood of developing allergic disease in an individual, however, is not constant over time and individuals with a vacant family history of atopy can develop AD. The genetic background of AD, however, cannot explain the obvious rapidly increasing frequency of AD in the short time span of the last few decades. Thus, it seems that other and still unrecognized factors in the environment can affect the occurrence of AD · in genetically susceptible persons.

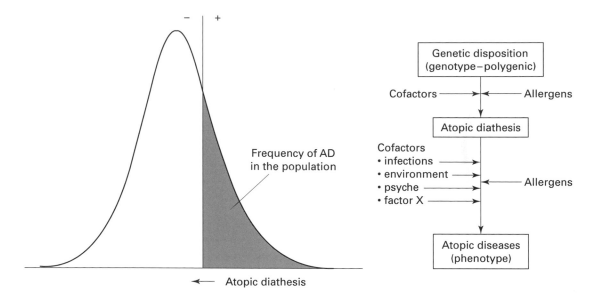

Fig. 7.5. A model of multifactorial inheritance in combination with a threshold is assumed for the inheritance of atopic diseases

Environmental factors may influence the phenotypic expression of AD and act as indicators of the genetic predisposition which is probably influenced by many alleles on several chromosomes. Under the hypothesis of a multifactorial pathogenesis with polygenetic inheritance, it seems plausible that a shift in the whole distribution of latent atopic disease might be responsible for the recent changes in disease prevalence, and the increase of the prevalence of AD might be caused by a shift of the whole distribution of the phenotype of atopic disorders (Figure 7.5).

In a recent paper it has been shown that, depending on the definition of the phenotype of atopy, different regions of potential linkage to autosomal markers on chromosomes 4, 6, 7, 11, 13 and 16 were detected (Daniels et al., 1996). The pleiotropy of phenotypes is consistent with the known variability of atopy and may be attributable to environmental events. Additionally, some markers showed significantly stronger maternal linkage. This maternal effect at several loci favours immunological interactions between mother and child. This hypothesis is also supported by the results of a study indicating a stronger familial aggregation of atopic diseases between siblings than between parents and siblings (Diepgen & Blettner, 1996). In this study, a higher odds ratio of AD between mothers and siblings than between fathers and siblings was also found. Family aggregation between mother and child may be explained by shared physical environment at home or environmental events that are passed on to the fetus in utero. It can be assumed that environmental factors will be shared more intensively between the mother and the child than between the father and the child. The familial aggregation of atopic dermatitis can also be explained by stronger maternal heritability, and would be consistent with atopic mothers carrying relatively more genes predisposing to disease than atopic fathers.

The hypothesis of environmental interactions is also supported by the observation of geographical differences and the results of migration studies.

Geographical differences and migration studies

Several studies of individuals belonging to the same ethnic group and having the same genetic back-

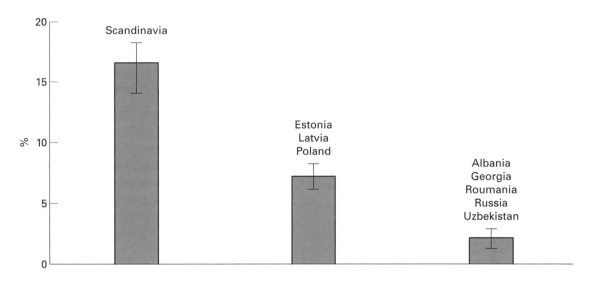

Fig. 7.6. The cumulative prevalence of flexural dermatitis among 13–14-year-old children participating in the International Study of Asthma and Allergy in Children (ISAAC) (modified according to Björkstén, 1997)

ground, but living under different conditions, have demonstrated that the incidence of atopic diseases is higher in industrialized countries than in former socialist countries of eastern Europe (ISAAC, 1998). For example, in northern and eastern Europe the highest one-year prevalence of flexural dermatitis was seen in Scandinavia; it was lower in the western part of the former socialist region, i.e. Estonia, Latvia and Poland, and lowest in those former socialist countries with a lifestyle even more different from that in western Europe, e.g. Albania, Georgia, Romania, Russia and Uzbekistan (Figure 7.6). Between eastern and western Germany similar differences were observed but are limited to the people born after 1961 (Wichmann, 1995; von Mutius et al., 1992). Similar data were observed between Estonia and Sweden (Jögi et al., 1996) and between Polish and Swedish schoolchildren (Braback et al., 1994). Additionally, in western and eastern countries the prevalence was higher in urban as opposed to rural areas (Braback et al., 1994).

Migrant studies also support the finding that envi-ronmental factors associated with 'urbanization' and 'development' are important in the aetiology of AD. The risk of AD is greater for Asian children born in Australia when compared with recently immi-grated Asian children (Leung & Ho, 1994). Polynesian immigrants to New Zealand have a higher prevalence of AD compared with similar genetic groups of their country of origin (Waite et al., 1980). London-born Black Caribbean children have been shown to be at higher risk of AD than their white counterparts (Williams et al., 1995). This sup-ports the theory that environmental factors seem to be at least as important as genetic factors in deter-mining the expression of AD.

Other interesting observations showed a 1.5–2-fold higher prevalence of AD in higher compared with lower socioeconomic groups (Bergmann et al., 1993; Schäfer et al., 1996; Williams, Strachan & Hay, 1994; Wüthrich, 1996), and in children in privately owned houses as compared with those in rented houses. There is also a greater risk of AD in smaller families (von Mutius et al., 1994).

In Table 7.5 epidemiological observations are summarized which support the role of urbanization, development and western lifestyle for the increasing prevalence of atopic diseases within the last few decades.

Table 7.5. Epidemiological observations supporting the role of urbanization, development and western lifestyle for the increasing prevalence of atopic diseases within recent decades

- Increasing prevalence over the last 30 years in industrialized western countries
- Prevalence higher in immigrants to western countries
- Prevalence higher in industrialized countries with a market economy
- Prevalence higher in urban than in rural areas
- Prevalence higher in privileged socioeconomic groups and smaller families
- Increase most obvious in children and young adults
- Increasing prevalence with increasing industrialization in developing countries

Environmental factors and lifestyle

In eastern Germany the prevalence of atopic sensitization increased after German unification. Between 1991 and 1996 there was a significant increase in the prevalence of hay fever, atopic sensitization and eczema in 9–11-year-old schoolchildren in Leipzig (von Mutius et al., 1998). In the former east Germany tremendous changes towards western lifestyle have occurred since unification. Which factors are associated with western lifestyle? The following factors have been proposed as potential explanations for the higher prevalence of atopic disorders in west European countries: smaller family size, high socioeconomic status, western diet, and increasing allergen exposure attributable to indoor and outdoor pollution. Changes in dietary habits have been implicated as a characteristic of societies with increasing affluence, and Black & Sharpe (1997) have postulated that high intake of certain polyunsaturated fatty acids, such as linoleic acid, may be a risk factor for the development of childhood asthma and allergies. Von Mutius et al. (1998) postulated that the increase in margarine consumption in eastern Germany might be a risk factor for the increase of allergic diseases. The relationship between increased versus unchanged margarine consumption and the prevalence of hay fever remained

significant in this study after adjustment for family history of atopic diseases, socioeconomic status, number of siblings, use of wood or coal for heating, and pet ownership (odds ratio 2.0, 95% CI 1.1–3.5). We can only speculate, however, about the role of environmental factors as we do not yet know whether these factors may enhance sensitization, trigger an allergic reaction in sensitized individuals, or act due to their physical properties. Can the increase of AD be at least partly explained by the exposure to new or higher concentrations of airborne or dietary antigens, and/or by environmental factors increasing the susceptibility to cutaneous irritation and sensitization? Epidemiological studies on environmental risk factors are difficult to perform because of the complexity and interrelationship of these factors. It is especially difficult to control for possible confounding factors and to find a real cause and effect relationship. Therefore, carefully designed studies are needed, and only a very limited number of questions can be answered with one study.

Environmental factors, such as exposure to allergens, and outdoor and indoor pollution (e.g. tobacco smoke, emissions from building material, ventilation), may enhance or trigger an atopic reaction in susceptible individuals. These factors have undergone major changes in recent decades. The discussion of the various environmental factors influencing atopic diseases, however, has mostly been limited to the possible effects of increased exposure to certain allergens (house dust mite, nutrition, airborne antigens, pets), deteriorating air quality (outdoor and indoor pollution) and poorly ventilated houses. Exposure to tobacco smoke is by far the best identified risk factor for the development of allergic diseases, but there is no convincing evidence that daily exposure to tobacco smoke results in an increased risk of developing AD (Mills et al., 1994). Outdoor pollution (SO_2, NO_2, diesel particles) may be one of the environmental factors behind the increased prevalence, but no clear relationship between air pollution and the prevalence of AD could be confirmed in different studies. Indoor concentrations of some pollutants may be far in excess

Table 7.6. Changes in lifestyle and environment after World War II in industrialized western countries (examples)

Factors	Changes
Urbanization	Higher exposure to air pollution, major changes in habits.
Lifestyle	Most time spent indoors.
	Extensive travelling and exposure to new environment.
	Smaller families.
	Higher income.
	More cars.
	More pets.
	Fewer infections.
Diet	A wider range of foods (many that are new).
	New food additives and preservatives.
	Foods processed by industry.
	Prolonged storage time of foods, genetic manipulation.
	No seasonal variation.
Buildings and homes	New building materials.
	More efficient isolation.
	Larger dwellings.
	New chemicals at home.
	Increased indoor humidity.

Table 7.7. Odds ratios for the occurrence and remission of atopic dermatitis in positive versus negative tuberculin responders by age according to multiple logistic regression analysis (adjusted for sex, lifestyle, nutritional status, environmental factors and family history) (according to Shirakawa et al., 1997). Only significant values are shown

Tuberculin response	Occurrence	Remission
Conversion to positive up to 6 years of age	0.50 (0.33–0.91)	1.6 (1.0–2.2)
Conversion to positive between 6 and 12 years of age	n.s.	6.7 (4.8–11.4)

n.s. = not significant.

Immunology and infections

The improved living standards and immunization programmes in western societies have induced a decline of many infectious diseases in developed countries. Can this medical progress be responsible for the increase of atopic diseases?

Epidemiological data support the possibility that diminished exposure to infections might prompt atopic responses (Von Mutius et al., 1994) and cross-infections from other siblings in larger families might have a protective role in atopic disease expression (Strachan, 1989). An interesting observation is that children with atopic dermatitis occasionally undergo spontaneous remission after severe bacterial or viral infections, although usually temporarily (Lacour, 1994). Epidemiological data from Guinea-Bissau show that a history of childhood measles infection was associated with a 50% decrease in the rate of positive atopic skin tests (Shaheen et al., 1996). Among Japanese schoolchildren, a strong inverse association between delayed hypersensitivity to *Mycobacterium tuberculosis* and atopy was recently reported (Shirakawa et al., 1997) (Table 7.7). Children with positive delayed hypersensitivity to tuberculin (DHT) had serum cytokine concentrations suggestive of predominant Th1 responses, in contrast to the Th2 profiles seen in

of the outdoor concentration (especially in rooms where people are smoking). The indoor environment probably plays a larger role for the development of AD. Modern, well isolated houses have been associated with an increased risk of development of sensitization and allergic manifestations (Lau et al., 1989).

'Environmental factors', however, are much more than emissions from traffic and industry, or exposure to mites and dander. The concept of 'lifestyle' seems to be more promising and tries to describe some major changes in our society within the last few decades. This concept includes, for example, dietary changes, the microbial environment, stress, new and better isolated houses, extensive travelling to new environments, etc. (Table 7.6).

children with negative DHTs. In this study no differences were found for possible confounding variables, such as lifestyle, environmental factors and nutritional status.

The primary immune responses to allergens are assumed to be different in atopic and nonatopic individuals. They are encountered during early life and include both Th1- and Th2-like immunity. With repeated exposure over time either type will become dominant. In nonatopic individuals the likelihood for Th1-type immunity to eventually prevail is high. In atopic individuals, however, Th2-type immunity associated with a continuing IgE antibody formation is common. This genetically determined propensity can be modified by infections and other microbial stimulation selecting for Th1-like immunity. If an individual has predominantly Th2 T cells, the Th2 phenotype interacts with the environmental allergens to produce atopic diseases. Infections may alter the balance between Th1 and Th2 phenotypes (Cookson & Moffatt, 1997). The clean living conditions of western societies with reduced incidence of infection may tip the balance toward the Th2 phenotype and predispose to atopic manifestations. Less microbial pressure exerted on young individuals in western societies during the maturation of the immune system would result in a lower, slower postnatal maturation of the immune system and thus the delayed achievement of an optimal balance between Th1- and Th2-like immunity (Holt, 1994). Helminth and other parasitic infections may protect against allergic diseases, despite up-regulation of Th2 responses. These findings could explain the lower prevalence of AD in rural regions and in developing countries.

The role of parasite, bacterial and viral infections in relation to AD needs to be further analysed in prospective studies, especially in AD, as most of the recent studies have been mainly focused on allergic asthma.

Future public health implications of increasing atopic dermatitis?

In conclusion, most of the studies support the notation that there has been a true increase in the prevalence of AD over the past three decades in industrialized countries with a market economy and a western lifestyle. However, the most important risk factor remains the genetic disposition. Therefore, a more detailed understanding of the factors responsible for the increase in atopic dermatitis and allergic diseases in western countries may be helpful in preventing atopic diseases in high-risk families. For a better understanding more carefully designed epidemiological studies on the role of potential risk factors would be useful, and for more effective primary and secondary prevention, well designed randomized intervention studies are needed. In developed countries atopic diseases should be ranked higher in public health programmes.

Also, in developing countries the public health implications for atopic diseases are high. A better understanding of the factors involved may help to prevent similar increases in developing countries which are undergoing rapid changes towards western lifestyle and economy.

More intensive research activities about the interrelationship between infections and sensitizations in our rapidly changing environment are needed. Comparative studies in developed and developing countries look promising. However, a good cooperation between epidemiology and fundamental biology will be necessary to answer the question 'why are atopic diseases increasing'?

Public health programmes have to be established for the prevention of atopic diseases. Family-orientated information about skin care and irritancy, allergen avoidance and diet should be available to high-risk individuals. Because of the magnitude of the problem, specific information should be released to the general population. General practitioners, gynaecologists, midwives, paediatricians and paediatric nurses should be primarily involved in such a programme. Dermatologists who frequently attend children with atopic dermatitis should be aware of the broad spectrum of allergic diseases. Physicians involved in disease management should not be limited to the prescribing of topical and systemic treatments; they should implement prophylactic measures. Later in life, counselling concerning professional occupation should be systematically given to AD patients, especially those with a history of hand dermatitis.

Summary of key points

- Due to methodological heterogeneities the comparison of separate individual cross-sectional studies and the extrapolation of data obtained from these studies in establishing secular trends in whole communities is fraught with uncertainty.
- Repeated cross-sectional studies using the same disease definition, questions, sampling frame and method suggest an increase in atopic dermatitis (AD), but these studies too tend to suffer from methodological problems.
- Sources of error for interpretation are differences in disease definition, study design and population, lack of validation (sensitivity, specificity, predictive value are often unknown), selection, information and recall bias.
- Further sources of misinterpretation are more public awareness and acceptability of allergy, improved diagnostic methods, and less ignoring of mild skin complaints.
- Collectively, most of the epidemiological studies indicate an increase in the prevalence of all atopic diseases (allergic asthma, allergic rhinitis and atopic dermatitis) among children.
- Studies of individuals belonging to the same ethnic group, but living under different conditions, have demonstrated that the prevalence of atopic diseases is higher in industrialized countries than in former socialist countries of eastern Europe. In eastern Germany the prevalence of atopic sensitization increased after German unification.
- Atopy is genetically determined but environmental factors may influence the phenotype expression of AD and act as indicators of the genetic predisposition.
- 'Environment' is much more than emission from traffic and industry, or exposure to mites and dander. The concept of 'lifestyle', which tries to describe some major changes in our society within the last few decades, seems to be more promising.
- Western lifestyle factors, such as smaller family size, high socioeconomic status, western diet, and increasing allergen exposure attributable to indoor and outdoor pollution, might play a role in the higher prevalence of atopic disorders in west European countries.
- Epidemiological studies on environmental risk factors, however, are difficult to perform because of the complexity and inter-relationship of these factors.
- Epidemiological data further support the possibility that diminished exposure to infections might prompt atopic responses, and cross-infections from other siblings in larger families might have a protective role in atopic disease expression.
- The role of parasitic, bacterial and viral infections in relation to AD need to be further analysed in prospective studies.
- For a better understanding of the increase in atopic diseases more carefully designed epidemiological studies and well designed randomized intervention studies are needed.
- Public health programmes need to be established for the prevention of atopic diseases.

References

Aberg, N. (1989). Asthma and allergies in Swedish conscripts. *Clin Exp Allergy*, **19**, 59–63.

Arbeiter, H.I. (1967). How prevalent is allergy among United States school children? A survey of findings in the Munster (Indiana) school system. *Clin Pediatr*, **6**, 140–2.

Austin, J. & Russell, G. (1997). Wheeze, cough, atopy, and indoor environment in the South Highlands. *Arch Dis Childh*, **76**, 22–6.

Barbee, R., Kaltenborn, W., Lebowitz, J. & Burrows, B. (1987). Longitudinal changes in allergen skin reactivity in a community population sample. *J All Clin Immunol*, **79**, 16–24.

Bergmann, K.E., Bergmann, R.L., Bauer, C.P., Dorsch, W., Forster, J., Schmidt, E., Schulz, J. & Wahn, U. (1993). Atopie in Deutschland. *Dt Ärztebl*, **90**, 28–32.

Björkstén, B. (1997). The environment and sensitisation to allergens in early childhood. *Pediat All Immunol*, **8** (Suppl. 10), 32–9.

Black, P.N. & Sharpe, S. (1997). Dietary fat and asthma: is there a connection? *Eur Resp J*, **10**, 6–12.

Braback, L., Breborowicz, A., Dreborg, S., Knutsson, A., Pieklik, H. & Björkstén, B. (1994). Atopic sensitizations and respiratory symptoms among Polish and Swedish school children. *Clin Exp Allergy*, **24**, 826–35.

Brereton, E.M., Carpenter, R.G., Rook, A.J. & Tyer, P.A. (1959). The prevalence and prognosis of eczema and asthma in Cambridgeshire school children. *Br Med J*, **11**, 317.

Burney, P. (1993). Epidemiology of asthma. *Allergy* **48**, 17–21.

Burr, M.L., Butland, B.K., King, S. & Vaughan-Williams, E. (1989). Changes in asthma prevalence: two surveys 15 years apart. *Arch Dis Child*, **64**, 1452–6.

Buser, K., Bohlen, F., Werner, P., Gernhuber, E. & Robra, B-P. (1993). Neurodermitis-Prävalenz bei Schulkindern im Landkreis Hannover. *Dtsch Med Wschr*, **118**, 1141–5.

Cookson, W.O.C.M. & Moffatt, M.F. (1997). Asthma: an epidemic in the absence of infection? *Science* **275**, 41–2.

Daniels, S.E., Bhattacharrya, S., James, A. et al. (1996). A genome-wide search for quantitative trait loci underlying asthma. *Nature* **383**, 247–50

Diepgen, T.L. & Fartasch, M. (1992). Recent epidemiological and genetic studies in atopic dermatitis. *Acta Dermatol Venereol (Stockh.)*, **176**, 13–18.

Diepgen, T.L., Fartasch, M. & Hornstein, O.P. (1989). Evaluation and relevance of atopic basic and minor features in patients with atopic dermatitis and in the general population. *Acta Dermatol Venereol (Stockh.)*, Suppl 144, 50–54.

Diepgen, T.L. & Blettner, M. (1996). Analysis of familial aggregation of atopic eczema and other atopic diseases by using odds ratio regression models. *J Invest Dermatol*, **106**, 977–81.

Diepgen, T.L., Sauerbrei, W. & Fartasch, M. (1996). Development and validation of diagnostic scores for atopic dermatitis incorporating criteria of data quality and practical usefulness. *J Clin Epidemiol*, **49**, 1031–8.

Ellsässer, G., Diepgen, T.L. & Gladitz, J. (1998). Risk factors for atopic diseases in primary-school children in Brandenburg. *Allergologie*, **21**, 296.

Engbaek, S. (1982). *The Morbidity of School Age*. Copenhagen: Laegeforeningens Forlag.

Eriksson-Lihr, Z. (1955). The incidence of allergic disease in childhood. *Acta Allergol*, **8**, 289–313.

Fergusson, D.M., Horwood, L.J. & Shannon, F.T. (1982). Risk factors in childhood eczema. *J Epidemiol Commun Hlth*, **36**, 118–22.

Freeman, G.L. & Johnson, S. (1964). Allergic diseases in adolescents. I. Description of survey: prevalence of allergy. *Am J Dis Child*, **107**, 549–59.

George, S., Berth-Jones, J. & Graham-Brown, R.A. (1997). A possible explanation of the increased referral of atopic dermatitis from the Asian community in Leicester. *Br J Dermatol*, **136**, 494–7.

Hanifin, J.M. & Rajka, G. (1980). Diagnostic features of atopic dermatitis. *Acta Dermatol Venereol (Stockh.)*, **92**, 44–7.

Hedberg, A. (1994). National Swedish Board of Welfare.

Holt, P.G. (1994). A potential vaccine strategy for asthma and allied atopic diseases during early childhood. *Lancet*, **344**, 456–8.

The International Study of Asthma and Allergies in Childhood (ISAAC) (1998). Worldwide variation in prevalence of symptoms of asthma, allergic rhinoconjunctivitis, and atopic eczema: ISAAC. *Lancet*, **351**, 1225–32.

Jögi, R., Jansson, C., Björnsson, E., Bomann, G. & Björkstén, B. (1996). The prevalence of asthmatic respiratory symptoms among adults in an Estonian and Swedish university town. *Allergology*, **51**, 331–6.

Kay, J., Gawkrodger, D.J., Mortimer, M.J. & Jaron, A.G. (1994). The prevalence of childhood atopic eczema in a general population. *J Am Acad Dermatol*, **30**, 35–9.

Kjellman, N-I.M. (1977). Atopic disease in seven-year-old children. *Acta Paediatr Scand*, **66**, 465–71.

Kuehr, J., Frischer, T., Karmaus, W., Meinert, R., Barth, R. & Urbanek, R. (1992). Clinical atopy and associated factors in primary-school pupils. *Allergy*, **47**, 650–5.

Lacour, M. (1994). Acute infections in atopic dermatitis: a clue for a pathogenic role of a Th1/Th2 imbalance? *Dermatology*, **188**, 255–7.

Larsson, P-A. & Lidén, S. (1980). Prevalence of skin diseases among adolescents 12–16 years of age. *Acta Dermatol Venereol (Stockh)*, **60**, 415–23.

Lau, S., Falkenhorst, G., Weber, A. et al. (1989). High mite-allergen exposure increases the risk of sensitisation in atopic children and young adults. *J All Clin Immunol*, **84**, 718–25.

Leung, R. & Ho, P. (1994). Asthma, allergy, and atopy in three south-east Asian populations. *Thorax*, **49**, 1205–10.

Mills, C.M., Srivastava, E.D., Harvey, I.M., Swift, G.L., Newcombe, R.G., Holt, P.J.A. & Rhodes, J. (1994). Cigarette smoking is not a risk factor in atopic dermatitis. *Int J Dermatol*, **33**, 33–4.

Von Mutius, E., Fritzsch, C., Weiland, S.K., Röll, G. & Magnussen, H. (1992). Prevalence of asthma and allergic disorders among children in united Germany: a descriptive comparison. *Br Med J*, **305**, 1395–9.

Von Mutius, E., Martinez, F.D., Fritzsch, C., Nicolai, T., Reitmeir, P. & Thiemann, H-H. (1994). Skin test reactivity and number of siblings. *Br Med J*, **308**, 692–5.

Von Mutius, E., Weiland, S.K., Fritzsche, C., Duhme, H. & Keil, U. (1998). Increasing prevalence of hay fever and atopy among children in Leipzig, East Germany. *Lancet*, **351**, 862–6.

Ninan, T.K. & Russell, G. (1992). Respiratory symptoms and atopy in Aberdeen schoolchildren: evidence from two surveys 25 years apart. *Br Med J*, **304**, 873–5.

Schäfer, T., Vieluf, D., Behrendt, H., Krämer, U. & Ring, J. (1996).

Atopic eczema and other manifestations of atopy: results of a study in East and West Germany. *Allergy*, **51**, 532–9.

Schultz Larsen, F. (1993). Atopic dermatitis. A genetic–epidemiologic study in a population-based twin sample. *J Am Acad Dermatol*, **28**, 719–23.

Schultz Larsen, F. & Hanifin, J.M. (1992). Secular change in the occurrence of atopic dermatitis. *Acta Dermatol Venereol (Stockh.)*, Suppl. 176, 7–12.

Schultz Larsen, F., Holm, N.V. & Henningsen, K. (1986). Atopic dermatitis. A genetic–epidemiologic study in a population-based twin sample. *J Am Acad Dermatol*, **15**, 487–94.

Schultz Larsen, F., Diepgen, T.L. & Svensson, A. (1996). The occurrence of atopic dermatitis in North Europe. An international questionnaire study. *J Am Acad Dermatol*, **34**, 760–4.

Service, W.C. (1939). The incidence of major allergic diseases in Colorado Springs, *J Am Med Ass*, **112**, 2034–7

Shaheen, S.O., Aaby, P., Hall, A.J. et al. (1996). Measles and atopy in Guinea-Bissau. *Lancet*, **347**, 1792–6.

Shirakawa, T., Enomato, T., Shimazu, S. & Hopkin, J.M. (1997). The inverse association between tuberculin response and atopic disorder. *Science*, **275**, 77–9.

Sibbald, B., Rink, E. & D'Souza, M. (1990). Is the prevalence of atopy increasing? *Br J Gen Pract*, **40**, 338–40.

Storm, K., Hahr, J. Kjellman, N-I.M. & Osterballe, O. (1986). The occurrence of asthma and allergic rhinitis, atopic dermatitis and urticaria in Danish children born in one year. *Ugeskr Laeger*, **148**, 3295–9.

Strachan, D.P. (1989). Hay fever, hygiene and household size. *Br Med J*, **299**, 1259–60.

Sugiura, H., Uchiyama, M., Omoto, M., Sasaki, K. & Uehara, M. (1997). Prevalence of infantile and early childhood eczema in a Japanese population: comparison with the disease frequency examined 29 years ago. *Acta Dermatol Venereol (Stockh.)*, **77**, 52–3.

Svensson, A., Edman, B. & Möller, H. (1985). A diagnostic tool for atopic dermatitis based on clinical criteria. *Acta Dermatol Venereol (Stockh.)*, **114**, 33–40.

Taylor, B., Wadsworth, J., Wadsworth, M. & Peckham, C. (1984). Changes in the reported prevalence of childhood eczema since the 1939–45 war. *Lancet*, **1**, 1255–7.

Turner, K.J., Rosman, D.L. & O'Mahony, J. (1974). Prevalence and familial association of atopic disease and its relationship to serum IgE levels in 1,061 school children and their families. *Int Arch Allergy*, **47**, 650–64.

Uehara, M., Horio, T. & Ofuji, S. (1975). Incidence of infantile eczema in the general population. *Acta Dermatol Kyoto*, **70**, 95–8.

Varjonen, E., Kalimo, K., Lammintausta, K. & Terho, P. (1992). Prevalence of atopic disorders among adolescents in Turku, Finland. *Allergy*, **47**, 234–48.

Varonier, H.S., de Haller, J. & Schopfer, C. (1984). Prévalence de l'allergie chez les enfants et les adolescents. *Helv Paediat Acta*, **39**, 129–36.

Waite, D.A., Eyles, E.F., Tonkin, S.L. & O'Donnell, T.V. (1980). Asthma prevalence in Tokelauan children in their environments. *Clin Allergy*, **10**, 71–5.

Walker, R.B. & Warin, R.P. (1956). The incidence of eczema in early childhood. *Br J Dermatol*, **68**, 182–3.

Wichmann, H. (1995). Environment, life-style and allergy: the German answer. *Allergol J*, **4**, 315–6.

Williams, H.C., Strachan, D.P. & Hay, R.J. (1994). Childhood eczema: disease of the advantaged? *Br Med J*, **308**, 1132–5.

Williams, H.C., Burney, P., Pembroke, A. & Hay, R.J. (1994). The UK working party's diagnostic criteria for atopic dermatitis. III: Independent hospital validation. *Br J Dermatol*, **131**, 406–16.

Williams, H.C., Pembroke, A.C., Forsdyke, H., Boodoo, G., Hay, R.J. & Burney, P.G.I. (1995). London-born black Caribbean children are at increased risk of atopic dermatitis. *J Am Acad Dermatol*, **32**, 212–7.

Williams, H.C., Burney, P., Pembroke, A. & Hay, R.J. (1996). Validation of the UK diagnostic criteria for atopic dermatitis in a population setting. *Br J Dermatol*, **135**, 12–17.

Wüthrich, B. (1996). Epidemiology and natural history of atopic dermatitis. *ACI International*, **8**, 77–82.

PART III

Analytical studies which point to causes of atopic dermatitis

8

Genetic epidemiology of atopic dermatitis

Finn Schultz Larsen

Family studies

The progress in the treatment of diseases caused by infection and malnutrition has changed the disease spectrum in developed and developing countries. Environmental diseases are nowadays being out-numbered by others which are entirely or partly genetically determined such as atopic dermatitis (AD), which has become one of the most common diseases of childhood (Schultz Larsen et al., 1996). Since the classical and comprehensive study of Cooke and van der Veer in 1916 it has been known that allergy runs in families. They found that if one parent was allergic, then nearly 50% of the children likewise had allergy; if both parents were allergic, then so too were 75% of their offspring. After the dis-covery of transmission of antibodies (reagins) in the 1920s, the road was opened for the definition of atopy and the underlining of the relationship of atopic dermatitis to the atopic diathesis. That common genes rather than common family envi-ronment causes this familial aggregation has been substantiated by several extensive publications (Edgren, 1943; Schwartz, 1952; Schnyder, 1960), but controversy has existed about the mode of inheri-tance. All types of Mendelian framework have been suggested, but in the 1960s the available data strongly indicated atopy as being polygenic and multifactorially determined, which means that several genes (polygenic) as well as genetic and envi-ronmental factors (multifactorial) determine the expression of the disease (Arsdel & Motulsky, 1959; Leigh & Marley, 1967). In addition, within this poly-genic system there are factors which increase the liability to atopy in general and which act side by side with other genes influencing the special 'end organ sensitivity', i.e. that among first degree rela-tives of asthmatics, respiratory atopy is much more frequent than AD, whereas among relatives of AD proband, affection of the skin prevails (Edfors-Lubs, 1971; Kjellman, 1977; Schultz Larsen, 1985; Dold et al., 1992). However, within this genetic system there might be a few major genes which explain most of the genetic variation. The majority of the family studies deal with the genetics of atopy in general; much less attention has been paid to AD in particu-lar. The literature on the subject reveals that about one-half to two-thirds of inpatients with AD had a single or double parental history of atopy, and the studies indicate that this percentage is higher when siblings are included (Schultz Larsen, 1991). A cross-sectional questionnaire study among 6665 German schoolchildren aged 9–11 years in 1989–1990 showed that, in families with a single positive history of atopy, 26% of the children developed AD at a time when the population frequency in Germany has been estimated to be about 11–13% (Dold et al., 1992; Buser et al., 1993; Schultz Larsen et al., 1996). This percentage rose to 46% of the children in fami-lies with a history of more than two affected first degree family members. However, as questionnaire studies tend to overestimate the occurrence of AD (Schultz Larsen et al., 1986; Bakke et al., 1990), this population-based survey shows that the percentage of AD in the offspring of atopic families is in general beyond 50%.

Polygenic mutifactorial inheritance

The following characteristics speak in favour of a polygenic, multifactorial inheritance: (1) atopic dermatitis is clearly familial with no distinct pattern of inheritance within the single family; (2) penetrance is reduced to less than 50% in the offspring; (3) the risk is higher when more than one family member is affected (Dold et al., 1992) – in contrast, for single gene disorders the risk to the next child remains unchanged; (4) the risk for the offspring in more severe cases is higher than the average risk; due to a greater liability the more severely affected inpatients have a higher degree of familial atopy than population-based subjects; (5) if a multifactorial disease is more frequent in one sex than in the other, the risk is higher for the relatives of patients of the less susceptible sex (Carter effect); although asthma is more common in boys it has recently been shown that asthma is more likely to occur in the families of affected girls (Happle & Schnyder, 1992; Schultz Larsen et al., 1996); (6) atopic dermatitis is a very common disease and has become even more common during one generation (Taylor et al., 1984; Ninan & Russell, 1992; Schultz Larsen, 1993); (7) as cases of discordant monozygotic twins definitely exist the disease must be susceptible to environmental factors (Schultz Larsen, 1993); (8) at present it seems unlikely to detect a single basal defect which fits a simple conception of the disease.

Box 8.1. Data favouring polygenic multifactorial inheritance

Familial aggregation
Reduced penetrance
Increased risk when more family members are affected
Increased risk in more severely affected families
Observation of Carter effect
Increased disease frequency in last decades
Existence of discordant monozygotic twins
No single aetiological defect

Recently, a complex genetic disease has been defined as a disease with a genetic aetiology but without Mendelian inheritance attributed to a single gene locus. Atopic diseases and many common disorders of adult life run in families but are neither single gene nor chromosomal in origin. Some of the problems or complexities are based on an unknown degree of incomplete and age-dependent penetrance and genetic heterogeneity. It has also to be stressed that any phenotypic misclassification severely threatens the validity of any genetic study. The hypothesis is that alleles in multiple loci are involved in the aetiology of AD, either directly (AD considered as a complex phenotype) or indirectly by the action of intermediate phenotypes, for example, specific immune response, serum IgE or atopy.

Twin studies

Another method to evaluate the role of genetics in complex diseases has been the study of twins. When the mode of inheritance is not simple Mendelian, the classical twin method is very helpful in estimating the weight of genetic influence. However, the classical twin method presupposes that the twin series is representative and that the diagnosis of zygosity is reliable. The outcomes of many older twin studies have been reviewed in detail elsewhere (Schultz Larsen, 1991). The most cited and extensive investigation of atopic diseases in twins originates in the older Swedish twin registry, which covers adult twin pairs born in Sweden during the period 1886–1925 and with both partners alive in 1961 (Edfors-Lubs, 1971). In 1967 a questionnaire was mailed to all the unbroken, like-sexed pairs of twins and 75%, or about 7000 pairs, completed and returned the questionnaire, which also contained questions designed to evaluate the type of zygosity by means of the similarity method. In order to diagnose AD the twins were asked about eczema in infancy. The pairwise concordance rate was calculated to be 15% for monozygotic and 5% for dizygotic twin pairs.

A possible explanation for the low concordance rates might be: (1) no validation of the consequences of 25% nonresponders and presumably missing data; (2) no sufficient evaluation of the replies to the vague questions about eczema, the answers to which may merely reflect skin problems in childhood; (3) recall bias in twins 42–81 years of age at the time they took part in the inquiry; and (4) the fact that the twins were asked more than 200 questions which served several other main purposes than the study of atopy. However, another interpretation might be that the concordance rates of this supposedly infrequent disease in the first decades of this century actually differ from what is recognized today.

In the late 1970s we initiated a Danish population-based twin study, the object of which was to encircle all living twins restricted to a well defined geographical area (the County of Fyn) and to a limited age group (birth cohort 1960–74) suitable for the study of AD (Schultz Larsen & Holm, 1983; Schultz Larsen, 1985; Schultz Larsen et al., 1986). The strategy for establishing the twin material rests upon the data content of the Danish identification number system. By means of demographic data and the follow-up of a relevant birth cohort, it was demonstrated that the identification method implies a deficiency of about 3–4% of twin pairs, both partners being alive. We compiled the probands by means of a one-page mailed questionnaire with an accompanying letter about AD defined in broad terms. The response rate surpassed 98%. An evaluation of the question of AD revealed very few false negative answers.

In the subsequent clinical examination of the affirmative responders attention was primarily directed to the diagnosis of AD, in which the criteria were adapted to the special clinical situation which allowed us to interview both the twins and the parents at the same time. In case of diagnostic doubt the twins were not included in the calculations. The diagnosis of zygosity was confirmed by an extensive system of polymorphic genetic markers (Schultz Larsen & Grunnet, 1987). The study revealed that the genetic component has a far greater weight on the phenotypic expression of AD than was presumed from the Swedish twin study (Edfors-Lubs, 1971), and the risk of 0.86 of developing the disease in a monozygotic twin having a twin partner with AD differs significantly from the risk

Table 8.1. Number of concordant and discordant twin pairs with atopic dermatitis and the pairwise concordance rate

	Zygosity	
	Monozygotic	Dizygotic
Concordant twin pairs	26	16
Discordant twin pairs	10	54
Pairwise concordance rate	0.72 (0.77)	0.23 (0.15)

The figures in parentheses refer to the twin study from 1986. χ^2 (without Yates' correction), $p<0.0001$.

run by the dizygotic twin partners (0.21). In order to expand and evaluate our previous findings a new twin study was conducted with the same technique in the same area in 1987 in the age group born between 1965 and 1979 (Schultz Larsen, 1993). The results are depicted in Table 8.1. Thus, it must be permissible to conclude that the pairwise concordance rate of AD nowadays is about 0.75 in monozygotic twin pairs and about 0.20 in dizygotic twin pairs, and there can be no doubt that genetic susceptibility plays a definite role in AD. Even though twin studies cannot provide further evidence for the mode of inheritance of complex diseases, it might be highly informative in the future to investigate discordant monozygotic twin pairs and monozygotic twins reared apart.

Newer genetic approaches

There is overwhelming evidence that both environmental and genetic factors are operative in atopic diseases. However, the characterization not only of the environment but also of the genetic component in complex disorders is difficult. We have to determine whether AD is caused by polygenes (several genes affect the disease, each by a small and additive amount), Mendelian major genes (one or more), or a mixed pattern with both polygenes and Mendelian major genes (Mendelian major genes acting on a residual, genetic background). The accessible genetic methods will be mentioned shortly.

Segregation studies

In segregation studies the fitting of different models to the observed inheritance pattern in the available pedigrees is compared. The best fit model (polygenic, Mendelian or mixed), or the model with the higher likelihood, suggest that this model is the most likely mode of inheritance. In successful cases computer programs provide evidence for dominant, codominant or recessive major genes. Recently, a two-locus model has been applied to the study of the inheritance of IgE (Xu et al., 1995). The next step would be to find out where this major gene is located on the genome. In practice, the only method which allows mapping of genes is linkage analysis using extended family pedigrees or affected sib pairs.

Genetic linkage studies

Genetic linkage is based on the process of inheritance of stretches of adjacent genes, or the tendency for alleles (genes) close together on the same chromosome to be transmitted as an intact unit. The gene with the unknown position can then be localized by a detection of linkage between the gene and a DNA marker or microsatellite with known position. The Lod score (log10 of the odds) is a measure for the probability of linkage, and is derived from the relative likelihood (the odds) of obtaining the observed data when two loci are linked, in comparison with the situation in which they are not linked. By convention a Lod score of more than 3 (or better 5) indicates linkage. The Lod score statistic is dependent on gene frequency, penetrance and the recombination fraction. If the two loci are close together then the cross over between them in meiosis will be rare, for example 1–2%, but if the loci are completely unlinked the recombination fraction rises to 50%. The value at which the Lod score is accepted as the best estimate is called the maximum likelihood estimate, and that estimate is at the same time the recombination fraction and a measure for the distance between the two loci (in centiMorgans). Finally, the results from linkage analysis might be confirmed in association studies as a case control design or ideally in isolated and homogenous populations or families.

Specific immune response

During recent decades several routes have been followed in the search for genes involed in atopic diseases. One of the earliest attempts was to define the specific immune response genetically. Ragweed sensitivity was an obvious model. The hypothesis at that time was that one or several genes which control the immune response may reside in the HLA region. Ragweed contains at least 22 clinically important allergens; *Amb a I* is the major purified ragweed allergen, and *Amb a V* is the smallest allergen with three epitopes and a molecular weight of 5 kDa to which approximately 10% of the ragweed allergic subjects respond. The specific immune response to *Amb a I* (at that time called antigen E) was first reported to be associated with HLA class I haplotype by Levine et al. in 1972. Because of the large size and the many epitopes of *Amb a I* most researchers had chosen to study the immune response of *Amb a V*. Recently, this purified allergen has been consistently noted to be strongly associated with HLA-DR2 (Huang et al., 1991), but there was no correlation between particular epitopes of *Amb a V* with the HLA class II allergens (Kim et al., 1994). Furthermore, *Amb a V*-sensitive and *Amb a V*-nonsensitive DR2-positive individuals did not differ with regard to the 45 amino acids sequence of *Amb a V* (Zwollo et al., 1991). Thus, current thinking indicates that the presence of a particular HLA class II molecule appears to provide a necessary, but not exclusive, factor involved in the responsiveness to a particular antigen. This also indicates that class II restrictions are not sufficient to account for individual differences in reactivity to allergens, and it is likely that other loci such as T-cell receptor or IL4 genes may contribute to the individual immune response.

Serum IgE level

As a high serum IgE level correlates with the clinical expression of both allergy and AD, this intermediate phenotype has been studied extensively. Bazarel et al. (1971) were the first to explore the genetics of IgE by measuring serum IgE levels in infants and their mothers. By ranking the values of IgE, the study revealed an apparent relationship of the IgE levels both to family history and to the reported allergic symptoms in six-month-old infants. The genetic basis of IgE was supported by a subsequent study in adult twins and twin children estimating the heritability to be 0.59 in adults and 0.79 in children (Bazarel et al., 1974). Although some criticism can be raised against the calculation of genetic variance and heritability it is remarkable that the within (intra) pair variance of log IgE in adult monozygotic and dizygotic twin pairs is of exactly the same magnitude as achieved later in a nonatopic control group (Schultz Larsen, 1985).

Some of the prerequisites in heritability estimates from twin data should be enumerated: (1) The effect of environment is similar for the two types of twins. This is one of the most troublesome assumptions in twin research. A higher common environmental covariance in monozygotic than in dizygotic twin pairs results in an overestimation of genetic variance. (2) There is no interaction between genotype and environment. If such a genotype–environmental covariance exists, it could influence twin partners differently in dizygotic twin pairs, inducing a further degree of overestimation in the calculation of genetic variance. (3) The trait is continuously distributed without variance due to dominance or epistasis. (4) Computation of the heritability requires knowledge of the total population variance for the trait under consideration. These obstacles in the computations of heritability estimates are not considered thoroughly in several twin studies in IgE (Bazarel et al., 1974; Sistonen et al., 1980; Lee et al., 1980; Al-Algidi, 1980; Wüthrich et al., 1981; Hopp et al., 1984). However, the studies indicate that the level of IgE in the peripheral blood is partly genetically determined, and that the heritability index is calculated to be around 0.60–0.70.

In the light of the aforementioned reservations this estimate is probably biased upwards and, in an attempt to overcome some of these problems, the serum IgE was measured in a nonatopic control group of twins (Schultz Larsen, 1985). The study showed that the genetic variance comprised about 50% of the total phenotypic variance of IgE and, furthermore, an analysis of variance of IgE indicated a greater environmental covariance in monozygotic than in dizygotic twin pairs and that dominance variance plays a role in the regulation of IgE, whereas the available data did not give any indiction of the presence of genotype–environmental interaction in serum IgE. Recently, Hansson et al. (1991) studied twins raised apart and compared them to twins raised together. This opportunity to investigate the effect of different environments on identical genotypes showed that twins reared apart were more similar than reared-together twins with regard to serum IgE. These data clearly indicate that common familial environment (common breeding) has very little effect on the IgE level.

Family studies have confirmed that genetic factors are operative in the regulation of IgE. By segregation analyses the heritability has been calculated to be 0.44 and 0.40, respectively (Billewicz et al., 1974; Grundbacher, 1975). The population study of Billewicz et al. (1974) from two villages in Gambia provides an outcome that is comparable to those of twin studies (Schultz Larsen, 1985). Despite differences in race and the mode of analysis the genetic variance and the phenotypic variance of IgE exhibit almost identical results in the two investigations (Table 8.2).

The twin studies and the family studies clearly demonstrate that a strictly environmental hypothesis can be rejected. Marsh et al. in 1974 provided the first segregation analyses, based on 28 mainly Maryland families having a total of 108 children. At least one of the children in each family was allergic to pollens. The analyses provided evidence for a major IgE-regulating gene. Gerrard et al. (1978) studied 174 white Canadian families, 145 randomly selected and 29 families with high prevalence of atopy. Computer-assisted complex segregation analyses supported the hypothesis of a major locus, as well as a significant polygenic influence of IgE regulation. The gene frequency for the r allele was 0.49

Table 8.2. Genetics of IgE. Heritability of quantitative traits is a statistical measure of the degree to which the total variance is determined by genetic variance

	Log IgE		
	Genetic variance	Total variance	Heritability
Twin studies:			
Bazarel et al. (1971)	0.11		0.59
Lee et al. (1980)	0.10		0.70
Schultz Larsen (1985)	0.16 (↓)	0.23 (↑)	0.50
Family studies:			
Billewicz et al. (1974)	0.14	0.24	0.44

(↓) indicates an overestimated value.
(↑) indicates an underestimated value.

in Saskatchewan, which was in close agreement with the value of 0.52 obtained by Marsh and his co-workers in Baltimore. However, subsequent studies of three large allergic families (Blumenthal et al., 1981), 23 randomly selected Amish families (Meyers et al., 1982) and and five Mormon pedigrees (Hasstedt et al., 1983) failed to prove the existence of a major IgE-regulating locus.

In the work of Blumenthal et al. (1981) the same model did not give the best fit for each pedigree, thus suggesting genetic heterogeneity. In 1987 Meyers et al. conducted a study of the IgE level in 42 nuclear families selected through a member working in a large corporation in Baltimore. Segregation analysis of these fairly randomly ascertained families once again indicated the existence of a major recessive high IgE gene, but in addition they observed, like previous researchers, a significant polygenic control over the IgE production. In a recent study of 50 Hispanic families and 241 nonHispanic white families Martinez et al. (1994) demonstrated a significant correlation of IgE levels among all family members and their segregation analyses, corrected for age and gender, gave no evidence of difference in the mode of inheritance between the two groups. In a Dutch study 92 atopic families were ascertained through a

parent with asthma diagnosed 25 years earlier (Meyers et al., 1994). The proband and their families have recently been re-evaluated. After correction for age and ascertainment bias sib-pair analyses gave significant evidence for linkage to a marker on chromosome 5q. However, the study also indicated that more than one loci influence IgE level, and there are several candidate genes (interleukins and colony-stimulating factors) in the region. Sib-pair analyses of 170 individuals from 11 Amish families also revealed linkage of markers in chromosome 5q with a gene controlling total serum IgE concentration (Marsh et al., 1994). Further analyses suggested that IL-4 receptor or a nearly located gene in the 5q region may regulate basal IgE levels. If this finding could be extended to other populations and the locus ultimately defined, then the relationship between basal IgE level and other intermediate or subphenotypes of AD must be a fruitful area of research. However, the strategy for future studies must include IgE measures in both cord blood and randomly ascertained nonethnically mixed probands taking due regard to age, sex, parasitic infection, smoking habits, the presumed period of minimal antigenic stimulation, recent allergen exposure and other possible confounding variables (Bjerke et al., 1994). Recently, the high-affinity receptor for IgE has been used as a candidate gene. Sandford et al. (1993), from the Oxford group, reported that the gene regulating the β chain of the high-affinity receptor for IgE lies on chromosome 11q13 in close genetic linkage with the gene for atopy (see below).

Atopy

As discussed previously the available genetic studies in the 1960s strongly indicated that the atopic disorders were both environmental and complex genetic diseases. It was therefore interesting that Cookson & Hopkin (1988) proposed that atopy was inherited as a single dominant gene with high penetrance and a few sporadic cases. They defined atopy as elevated serum IgE level and/or elevated specific IgE to common allergens measured by RAST or skin prick test. The atopic families were collected through clinics and media appeal. In a random search by the use of only 17 markers (probes), they were fortunate enough to indentify an apparent genetic linkage in their last probe to the long arm of chromosome 11 in an area designated 11q13. They reported a Lod score of 5.58 to a DNA marker at a recombination fraction of 0.105 (Cookson & Hopkin, 1988; Cookson et al., 1989) under the assumption of a gene frequency of 0.2 corresponding to the prevalence of atopy in the material. A second study on 64 young nuclear families gave a Lod score of 3.80 with 0.007 recombination (Young et al., 1992). However, a number of investigators outside the Oxford group have failed to replicate these findings (Rich et al., 1992; Lympany et al., 1992; Hizawa et al., 1992; Amelung et al., 1992). How could these conflicting results be explained? In the original report of Cookson et al. (1989) a significant amount of the Lod score value (3.14) came from only one family. In continuation of these studies Coleman et al. (1993) investigated 95 nuclear families with at least two first-degree relatives with AD ascertained through an affected child. Linkage analyses between AD and the same markers on chromosome 11q13 excluded a major gene in this region. Thus, for the time being we have to say that it remains possible that loci in the region of 11q13 contribute to the atopic phenotype in some, but certainly not in all, populations.

T-cell receptor

In our current understanding of the initial process of sensitization the antigen is taken up by an antigen-presenting cell and broken down to peptides which become associated with a class II HLA molecule. The antigen–peptide–HLA complex then interacts with lymphocytes of the T-helper (TH) clones, which have T-cell receptors (TCR) specific for the class II peptide–HLA complex. In atopics there appears to be an augmented number of TH2 cells (and TH2 signals or interleukins) in relation to TH1 cells that interact with the antigen. Many of these steps may be under genetic control. Using 66 nuclear families and five extended pedigrees Moffatt et al. (1994) have recently presented evidence indicating linkage

of microsatellites from the TCR-α/δ region and specific immune response to house dust mite antigens. The locus for the TCR-α/δ chain is located on chromosome 14, which may be important in the specific immune response of atopic individuals. However, replication among other populations in other laboratories using the same or adjacent markers remains the only way to validate this suggested linkage from the Oxford group.

HLA system

As the specific immune response is associated with the HLA system, especially the DR region, several investigators have studied the distribution of HLA antigens in AD. In the first publication Krain & Terasaki in 1973 reported an enhanced frequency of HLA-A3 and HLA-A9 in a study comprising 45 patients with AD and 870 controls. This association could not be detected in later French studies in a rather limited study population of 30 patients (Desmons et al., 1976). They found that HLA-B35 was statistically significantly increased with the disease. However, a simultaneous, but less detailed, reported study revealed no difference in the antigen frequency of 26 HLA types in 103 patients with AD (Scholtz et al., 1977). Similar negative observations have been made in the Japanese population (Ohikido et al., 1977) and in a population-based nonethnically mixed group of 68 Caucasians with AD (Schultz Larsen & Grunnet, 1987). The calculated p-values in all the positive studies are not below the level of 0.01, which is considered necessary in order to demonstrate an association between an HLA antigen and a disease. Other sources of biases may be attributed to stratification effects owing to data collected from ethnically mixed groups and hospital-based control materials in which the tested individuals have been HLA-typed due to suspected HLA-associated diseases.

Some early studies reported an augmented prevalence of the HLA-A1,B8 haplotype in childhood asthma (Thorsby et al., 1971), and in 1977 Turner et al. undertook an investigation of HLA-A1,B8 in combined atopy. They found an increased frequency in

18 patients with combined atopy characterized by bronchial asthma, allergic rhinitis and AD. Later works have been unable to confirm this finding, both in 43 cases of combined atopy (Svejgaard et al., 1985) and in an AD group as a whole – 61 with pure AD and 7 with combined atopy (Schultz Larsen & Grunnet, 1987). In a report on HLA-DR antigens Svejgaard et al. (1985) mentioned a strikingly low frequency of HLA-DR7 in 34 cases of both pure AD and combined atopy. However, the decrease was not statistically significant even before correcting for the number of studied antigens. Thus, population studies in the field of HLA and AD have not provided any conclusive observations, nor have the few family studies (Mackie & Dick, 1979; Schultz Larsen et al., 1980), although the last-mentioned study revealed an astonishing, but possible coincidental, linkage between haplotype A2,Bw35,Cw2 and AD in five family members in three generations. The segregation of HLA haplotype has recently been studied in 20 families with mite-sensitive allergic asthma using the affected sib-pair method (Carabello & Hernandez, 1990). Their study indicated the existence of an HLA-linked gene controlling the specific IgE responsiveness to mite allergens. Within the short arm of chromosome 6 there are HLA-linked loci such as C2, C4a and C4b and, together with the HLA system, they form extended haplotypes. The association of ragweed allergic rhinitis and asthma with such extended haplotypes has recently been investigated in nuclear families (Blumenthal et al., 1992). The frequency of HLA-DR2 and the extended haplotype B7, SC31, DR2 was significantly increased among patients with asthma and a high level of specific IgE to *Amb a V*, and the authors suggest that certain combinations of alleles, especially of the DR and complement loci, are associated with susceptibility to diseases, including atopy, or in this case that HLA-linked gene or genes on this extended haplotype are controlling the specific IgE response to ragweed *Amb a V* and predisposing to asthma. At the present time the genetics of AD has not been analysed as a function of any extended haplotypes. It remains possible that the discrepancies in the HLA studies are due to a hitherto undetected segregation of certain immune response-containing extended haplotypes.

Maternal effect and genomic imprinting

In recent years there has been an increasing awareness that mothers seem to transmit atopic disorders more frequently than fathers. In 1980 Michel et al. noticed that cord blood IgE was significantly higher when maternal (but not paternal) IgE surpassed a certain limit. Another study of 288 unselected newborns showed that maternal atopy influenced cord IgE levels whereas paternal atopy did not (Magnusson, 1988). The specific IgE responses have recently been studied in 302 randomly selected schoolchildren and their families (Kuehr et al., 1992). Sensitization to common allergens (grass, birch, cat) occurred significantly more often in children whose mothers were sensitized to the same antigens, whereas there was no augmented risk following paternal sensitization. The first study to explore the influence of maternal atopy on the development of AD was reported from London in 1992 (Ruiz et al., 1992). In a hospital study of 19 atopic mothers and 20 atopic fathers diagnosed by positive skin prick tests, seven infants of atopic mothers and two infants of atopic fathers developed AD during the first year of life ($p = 0.02$). Although the numbers were relatively small the authors compared several confounding factors. In the previously mentioned large-scale population-based study of the genetic risk of atopy in schoolchildren in Germany (Dold et al., 1992), the tables reveal that, in families with mothers with AD, the risk of the children developing AD was increased with an odds ratio (OR) of 3.9 (95% confidence interval 2.9–5.2) versus an OR of 2.5 (1.5–3.9) in families with paternal AD. The same tendency has recently been published from another area of the southern part of Germany (Diepgen & Blettner, 1996). They compared data from the relatives of 426 patients with AD with data from 628 controls, and found a higher odds ratio of AD between mothers and siblings (OR = 2.7 (1.5–4.9)) than between fathers and siblings (OR = 1.3 (0.7–1.9)). This maternal effect might be explained in several ways. It might be assumed that mothers and children share a higher degree of home environment, and/or that environmental influences affect the fetus in utero. Furthermore, recall bias from informant mothers may underestimate paternal atopy. In one of the studies from Germany 80% of the questionnaires were filled out by the mothers (Dold et al., 1992).

However, the presence of increased maternal influence raises the possibility of what is called genomic imprinting, which implies that genetic material (in our case paternal genes) is modified and suppressed during spermatogenesis (as is seen in mice associated with differences in DNA methylation patterns). This modification is not a mutation nor an allele of the particular gene, but rather a temporary change in function which may, however, have a profound, longlasting effect for the individual in question. A popular explanation or hypothesis is that another layer of meaning – an imprint – is added to the genes. It has been known for some years that the severity of von Recklinghausen's disease (NF 1) is increased with maternal transmission, but so far there has been no clear evidence for imprinting in complex diseases. However, in 1992 the Oxford group suggested, on the basis of IgE measurements and the simple affected sib-pair method, that the transmission of high IgE was detectable only when the affected sib pairs shared the maternal 11q13 allele (Cookson et al., 1992). They proposed that the results could be due to paternal genomic imprinting, but at the time of writing their findings have not been confirmed.

Conclusions

It is clear that the task of unravelling the genetic component of complex diseases such as AD is much more difficult than solving the single-gene or chromosomal diseases. The work is still in its infancy, and the search for genes involved in the control of allergy and IgE is just beginning. We know that the immune response to certain aeroallergens is genetically determined by genes located to DR loci on chromosome 6; and that the regulation of IgE is partly heritable and due to at least one major gene that is located to chromosome 5q; and that the high-affinity receptor for IgE may be under genetic control and related to atopy. How should we proceed in the future in this challenging field? Two basic strategies have been followed. The first is segregation analysis followed by linkage analysis using the genetic model indentified from the segregation study. The second and more promising approach is linkage analysis on affected sib pairs without any underlying model, using candidate genes selected through their likely function to influence disease processes, together with multiple markers (microsatellite, restriction fragment length polymorphism) against adjacent stretches of the genome.

Perspectives

Clearly, mapping the genes of complex diseases is a laborious area of medicine, but may prove to be very important to our understanding of the nature of atopic disorders and the designing of new treatments. If AD requires the combined presence of certain modifying genetic sequences and environmental triggers, then those who have inherited the susceptible allele can strive to avoid the precipitating events. Furthermore, those who already have the disease might be treated with genes which correct, for example, the TH1/TH2 imbalance. Nowadays, gene therapy is not just an idea. Today genes are already used to fight rare inborn errors of metabolism, such as adenosine deaminase deficiency, and it is highly probable that some form of gene therapy of complex diseases will be part of our future.

Summary of key points

- Atopic dermatitis (AD) is a complex disease caused by several genes and environmental triggers.
- The specific immune response is partly governed by HLA class II antigens or HLA extended haplotypes on chromosome 6.
- The genetic variance of serum IgE constitutes about 50% of the phenotypic variance. One of the

loci influencing the IgE level is located on chromosome 5. A nonconfirmed report suggests that another loci is located on chromosome 11 (high-affinity receptor of IgE).

• Maternal atopy causes a greater risk of atopic disorders in the offspring than paternal atopy.

References

Al-Algidi, S. (1980). Serum immunoglobin levels in Iraqi twins. *Hum Biol*, **52**, 393–9.

Amelung, P.J., Panhuysen, C.I.M., Postma, D.S. et al. (1992). Atopy and bronchial hyperresponsiveness: exclusion of linkage to markers on chromosomes 11q and 6p. *Clin Exp Allergy*, **12**, 1077–84.

Arsdel, P.P. van & Motulsky, A.G. (1959). Frequency and heritability of asthma and allergic rhinitis in college students. *Acta Genet (Basel)*, **9**, 101–14.

Bakke, P., Eide, G.E. & Gulsvik, A. (1990). Hay fever, eczema and urticaria in Southwest Norway. Lifetime prevalences, association with sex, age, smoking habits, occupational airborne exposure and respiratory symptoms. *Allergy*, **45**, 515–22.

Bazarel, M., Orgel, H.A. & Hamburger, R.N. (1971). IgE levels in normal infants and mothers and an inheritance hypothesis. *J Immunol*, **107**, 794–801.

Bazarel, M., Orgel, H.A. & Hamburger, R.N. (1974). Genetics of IgE and allergy: serum IgE levels in twins. *J All Clin Immunol*, **54**, 288–304.

Billewicz, W.Z., McGregor, I.A., Roberts, D.F., Rowe, D.S. & Wilson, R.J.M. (1974). Family studies in immunoglubulin levels. *Clin Exp Immunol*, **16**, 13–22.

Bjerke, T., Hedegaard, M., Henriksen, T.B., Nielsen, B.W. & Schiøtz, P.O. (1994). Several genetic and environmental factors influence cord blood IgE concentration. *Pediat All Immunol*, **5**, 88–94.

Blumenthal, M.N., Namboodiri, K., Mendell, N., Gleich, G., Elston, R.C. & Yunis, E. (1981). Genetic transmission of serum IgE levels. *Am J Med Genet*, **10**, 219–28.

Blumenthal, M.N., Marcus-Bagley, D., Adweh, Z. et al. (1992). Extended major: HLA-DR2, [HLA-B7,SC31,DR2] and [HLA-B8,SC01,DR3] haplotypes distinguish subjects with asthma from those with only rhinitis in ragweed pollen allergy. *J Immunol*, **148**, 411–16.

Buser, K., von Bohlen, P., Werner, P., Gernhuber, E. & Robra, B-P. (1993). Neurodermitis-Prävalenz bei Schulkindern im Landkreis Hannover. *Dtsch Med Wschr*, **118**, 1141–5.

Carabello, L.R. & Hernandez, M. (1990). HLA haplotype segregation in families with allergic asthma. *Tissue Antigens*, **35**, 182–6.

Coleman, R., Trembath, R. & Harper, J.I. (1993). Chromosome 11q13 and atopy underlying atopic eczema. *Lancet*, **341**, 1121–2.

Cooke, R.A. & van der Veer, A. (1916). Human sensitization. *J Immunol*, **1**, 201–305.

Cookson, W.O.C.M. & Hopkin, J.M. (1988). Dominant inheritance of atopic immunoglobulin-E responsiveness. *Lancet*, **i**, 86–8.

Cookson, W.O.C.M., Sharp, P.A., Faux, J.A. & Hopkin, J.M. (1989). Linkage between immunoglobulin E responses underlying asthma and rhinitis and chromosome 11q. *Lancet*, **i**, 1292–5.

Cookson, W.O.C.M., Young, R.P., Sandford, A. et al. (1992). Maternal inheritance of atopic IgE responsiveness on chromosome 11q. *Lancet*, **340**, 381–4.

Desmons, F., Delmas-Marsalet, Y. & Goudemand, J. (1976). HLA antigens in atopic dermatitis. *Allergol Immunopathol (Madr.)*, **4**, 29–38.

Diepgen, T.L. & Blettner, M. (1996). Analysis of familial aggregation of atopic eczema and other diseases by odds ratio regression models. *J Invest Dermatol*, **106**, 977–81.

Dizier, M.H., Hill, M. James, A. et al. (1993). Genetic control of basal IgE level accounting for specific atopy. *Genet Epidemiol*, **10**, 33–34 (abstract).

Dold, S., Wjst, M., von Mutius, E., Reitmeir, P. & Stiepel, E. (1992). Genetic risk for asthma, allergic rhinitis, and atopic dermatitis. *Arch Dis Child*, **67**, 1018–22.

Edfors-Lubs, M-L. (1971). Allergy in 7000 twin pairs. *Acta Allergol*, **26**, 249–85.

Edgren, G. (1943). Prognose und Erbliebkeitsmomente bei Ekzema Infantum. Eine Klinisch-statistiche Untersuchung von Allergieerscheinungen. *Acta Paediatr (Scand.)*, **30** (Suppl. 2), 1–204.

Gerrard, J.W., Rao, D.C. & Morton, N.E. (1978). A genetic study of immunoglobulin E. *Am J Hum Genet*, **30**, 46–58.

Grundbacher, F.J. (1975). Causes of variation in serum IgE levels in normal populations. *J All Clin Immunol*, **56**, 104–11.

Hansson, B., McGue, M., Roitman-Johnson, B., Segal, N.L., Bouchard, T.J. & Blumenthal, M.N. (1991). Atopic disease and immunoglobin E in twins reared apart and together. *Am J Hum Genet*, **48**, 873–9.

Happle, R. & Schnyder, U.W. (1992). Evidence for the Carter effect in atopy. *Int Arch All Appl Immunol*, **68**, 90–92.

Hasstedt, S.J., Meyers, D.A. & Marsh, D.G. (1983). Inheritance of immunoglobulin E: genetic model fitting. *Am J Med Genet*, **14**, 61–6.

Hizawa, N., Yamaguchi, E., Ohe, M. et al. (1992). Lack of linkage between atopy and locus 11q13. *Clin Exp Allergy*, **22**, 1065–9.

Hopp, R.J., Bewtra, A.K., Watt, G.D., Nair, N.M. & Townley, R.G. (1984). Genetic analysis of allergic disease in twins. *J All Clin Immunol*, **73**, 265–70.

Huang, S., Zwollo, P. & Marsh, D.G. (1991). Class II major histo-compatibility complex restriction of human T cell responses to short ragweed allergen Amb a V. *Eur J Immunol*, **21**, 1469–73.

Kim, K.E., Rosenberg, A. & Blumenthal, M.N. (1994). Regulation of IgE response to Amb a V by a gating mechanism (abstr). *J All Clin Immunol*, **93**, 252–3.

Kjellman, N-I.M. (1977). Atopic disease in seven-year-old children. *Acta Paediatr (Scand.)*, **66**, 465–71.

Krain, L.S. & Terasaki, P.I. (1973). HLA types in atopic dermatitis. *Lancet*, **i**, 1059–60.

Kuehr, J., Karmaus, W., Foster, J. et al. (1992). Sensitization to four common inhalant allergens within 302 nuclear families. *Clin Exp Allergy*, **23**, 600–5.

Lee, S.K., Metrakos, J.D., Tanaka, K.R. & Heiner, D.C. (1980). Genetic influence on serum IgD levels. *Pediatr Res*, **14**, 60–63.

Leigh, D. & Marley, E. (1967). *Bronchial Asthma. A Genetic, Population and Psychiatric Study*. Oxford: Pergamon Press.

Levine, R.B., Stember, R.H. & Fotino, M. (1972). Ragweed hay fever: genetic control and linkage to HJA haplotypes. *Science*, **178**, 1201–3.

Lympany, P., Welsh, K.I., Cochrane, G.M., Kemeny, D.M. & Lee, T.H. (1992). Genetic analysis of the linkage between chromosome 11q and atopy. *Clin Experim Allergy*, **22**, 1085–92.

MacKie, R.M. & Dick, H.M. (1979). A study of HLA antigen distribution in families with atopic dermatitis. *Allergy*, **34**, 19–23.

Magnusson, C.G.M. (1988). Cord serum IgE in relation to family history and as predictor of atopic disease in early infancy. *Allergy*, **43**, 241–51.

Marsh, D.G., Bias, W.B. & Ishizaka, K. (1974). Genetic control of basal serum immunoglobulin E level and its effect on specific reaginic sensitivity. *Proc Natl Acad Sci USA*, **71**, 3588–92.

Marsh, D.G., Neely, J.D., Breazeale, D.R. et al. (1994). Linkage analysis of IL4 and other chromosome 5q31.1 markers and total serum immunoglobin E concentrations. *Science*, **264**, 1152–6.

Martinez, F.D., Holberg, C.J., Halonen, M., Morgan, W.J., Wright, A.L. & Taussig, L.M. (1994). Evidence of Mendelian inheritance of serum IgE levels in Hispanic and non-Hispanic white families. *Am J Hum Genet*, **55**, 555–5.

Meyers, D.A., Bias, W.B. & Marsh, D.G. (1982). A genetic study of total IgE in the Amish. *Hum Hered*, **32**, 15–23.

Meyers, D.A., Hasstedt, S.J. & Marsh, D.G. (1983). The inheritance of immunoglobulin E: linkage analysis. *Am J Med Genet*, **16**, 575–872.

Meyers, D.A., Beaty, T.H., Freidhoff, L.R. & Marsh, D.G. (1987). Inheritance of total IgE (basal levels) in man. *Am J Hum Genet*, **41**, 51–62.

Meyers, D.A., Postma, D.S., Panhuysen, J. et al. (1994). Evidence for a locus regulating IgE levels mapping to chromosome 5. *Genomics*, **23**, 464–70.

Michel, F.B., Bousquet, J., Greillier, P., Robinet-Levy, M. & Coulomb, Y. (1980). Comparison of cord blood immunoglobulin E concentrations and maternal allergy for prediction of atopic diseases in infancy. *J All Clin Immunol*, **65**, 422–30.

Moffatt, M.F., Hill, M.R., Cornelis, J., Schou, C. et al. (1994). Genetic linkage of T-cell α/δ complex to specific IgE responses. *Lancet*, **343**, 1597–600.

Ninan, T.K. & Russell, G. (1992). Respiratory symptoms and atopy in Aberdeen schoolchildren: evidence from two surveys 25 years apart. *Br Med J*, **304**, 873–5.

Ohikido, M., Ozawa, A., Matsuo, I. et al. (1977). HLA antigens and susceptibility to atopic dermatitis. *Monogr Allergy*, **11**, 36–43.

Rich, S.S., Roitman-Johnson, B., Greenberg, B., Roberts, S. & Blumenthal, M.N. (1992). Genetic analysis of atopy in three large kindreds: no evidence of linkage to D11S97. *Clin Exp Allergy*, **22**, 1070–6.

Ruiz, R.G.G., Kemeny, D.M. & Price, J.F. (1992). Higher risk of infantile atopic dermatitis from maternal atopy than from paternal atopy. *Clin Exp Allergy*, **22**, 762–6.

Sandford, A.J., Shivakawa, T., Moffat, M.F., Daniels, S.E., Faux, J.A., Young, R.P., Cookson, W.O.C.M. et al. (1993). Localization of atopy and β subunit of high-affinity IgE receptor (FcϵRI) on chromosome 11q. *Lancet*, **341**, 332.

Schnyder, U.W. (1960). Neurodermitis – Asthma – Rhinitis. Eine genetisch-allergologische Studie. *Acta Genet Stat Med*, **10** (Suppl. 18), 1–106.

Scholtz, S., Ziegler, E., Wünster, H., Braun-Falco, O. & Albert, E.D. (1977). HLA family studies in patients with atopic dermatitis. *Monogr Allergy*, **11**, 44.

Schultz Larsen, F. (1985). Atopic dermatitis. Etiological studies based on a twin population. Thesis, University of Odense, Lægeforeningens Forlag, Copenhagen.

Schultz Larsen, F. (1991). Genetic aspects of atopic eczema. In: Ruzicka, T., Ring, J. & Przybilla, B. (eds.) *Handbook of Atopic Eczema*, pp. 15–26. Berlin: Springer.

Schultz Larsen, F. (1993). Atopic dermatitis: a genetic–epidemiologic study in a population-based twin sample. *J Am Acad Dermatol*, **28**, 719–23.

Schultz Larsen, F. & Holm, N.V. (1983). Evaluation of an identification method of twin pairs based on the personal numbering system in Denmark. *Dan Med Bull*, **30**, 424–7.

Schultz Larsen, F. & Grunnet, N. (1987). Genetic investigations in atopic dermatitis. *Tissue Antigens*, **29**, 1–6.

Schultz Larsen, F., Grunnet, N. & Vase, P. (1980). HLA antigens in atopic dermatitis. A family study. *Dermatologica*, **160**, 17–20.

Schultz Larsen, F., Holm, N.V. & Henningsen, K. (1986). Atopic dermatitis. A genetic–epidemiologic study in a population-based twin sample. *J Am Acad Dermatol*, **15**, 487–94.

Schultz Larsen, F., Diepgen, T.L. & Svensson, Å. (1996). The occurrence of atopic dermatitis in North Europe: an international questionnaire study. *J Am Acad Dermatol*, **34**, 760–4.

Schwartz, M. (1952). Heredity in bronchial asthma. Thesis, University of Copenhagen, Munksgård, Copenhagen.

Sistonen, P., Johnsson, V., Koskenvuo, M. & Aho, K. (1980). Serum IgE levels in twins. *Hum Hered*, **30**, 155–8.

Svejgaard, E., Jakobsen, B. & Svejgaard, A. (1985). Studies of HLA-ABC and DR antigens in pure atopic dermatitis and atopic dermatitis combined with allergic respiratory disease. *Acta Derm Venereol (Stockh.)*, Suppl. **114**: 72–6.

Taylor, B., Wadsworth, M., Wadsworth, J. et al. (1984). Changes in the reported prevalence of childhood eczema since the 1939–45 war. *Lancet*, **ii**, 1255–8.

Thorsby, E., Engeset, A. & Lie, S.O. (1971). HL-A antigens and susceptibility to diseases. A study of patients with acute lymphoblastic leukaemia, Hodgkin's disease, and childhood asthma. *Tissue Antigens*, **1**, 147–52.

Turner, M.W., Brostoff, J., Wells, R.S., Stokes, C.R. & Soothill, J.F. (1977). HLA in eczema and hay fever. *Clin Exp Immunol*, **27**, 43–7.

Wüthrich, B., Baumann, E., Fries, R.A. & Schnyder, U.W. (1981). Total and specific IgE (RAST) in atopic twins. *Clin Allergy*, **11**, 147–54.

Xu, J., Levitt, R.C., Panhuysen, C.I.M. et al. (1995). Evidence of two unlinked loci regulating total serum IgE levels. *Am J Hum Genet*, **57**, 425–30.

Young, R.P., Sharp, P.A., Lynch, J.R. et al. (1992). Confirmation of genetic linkage between atopic IgE responses and chromosome 11q13. *J Med Genet*, **29**, 236–8.

Zwollo, P., Erlich Kautsky, E., Scharf, S. et al. (1991). Sequences of HLA D in responders and nonresponders to short ragweed Amb a V. *Immunogenetics*, **33**, 141–51.

9

Fetal and perinatal origins of atopic dermatitis

Keith Godfrey

Introduction

We have become accustomed to the idea that many disorders of adult life such as noninsulin-dependent diabetes, hypertension and obstructive airways disease arise through an interaction between a genetically determined susceptibility and influences in the current environment including diet, obesity, smoking and allergen exposure. Recent research, however, suggests that the fetal and early infant environment may play a critical role in programming a lifelong predisposition to a number of common adult diseases. As yet, there is only limited and indirect evidence to suggest major long-term effects of the fetal and perinatal environment in relation to atopic dermatitis (AD). Research into this hypothesis, however, is in its very earliest stages and future epidemiological studies of the fetal environment may provide important insights into the aetiology of AD.

The concept of programming during early development

In fetal life and early infancy different tissues of the body grow during periods of rapid cell division, so-called 'critical' periods (Widdowson & McCance, 1975). The timing of these critical periods differs for different tissues; a critical period for reproductive tract development exists, for example, very early in development (Beral & Colwell, 1981), as compared with one for kidney development later in gestation between 26 and 34 weeks of pregnancy (Konje et al.,

1996). Growth depends on nutrients and oxygen, and the fetus's main adaptation to the lack of these is to slow its rate of cell division, especially in those tissues which are undergoing critical periods at the time. Even brief periods of undernutrition may permanently reduce the number of cells in particular organs and hence 'programme' the body. Other lasting memories of fetal undernutrition include changes in the distribution of cell types, hormonal feedback, metabolic activity and organ structure (Barker, 1995). Only recently, however, has it become apparent that some of the body's memories of early undernutrition become translated into pathology and thereby determine disease in later life. Rickets serves as an unquestionable example of the fact that the structure of the human body can be programmed by undernutrition.

Numerous examples of programming have been described in animal studies, including permanent effects on growth, on relative organ size, on immune function and on lipid metabolism (Lucas, 1991; Barker & Sultan, 1994). Alterations in the balance of macronutrients in the mother's diet during pregnancy have, for example, been shown to have life-long effects on the offspring. Thus, feeding pregnant rats a diet with a low ratio of protein to energy permanently alters the balance between glucose production and utilization in the liver of the offspring. The same low protein diet during postnatal life has no effect on glucose metabolism in the liver (Desai et al., 1995).

For many years ideas about the aetiology of AD and other atopic diseases have been dominated by

Table 9.1. Twin concordance rates for tuberculosis (Kallman & Reisner, 1943)

Relationship to 'index case'	% with disease
One-egg twin	87.0
Two-egg twin	25.6
Other brother and sister	25.5
Marriage partner	7.0

the apparently overwhelming importance of genetic influences inferred from high concordance rates in monozygotic twins (Larsen, Holm & Henningsen, 1986). The demonstration of programming by the intra-uterine environment, however, has recently led to the suggestion that classical twin studies may have overestimated the genetic contribution to many diseases (Phillips, 1993). Most monozygotic twins share a common placenta and higher disease concordance rates in monozygotic than dizygotic twins may in part reflect effects of nutrient supply to the developing fetus. One example of the potential for overinterpretation of classical twin studies is shown in Table 9.1. These twin concordance rates (Kallman & Reisner, 1943) are strikingly similar to those which have been produced for AD (Larsen, Holm & Henningsen, 1986). The data in the table, however, relate to tuberculosis which, prior to the discovery of the tubercle bacillus, was firmly held to be a simple genetic disorder.

The familial clustering of atopic diseases has also been interpreted as indicating that atopy is largely genetic in origin. It is now known, however, that environmental influences can be transmitted vertically over several generations through intergenerational effects on fetal growth (Stewart, Preece & Sheppard, 1975; Lumey, 1992; Emanuel et al., 1992; Godfrey et al., 1997). Such effects may account for the results of rat studies in which maternal undernutrition in one generation has affected immune function in the next two generations (Chandra, 1975). A substantial environmental contribution to the aetiology of atopic diseases is also consistent with the considerable rise in the incidence of AD and asthma over recent decades in the absence of a change in genetic stock (see Chapter 7). Whilst hereditability has traditionally formed part of the basis of the definition of atopic diseases, it is clear from the changes over recent decades that the environment must have had a major influence on phenotype. If this population shift is to be reversed, then detailed study of the environmental causes is essential. The identity of the key factors and their relative importance is still unclear and long-term cohort studies over many years will be required to establish which of the many possible factors are critical in the development of AD and other allergic disorders. The inability of currently recognized risk factors to account for the rise of atopic diseases indicates the need for a broad perspective in epidemiological research into their aetiology (Strachan, 1995).

Lessons from the programming of nondermatological disease

Attempts to understand many chronic diseases, including coronary heart disease, noninsulin-dependent diabetes, hypertension and obstructive airways disease, have hitherto focused on a 'destructive' model for the disease, in which influences acting in adult life, such as diet, obesity, smoking and allergen exposure, lead to tissue damage and hence disease. Babies who are small or disproportionate at birth, however, are now known to be at an increased risk of developing coronary heart disease, hypertension and noninsulin-dependent diabetes during adult life (Barker, 1994, 1995). These observations, linking impaired fetal growth with common adult diseases, suggest that a 'developmental' model may be more appropriate and point to a new focus for disease prevention.

Evidence that coronary heart disease, hypertension and diabetes are programmed came initially from longitudinal studies of 25 000 British men and women where size at birth was related to the occurrence of the disease in middle age (Barker, 1995). Death rates from coronary heart disease fell progressively between those who weighed less than 5.5 lb (2.5 kg) at birth and those who were 9.5 lb (4.31 kg) or more. These findings have recently been repli-

Table 9.2. Tissues and systems for which evidence of programming exists in humans

Tissue/system	Examples of programming	Reference
Cardiovascular system	Vascular compliance	Martyn et al. (1995a)
	Left ventricular thickness	Vijayakumar et al. (1995)
Respiratory system	Lung volumes	Shaheen & Barker (1994)
Endocrine system	Hypothalamic–pituitary–adrenal axis	Clark et al. (1996)
	Glucose–insulin metabolism	Barker et al. (1993b)
	Growth hormone–IGF-I axis	Fall et al. (1995)
Skeletal muscle	Insulin resistance	Phillips (1996)
	Glycolysis during exercise	Taylor et al. (1995)
Kidney	Renin–angiotensin system	Martyn, Lever & Morton (1996)
Liver	Cholesterol metabolism	Barker et al. (1993c)
	Fibrinogen and factor VII synthesis	Martyn et al. (1995b)
Immune system	Thyroid autoantibodies	Phillips et al. (1993)

cated by studies in Sweden and the United States (Rich-Edwards et al., 1995; Curhan et al., 1996; Lithell et al., 1996). A study of people in Sheffield, England, showed that these relations are independent of the duration of gestation, suggesting that cardiovascular disease is linked to impaired fetal growth and development rather than to premature birth (Barker et al., 1993a).

Consistent with the thesis that programming reflects a general principle of developmental biology, follow-up studies of children and adults have shown that a wide range of organs and systems may be programmed by the intra-uterine environment in humans, just as in animals. Table 9.2 lists a number of key tissues and systems for which evidence exists in humans pointing to programming by the nutrient and hormonal milieu of the fetus. A number of these lifelong effects are thought to result from persisting consequences of fetal adaptations to undernutrition that are beneficial in the short term but detrimental in the long term (Barker, 1995). These adaptations appear to contribute in a substantial way to the remarkable diversity in the size and shape of the human fetus (Figure 9.1) and to underlie the associations between a baby's birth proportions and later disease. As yet, the extent to which fetal programming plays an important role in the aetiology of AD is unknown. Attempts to address

this issue should be performed in the knowledge that a baby's size at birth is a crude summary measure of its intra-uterine experience and many of the influences shown to programme physiology and metabolism in animals do so without having substantial effects on weight at birth (Barker & Sultan, 1994). Clues to the possibility of a fetal and perinatal origin for AD should be sought within a more sophisticated framework that takes account of a number of principles thought to underlie programming (Table 9.3).

Atopy – effects of fetal growth and of maternal nutrition

Given the paucity of published epidemiological studies specifically addressing fetal and perinatal risk factors for AD, a background knowledge of the asthma literature is of interest. However, it is crucial to be aware that, although asthma and AD co-exist in a proportion of the population, they exhibit differing epidemiological associations (see Chapter 17). This observation may in itself be of importance in understanding the aetiology of AD and serves to illustrate that great caution should be exercised in extrapolating directly from atopy or asthma to AD itself.

Population-based studies which have addressed the relationship between birth weight and later

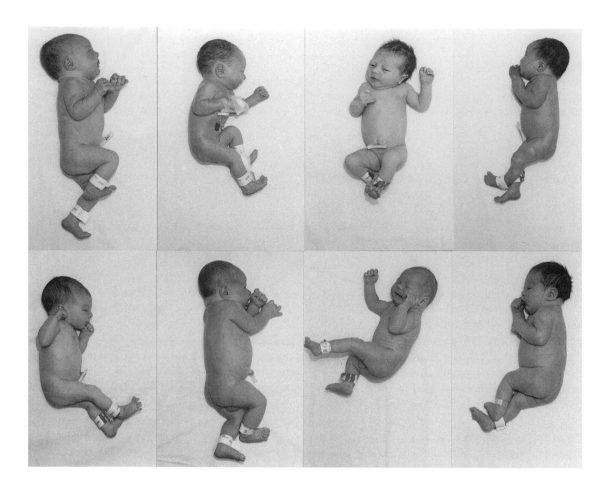

Fig. 9.1. Fetal adaptations to undernutrition result in alterations of the baby's size and shape, and have long-term effects on susceptibility to common adult diseases

asthma or recurrent wheeze are shown in Table 9.4. Weak associations between low birth weight and later asthma and wheezing have been demonstrated in substantial studies in Finland (Alho et al., 1990), Britain (Arshad, Stevens & Hide, 1993; Lewis et al., 1996), the United States (Schwartz et al., 1990) and Israel (Seidman et al., 1991); smaller case-control (Chan et al., 1989) and follow-up studies (Barker et al., 1991) have not shown statistically significant associations (Table 9.4). One sample of English and Scottish primary schoolchildren (Rona, Gulliford & Chinn, 1993) found that childhood wheezing was related to prematurity rather than low birth weight for gestational age. No comparable association between prematurity and asthma or wheezing in childhood, adolescence or early adult life was found, however, in recent analyses of the 1958 National Health and Development Study cohort (Strachan, Butland & Anderson, 1996).

Table 9.4 also shows data from three studies which have examined the possibility of an association between birth weight and AD. Although no significant association between low birth weight and AD at the age of two years was found in a cohort of infants born on the Isle of Wight, England, there was a weak tendency, in contrast to asthma, for low birth weight children to have a reduced prevalence of AD

Table 9.3. Principles underlying programming by the early life environment

(1) Alterations in the nutrient and hormonal milieu of the fetus and neonate can alter its gene expression leading to permanent changes (Barker, 1994)

(2) Alterations in the nutrient and hormonal milieu have different effects at different times in early life (Barker et al., 1993d).

(3) Rapidly growing fetuses and neonates have greater nutrient requirements than those growing more slowly, and are paradoxically more vulnerable to undernutrition (Harding et al., 1992).

(4) Fetal undernutrition results from inadequate maternal intake, transport or transfer of nutrients (Godfrey & Barker, 1995).

(5) The permanent effects of alterations in the early nutrient and hormonal milieu include changes in cell number and type, altered organ structure and resetting of hormonal axes (Barker, 1995).

(Arshad et al., 1993). Likewise, analyses of the 1970 British birth cohort also showed a reduced prevalence of AD at the age of five years in low birth weight infants (Golding & Peters, 1986, 1987); this association, however, was weakened after taking into account the duration of the second stage of labour and whether or not the mother had used any method of contraception prior to the pregnancy (Peters & Golding, 1987). When birth weight was analysed as a continuous variable a rising prevalence of AD with increasing birth weight has been shown in both the 1970 British birth cohort (Peters & Golding, 1987) and in a group of children in Denmark (Braae Olesen et al., 1997).

Against this background of a weak association between higher birth weight and increased AD one recent study has suggested that accelerated but disproportionate fetal growth might be associated with altered fetal immune development and a lifelong predisposition to atopic disease (Godfrey, Barker & Osmond, 1994). Thus, among 280 men and women aged 50 years whose size at birth had been measured in detail, those with a raised total serum IgE concentration in adult life had had a larger head circumference at birth but were of similar crown–heel length to those with a normal adult IgE concentration. Odds ratios of a raised IgE rose progressively to more than 4 as head circumference at birth increased from 13 inches or less, to more than 14 inches (Godfrey et al., 1994). This association with disproportionate growth of the fetal head in relation to the trunk and limbs was independent of the mother's pelvic size and parity, and of adult physique, social class and smoking, and was similar in men and women.

In subsequent, as yet unpublished, studies, however, there has been some inconsistency in the association betweeen accelerated fetal growth and later atopy, suggesting that a confounding influence generally, but not invariably, associated with large babies might be operating. Large babies, for example, have greater nutrient requirements and are more likely to make their mothers anaemic during pregnancy (Howe, 1995), leading to iron and folate supplementation. Follow-up studies of the Hungarian randomized controlled trial of folate and iron supplementation in the prevention of neural tube defects support the possibility of such effects, with a 3–4-fold excess prevalence of AD and asthma in those whose mothers received iron and folate supplements (Czeizel & Dodo, 1994). Preliminary data from a prospective observational study of pregnancies in Southampton, England, found strong evidence of a similar, graded effect of dietary and supplemental iron intakes (Godfrey, Osmond & Hammond, 1995).

Whilst these observations must necessarily be regarded as preliminary and in need of extensive replication, consideration of potential mechanisms which might underlie them nonetheless serves to increase the likelihood of future epidemiological studies being informative. One possible mechanism relates to feto-maternal essential fatty acid (EFA) metabolism. Thus, alterations in fetal growth have been associated with differences in maternal dietary EFA intake in pregnancy (Crawford et al., 1989), and

Table 9.4. Population studies of asthma, wheezing and atopic dermatitis in relation to birth weight

Study population and reference	Finding
Asthma/wheezing	
Random sample of Finnish children aged 2 years ($n = 2512$) (Alho et al., 1990)	Odds-ratio (95% CI) for wheezy bronchitis; 1.7 (1.0 to 2.3) for birth weight ≤ 2500 g
Birth cohort of infants born on the Isle of Wight, England, aged 2 years ($n = 1174$) (Arshad et al., 1993)	Odds-ratio (95% CI) for asthma; 3.0 (1.4 to 6.5) for birth weight ≤ 2500 g
National sample of English and Scottish schoolchildren aged 5–11 years ($n = 5573$) (Rona, Gulliford & Chinn, 1993)	No association between birth weight for gestational age and wheezing
Case-control study of low birth weight children aged 7 years ($n = 130$ cases) (Chan et al., 1989)	No association between birth weight < 2000 g and wheezing
Nationally representative US cohort aged 6 months to 11 years (NHANES II; $n = 5672$) (Schwartz et al., 1990)	Odds-ratios (95% CI) for a 2-SD birth weight decrease asthma 1.31 (1.00 to 1.72) wheeze 1.33 (1.08 to 1.65)
Nationally representative UK cohorts aged 16 years (1958 NCDS and 1970 BCS; $n = 20528$) (Lewis et al., 1996)	Odds-ratios of asthma for birth weight groupings < 2000 g, 2000–2500 g, 2500–3000 g, > 3000 g; 1.00 (referrent), 0.77, 0.78, 0.64 respectively
Male recruits to the Israeli army aged 17 years ($n = 20312$) (Seidman et al., 1991)	Odds-ratios* (95% CI) for asthma 1.44 (0.79 to 2.62) for birth weight < 2000 g 1.49 (1.05 to 2.12) for birth weight 2000–2499 g
Men born in Hertfordshire, England, aged 60 years ($n = 825$) (Barker et al., 1991)	Odds-ratios† (95% CI) for wheeze 1.38 (0.88 to 2.17) for birth weight ≤ 6.5 pounds 1.11 (0.73 to 1.69) for birth weight 6.5–8.5 pounds
Atopic dermatitis	
Birth cohort of infants born on the Isle of Wight, England ($n = 1174$) (Arshad et al., 1993)	Prevalence (%) of atopic dermatitis not significantly related to low birth weight birth weight ≤ 2500 g = 7.9%, > 2500 g = 12.5%
Nationally representative UK cohort (1970 BCS; $n = 12555$) (Golding & Peters, 1986)	Prevalence (%) of atopic dermatitis lower in children with a low birth weight ($p < 0.01$); birth weight ≤ 2500 g = 8.8%, > 2500 g = 12.5%
Birth cohort of Danish children aged 5.5 to 9.5 years ($n = 7862$) (Braae Olesen et al., 1997)	High birth weight for sex and gestational age associated with a higher risk of atopic dermatitis diagnosed by a doctor ($p = 0.02$), but not that diagnosed by a specialist

Note:
Compared with: * birth weight 3000–3499 g and † birth weight > 8.5 lb.

cord blood IgE concentrations and infantile AD with differences in the mother's and infant's EFA status in the neonatal period (Strannegard, Svennerholm & Strannegard, 1987; Businco et al., 1993). Experimental studies in animals have shown that alterations in fetal and neonatal nutrition exert profound effects on thymic development (Winick & Noble, 1966). The action of these during a critical period late in fetal development has been hypothesized to result in a propensity to a persistent IgE response to common environmental antigens (Godfrey et al., 1994). Since postmaturity is also known to be associated with marked wasting of the thymus (Gruenwald, 1975), such a hypothesis is also in accord with the tendency for increased gestational age at birth to be associated with a higher risk of later AD (Braae Olesen et al., 1997) and a raised IgE concentration in adult life (Godfrey et al., 1994).

Pointers to the possibility of programming by other maternal influences

The offspring of atopic parents are widely recognized to be at increased risk of themselves developing atopy. Intriguingly, a number of studies have raised the possibility of preferential inheritance through the maternal line (Bray, 1931; Cookson et al., 1992; Ruiz, Kemeny & Price, 1992; Arshad et al., 1993). Much of the evidence suggesting such an effect has come from small studies or those involving selected populations (Doull, 1996) with conflicting findings coming from the largest study (Dold et al., 1992) and from a group of families randomly selected without regard to atopy (Watson et al., 1995). With specific respect to AD, while two studies have found AD in infancy and early childhood to be more common in the offspring of atopic mothers than in those of atopic fathers (Arshad et al., 1993; Ruiz et al., 1992), three studies of older children have failed to demonstrate a substantially stronger effect of maternal family history (Dold et al., 1992; Coleman, Trembath & Harper, 1993; Watson et al., 1995). This has led to the suggestion that preferential inheritance of atopy through the maternal line might only apply to cord IgE and AD in early life (Doull, 1996).

Against this background of conflicting data, initial claims (Cookson et al., 1992) of a common maternally inherited major gene for atopy on chromosome 11q13 have not been substantiated (Watson et al., 1995). Paternal genomic imprinting at a different genetic locus nonetheless remains a possibility. If preferential inheritance of AD through the maternal line is confirmed, genomic imprinting is not the only possible explanation of such a phenomenon. Alternatively, it has been proposed that this could reflect nongenetic factors such as fetal programming or transplacental passage of maternally derived cytokines (Doull, 1996).

Other pointers to the possibility of important maternal environmental effects on atopy have come from studies linking young maternal age with asthma (Lewis et al., 1996) and older maternal age with AD (see Chapter 11), and from further detailed analyses of the 1958 and 1970 UK National birth cohorts (Peters & Golding, 1987; Strachan et al., 1996). These latter analyses have linked maternal vaginal bleeding and albumenuria during pregnancy with asthma in adolescence and adulthood (Strachan et al., 1996), and have suggested that maternal contraceptive use prior to pregnancy may be a risk factor for AD in early childhood (Peters & Golding, 1987). Given the multiplicity of associations examined in these wonderfully well characterized cohorts, replication of these results is necessary before they can be regarded as secure. Fetal programming, for example of thymic development (Godfrey et al., 1994) consequent upon changes in the fetal growth trajectory induced by the periconceptional sex steroid balance (Kleeman, Walker & Seamark, 1994), nonetheless offers a potential mechanism linking such maternal influences with later AD.

Two other maternal influences that have been much studied in relation to atopy are smoking in pregnancy and breast feeding. An initial case-control study found that children of mothers who smoke have increased admission rates with AD in childhood (Rantakallio, 1978). While two subsequent surveys suggested that maternal smoking is associated with a marginally *lower* prevalence of AD in the offspring (Peters & Golding, 1987; Arshad et al., 1993), neither showed a statistically significant effect independently of other influences. The possibility that breast feeding might protect infants against the later development of AD and other atopic diseases has been addressed in a multitude of observational studies following on from the initial observations of Grulee & Sanford (1936). Mothers who choose to breast feed and formula feed their infants, however, do differ in several important risk factors for atopy (Sauls, 1979). Whilst some authors have strongly advocated a beneficial effect of breast feeding (Saarinen & Kajosaari, 1995), a systematic review of the literature has suggested little or no benefit (Kramer, 1988). One randomized trial in preterm infants has shown that, compared with preterm formula, breast milk reduced the risk of later AD, but only in babies with a family history of atopy (Lucas et al., 1990).

The hypothesis that maternal intakes of dietary allergens during pregnancy and lactation may be important determinants of later atopy in the offspring have led to a number of interventional studies in women at high risk for atopic offspring. A systematic review of the few controlled trials of maternal allergen avoidance *during pregnancy* concluded, however, that this intervention is unlikely to reduce substantially the risk of giving birth to an atopic child (Kramer, 1996a). Perhaps materno-fetal immunological priming (Warner et al., 1996) or placental permeability (Boyd, D'Souza & Sibley, 1994) to antigens may prove to be more important determinants of fetal sensitization than the mother's dietary intakes. Whilst systematic review of controlled trials examining the effects of maternal allergen avoidance *during lactation* suggested the possibility of a protective effect against atopic eczema, caution has been urged in interpreting these findings as a result of methodological shortcomings in the studies concerned (Kramer, 1996b).

Cord blood predictors of later atopic disease

The concentration of total IgE in umbilical cord blood has been shown to predict the later development of atopy in several studies, especially in infants with a family history of atopy (Michel et al., 1980; Businco et al., 1983; Croner et al., 1984; Chandra, Puri & Cheema, 1985; Martinez et al., 1995). Interferon-γ downregulates IgE production, and reduced secretion of this inhibitory cytokine at birth has also been shown to predict later atopy (Tang et al., 1994). Seven-year follow-up of a Swedish cohort of 1651 unselected infants ascertained that obvious atopic disease developed in 20%, of whom 58% had a raised cord blood IgE and 14% a low cord blood IgE (Kjellman & Croner, 1984). These studies generated interest in the concept that a combination of the family history and cord blood IgE concentration might be used to derive a 'family allergy score' that gave an indication of the probability that an infant would develop later atopy. Such a score could then be used to identify a group of 'high risk' infants in whom to study preventive regimens. Subsequent studies, including some with longer follow-up, however, have failed to substantiate the value of cord blood IgE in the prediction of later AD (Merrett et al., 1988; Hide et al., 1991; Ruiz et al., 1991). Thus, although a raised cord blood IgE is a reasonably specific indicator of later atopy, it is currently thought to be too insensitive to have value as a predictive test.

Notwithstanding these considerations of cord IgE as a predictive test, it is nonetheless a useful pointer suggesting that intra-uterine influences bear on the later risk of atopic disease. The IgE in cord blood is not specifically directed against antigens thought to be relevant to allergic disease, and may be acting as a general marker of immune development and allergic responsiveness. A number of environmental influences, including maternal progesterone and metoprolol treatment (Michel et al., 1980; Bjorksten, Finnstrom & Wichman, 1988), maternal alcohol ingestion (Bjerke et al., 1994) and high cord blood linoleic acid levels (Strannegard et al., 1987) have been associated with an increased cord blood IgE concentration. The relevance of these maternal influences to later AD, however, is unclear.

In contrast to studies of cord blood IgE affinities, evidence that allergen-specific immune responses *do* develop in utero has come from detailed studies of peripheral mononuclear cells isolated from umbilical cord blood (Kondo et al., 1992; Piccinni et al., 1993; Warner et al., 1994). These indicate that latent allergen-specific immune responses can be unmasked by stimulation of cord blood mononuclear cells with dietary antigens and aeroantigens. Initial studies have, moreover, shown that a higher proliferative response and a lower interferon-γ production following beta-lactoglobulin or ovalbumen stimulation was associated with an increased prevalence of AD in infancy (Kondo et al., 1992; Warner et al., 1994). As yet, however, these studies have been confined to small groups of 'high-risk' infants both of whose parents are atopic. If such observations are replicated in larger studies and in unselected populations they will facilitate the identification of maternal influences leading to fetal sensitization, and could lead to predictive tests of value in research and clinical practice.

Month of birth

Much attention has been focused on the thesis that allergen load during a 'susceptible' period in early infancy may programme long-term effects on sensitization. Such a hypothesis predicts that exposure to seasonal allergens at a time when a maturational immune response defect may be present would result in an association between month of birth and lifelong sensitization. The published literature examining the relationship between an individual's month of birth and later allergic disease does contain inconsistencies, however, and concern has been raised that publication bias might contribute to the rather confusing picture (Strachan, 1994).

Thus, whilst some studies have suggested that exposure to seasonal allergens in the initial months following birth may lead to aeroallergen sensitization and respiratory allergy (Bjorksten, Suoniemi & Koski, 1980; Kemp, 1979; Businco et al., 1988), others have failed to find significant associations (Reed & Corvallis, 1958; David & Beards, 1985). Figure 9.2 gives an example of the inconsistent results that have been found for grass pollen sensitivity. With

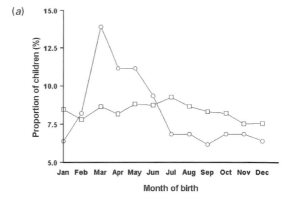

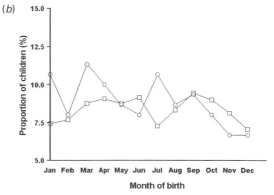

Fig. 9.2. Proportions of subjects with sensitization to grass pollen (○) and of controls (□) according to their month of birth in: (a) an Italian study (Buscino et al., 1988); and (b) a US study (Reed & Corvallis, 1958)

specific regard to AD, initial studies provided weak evidence suggesting differing associations between birth month and later AD (Soothill et al., 1976; Beck & Hagdrup, 1987). Subsequently population-based studies of larger groups, however, have found no association between the child's month of birth and a later history of eczema (Anderson, Bailey & Bland, 1981; Schafer et al., 1993).

Overall, population studies provide only limited support for the hypothesis that seasonal variations in the early postnatal environment may have long-term effects on allergen sensitization and allergic disease. Any such effects appear confined to childhood and adolescence, and are not manifest in adults (Bjorksten et al., 1980; Sibbald & Rink, 1990). Allergic contact dermatitis serves to illustrate that many individuals only become sensitized when exposed to common allergens in adult life. Furthermore, it is as yet unclear whether interventional studies reducing allergen exposure in the first months after birth are simply delaying sensitization, rather than completely preventing it (Zeiger et al., 1992; Hide et al., 1994). One further note of caution is made necessary by the observation of a strong association between month of birth and sensitization to 'nonseasonal' allergens (Aalberse et al., 1992). In addition to aeroallergens, seasonal variations exist in a wide variety of other exposures, including maternal ovulatory patterns, vitamin D status and viral infections, and the possible importance of these in fetal immune development may well prove substantial.

Conclusions

Diverse research approaches have indicated that early life events may play an important role in the genesis of AD and other atopic disorders. Initial epidemiological studies suggest that environmental influences acting during fetal life and early infancy could programme the later development of AD. Such influences include fetal nutrition and immunological priming of the fetus and neonate. Secure identification of the critical factors, and elucidation of the mechanisms through which they operate, offers the real prospect of defining effective interventions to reverse the increase in AD over recent decades.

Summary of key points

- The fetal and early infant environment may play a critical role in programming a lifelong predisposition to common adult diseases, including coronary heart disease and noninsulin-dependent diabetes mellitus.
- Effects of the intra-uterine environment may have resulted in classical twin studies overestimating the genetic contribution to many diseases, including atopic dermatitis (AD).
- Some studies suggest a weak association between higher birth weight and AD.

- Recent studies have found associations between disproportionate fetal growth and adult IgE concentration, and between increased iron intake in pregnancy and AD in the offspring.
- These associations could reflect effects on essential fatty acid metabolism or inability of the maternal supply line to match fetal nutrient requirements during a critical period in thymic development.
- Some studies suggest that maternal age and prior contraceptive use are linked to later AD.
- A systematic review of the literature has suggested little or no benefit from breast feeding.
- Raised cord blood IgE is a reasonably specific indicator of later atopy, although too insensitive to be useful as a predictive test.
- Studies of mononuclear cells in cord blood have shown links between allergen-specific immune responses and increased AD.
- The evidence linking month of birth with AD is weak and conflicting.
- Identification of materno-fetal predictors of AD offers real hope of prevention of sensitization and clinical disease.

References

Aalberse, R.C., Nieuwenhuys, E., Hey, M. & Stapel, S.O. (1992). 'Horoscope effect' not only for seasonal but also for non-seasonal allergens. *Clin Exp Allergy*, **22**, 1003–6.

Alho, O.P., Koivu, M., Hartikainen-Sorri, A.L., Sorri, M., Kilkku, O. & Rantakallio, P. (1990). Is a child's history of acute otitis media and respiratory infection already determined in the antenatal and perinatal period? *Int J Pediat Otorhinolaryngol*, **19**, 129–37.

Anderson, H.R., Bailey, P.A. & Bland, J.M. (1981). The effect of birth month on asthma, eczema, hayfever, respiratory symptoms, lung function, and hospital admissions for asthma. *Int J Epidemiol*, **10**, 45–51.

Arshad, S.H., Stevens, M. & Hide, D.W. (1993). The effect of genetic and environmental factors on the prevalence of allergic disorders at the age of two years. *Clin Exp Allergy*, **23**, 504–11.

Barker, D.J.P. (ed.) (1994). *Mothers, Babies and Disease in Later Life*. London: BMJ Publications.

Barker, D.J.P. (1995). Fetal origins of coronary heart disease. *Br Med J*, **311**, 171–4.

Barker, D.J.P. & Sultan, H.Y. (1994). Programming the baby. In: Barker, D.J.P. (ed.) *Mothers, Babies and Disease in Later Life.* London: BMJ Publications.

Barker, D.J.P., Godfrey, K.M., Fall, C., Osmond, C., Winter, P.D. & Shaheen, S.O. (1991). Relation of birth weight and childhood respiratory infection to adult lung function and death from chronic obstructive airways disease. *Br Med J*, **303**, 671–5.

Barker, D.J.P., Osmond, C., Simmonds, S.J. & Wield, G.A. (1993a). The relation of head size and thinness at birth to death from cardiovascular disease in adult life. *Br Med J*, **306**, 422–6.

Barker, D.J.P., Hales, C.N., Fall, C.H.D., Osmond, C., Phipps, K. & Clark, P.M.S. (1993b). Type 2 (non-insulin-dependent) diabetes mellitus, hypertension and hyperlipidaemia (syndrome X): relation to reduced fetal growth. *Diabetologia*, **36**, 62–7.

Barker, D.J.P., Martyn, C.N., Osmond, C., Hales, C.N. & Fall, C.H.D. (1993c). Growth in utero and serum cholesterol concentrations in adult life. *Br Med J*, **307**, 1524–7.

Barker, D.J.P., Gluckman, P.D., Godfrey, K.M., Harding, J., Owens, J.A. & Robinson, J.S. (1993d). Fetal nutrition and cardiovascular disease in adult life. *Lancet*, **341**, 938–41.

Beck, H-I. & Hagdrup, H.K. (1987). Atopic dermatitis, house dust mite allergy and month of birth. *Acta Dermatol Venereol (Stockh.)*, **67**, 448–51.

Beral, V. & Colwell, L. (1981). Randomised trial of high doses of stilboestrol and ethisterone therapy in pregnancy: long-term follow-up of the children. *J Epidemiol Commun Hlth*, **35**, 155–60.

Bjerke, T., Hedegaard, M., Henriksen, T.N., Nielson, B.W. & Schiotz, P.O. (1994). Several genetic and environmental factors influence cord blood IgE concentration. *Pediat Allergy Immunol*, **5**, 88–94.

Bjorksten, F., Suoniemi, I. & Koski, V. (1980). Neonatal birch pollen contact and subsequent allergy to birch pollen. *Clin Allergy*, **10**, 581–91.

Bjorksten, B., Finnstrom, O. & Wichman, K. (1988). Intrauterine exposure to the beta-adrenergic receptor-blocking agent metoprolol and allergy. *Int Arch Allergy Immunol*, **87**, 59–62.

Boyd, R.D.H., D'Souza, S.W. & Sibley, C.P. (1994). Placental transfer. In: Ward, R.H.T., Smith, S.K. & Donnai, D. (eds.) *Early Fetal Growth and Development*, pp. 211–21. London: RCOG Press.

Braae Olesen, A., Ringer Ellingsen, A., Olesen, H., Juul, S., Thestrup-Pedersen, K. (1997). Atopic dermatitis and birth factors: historical follow up by record linkage. *Br Med J*, **314**, 1003–8.

Bray, G.W. (1931). The hereditary factor in hyperresponsiveness, anaphylaxis and allergy. *J Allergy*, **2**, 205–24.

Businco, L., Marchetti, F., Pellegrini, G. & Perlini, R. (1983). Predictive value of cord blood IgE levels in 'at risk' newborn babies and influence of type of feeding. *Clin Allergy*, **13**, 503–8.

Businco, L., Cantani, A., Farinella, F. & Businco, E. (1988). Month of birth and grass pollen or mite sensitisation in children with respiratory allergy: a significant relationship. *Clin Allergy*, **18**, 269–74.

Businco, L., Ioppi, M., Morse, N.L., Nisini, R. & Wright, S. (1993). Breast milk from mothers of children with newly developed atopic eczema has low levels of long chain polyunsaturated fatty acids. *J Allergy Clin Immunol*, **91**, 1134–9.

Chan, K.N., Noble-Jamieson, C.M., Elliman, A., Bryan, E.M. & Silverman, M. (1989). Lung function in children of low birth weight. *Arch Dis Childh*, **64**, 1284–93.

Chandra, R.K. (1975). Antibody generation in the first and second generation offspring of nutritionally deprived rats. *Science*, **190**, 289–90.

Chandra, R.K., Puri, S. & Cheema, P.S. (1985). Predictive value of cord blood IgE in the development of atopic disease and the role of breast-feeding in its prevention. *Clin Allergy*, **15**, 517–22.

Clark, P.M.S., Hindmarsh, P.C., Shiell, A.W., Law, C.M., Honour, J.W. & Barker, D.J.P. (1996). Size at birth and adrenocortical function in childhood. *Clin Endocrinol*, **45**, 721–6.

Coleman, R., Trembath, R.C. & Harper, J.I. (1993). Chromosome 11q and atopy underlying atopic eczema. *Lancet*, **341**, 1121–2.

Cookson, W.O.C.M., Young, R.P., Sandford, A.J. et al. (1992). Maternal inheritance of atopic IgE responsiveness on chromosome 11q. *Lancet*, **340**, 381–4.

Crawford, M.A., Doyle, W., Drury, P., Lennon, A., Costeloe, K. & Leighfield, M. (1989). N-6 and n-3 fatty acids during early human development. *J Int Med*, **225** (Suppl. 1), 159–69.

Croner, S., Kjellman, N-I.M., Eriksson, B. & Roth, A. (1984). IgE screening in 1701 newborn infants and the development of atopic disease during infancy. *Arch Dis Childh*, **57**, 364–8.

Curhan, G.C., Willett, W.C., Rimm, E.B. & Stampfer, M.J. (1996). Birth weight and adult hypertension and diabetes in US men. *Am J Hypertension*, **9**, 11A.

Czeizel, A.E. & Dodo, M. (1994). Postnatal somatic and mental development after periconceptual multivitamin supplementation. *Arch Dis Childh*, **70**, 229–33.

David, T.J. & Beards, S.C. (1985). Asthma and the month of birth. *Clin Allergy*, **15**, 391–5.

Desai, M., Crowther, N.J., Ozanne, S.E., Lucas, A. & Hales, C.N. (1995). Adult glucose and lipid metabolism may be programmed during fetal life. *Biochem Soc Trans*, **23**, 331–5.

Dold, S., Wjst, M., Mutius, E.V., Reitmeir, P. & Stiepel, E. (1992). Genetic risk for asthma, allergic rhinitis, and atopic dermatitis. *Arch Dis Childh*, **67**, 1018–22.

Doull, I.J.M. (1996). Maternal inheritance of atopy? *Clin Exp Allergy*, **26**, 613–5.

Emanuel, I., Filakti, H., Alberman, E. & Evans, S.J.W. (1992).

Intergenerational studies of human birthweight from the 1958 birth cohort. 1. Evidence for a multigenerational effect. *Br J Obstet Gynaecol*, **99**, 67–74.

Fall, C.H.D., Pandit, A.N., Law, C.M., Yajnik, C.S., Clark, P.M.S., Breier, B., Osmond, C., Shiell, A.W., Gluckman, P.D. & Barker, D.J.P. (1995). Size at birth and plasma insulin-like growth factor-1 concentrations. *Arch Dis Childh*, **73**, 287–93.

Godfrey, K.M. & Barker, D.J.P. (1995). Maternal nutrition in relation to fetal and placental growth. *Europ J Obstet Gynecol Reprod Biol*, **61**, 15–22.

Godfrey, K.M., Barker, D.J.P. & Osmond, C. (1994). Disproportionate fetal growth and raised IgE concentration in adult life. *Clin Exp Allergy*, **24**, 641–8.

Godfrey, K.M., Osmond, C. & Hammond, J. (1995). Maternal nutrition during pregnancy in relation to atopic eczema in the first nine months of life. *Br J Dermatol*, **133**, 1006.

Godfrey, K.M., Barker, D.J.P., Robinson, S. & Osmond, C. (1997). Mother's birthweight and diet in pregnancy in relation to the baby's thinness at birth. *Br J Obstet Gynaecol*, **104**, 663–7.

Golding, J. & Peters, T. (1986). Eczema and hay fever. In: Butler, N.R. & Golding, J. (eds.) *From Birth to Five*, pp. 171–86. Oxford: Pergamon Press.

Golding, J. & Peters, T.J. (1987). The epidemiology of childhood eczema: I. A population based study of associations. *Paediat Perinatal Epidemiol*, **1**, 67–79.

Gruenwald, P. (1975). Pathology of the deprived fetus and its supply line. In: Elliott, K. & Knight, J. (eds.) *Size at Birth*, pp. 3–19. Ciba Foundation Symposium No. 27. Amsterdam: Elsevier.

Grulee, C.G. & Sanford, H.N. (1936). The influence of breast and artificial feeding on infantile eczema. *J Pediat*, **9**, 223–5.

Harding, J.E., Liu, L., Evans, P., Oliver, M. & Gluckman, P.D. (1992). Intrauterine feeding of the growth retarded fetus: can we help? *Early Hum Developm*, **29**, 193–7.

Hide, D.W., Arshad, S.H., Twiselton, R. & Stevens, M. (1991). Cord serum IgE: an insensitive method for prediction of atopy. *Clin Exp Allergy*, **21**, 739–43.

Hide, D.W., Matthews, S.S., Matthews, L., Stevens, M., Ridout, S., Twiselton, R., Grant, C. & Arshad, S.H. (1994). Effect of allergen avoidance in infancy on allergic manifestations at age 2 years. *J Allergy Clin Immunol*, **93**, 842–6.

Howe, D. (1995). Maternal haemoglobin and birth weight in different ethnic groups. *Br Med J*, **310**, 1601.

Kallman, F.J. & Reisner, D. (1943). Twin studies on genetic variation in resistance to tuberculosis. *J Hered*, **34**, 269–76.

Kemp, A.S. (1979). Relationship between the time of birth and the development of immediate hypersensitivity to grass pollen antigens. *Med J Aust*, **1**, 263–4.

Kjellman, N-I.M. & Croner, S. (1984). Cord blood IgE determination for allergy prediction – a follow-up to seven years of age in 1651 children. *Ann Allergy*, **53**, 167–71.

Kleeman, D.O., Walker, S.K. & Seamark, R.F. (1994). Enhanced growth in sheep administered progesterone during the first three days of pregnancy. *J Reprod Fertil*, **102**, 411–7.

Kondo, N., Kobayashi, Y., Shinoda, S. et al. (1992). Cord blood lymphocyte responses to food antigens for the prediction of allergic disorders. *Arch Dis Childh*, **67**, 1003–7.

Konje, J.C., Bell, S.C., Morton, J.J., De Chazal, R. & Taylor, D.J. (1996). Human fetal kidney morphometry during gestation and the relationship between weight, kidney morphometry and plasma active renin concentration at birth. *Clin Sci*, **91**, 169–75.

Kramer, M.S. (1988). Does breast feeding help protect against atopic disease? Biology, methodology and a golden jubilee of controversy. *J Pediat*, **112**, 181–90.

Kramer, M.S. (1996a). Maternal antigen avoidance in pregnancy in women at high risk for atopic offspring. In: Neilson, J.P., Crowther, C.A., Hodnett, E.D., Hofmeyr, G.J. & Keirse, M.J.N.C. (eds.) *Pregnancy and Childbirth Module of The Cochrane Database of Systematic Reviews*. Oxford: The Cochrane Collaboration.

Kramer, M.S. (1996b). Maternal antigen avoidance during lactation in women at high risk for atopic offspring. In: Neilson, J.P., Crowther, C.A., Hodnett, E.D., Hofmeyr, G.J. & Keirse, M.J.N.C. (eds.) *Pregnancy and Childbirth Module of The Cochrane Database of Systematic Reviews*. Oxford: The Cochrane Collaboration.

Larsen, F.S., Holm, N.V. & Henningsen, K. (1986). Atopic dermatitis: a genetic–epidemiologic study in a population-based twin sample. *J Am Acad Dermatol*, **15**, 487–94.

Lewis, S., Butland, B., Strachan, D., Bynner, J., Richards, D., Butler, N. & Britton, J. (1996). Study of the aetiology of wheezing illness at age 16 in two national British cohorts. *Thorax*, **51**, 670–6.

Lithell, H.O., McKeigue, P.M., Berglund, L., Mohsen, R., Lithell, U-B. & Leon, D.A. (1996). Relation of size at birth to non-insulin dependent diabetes and insulin concentrations in men aged 50–60 years. *Br Med J*, **312**, 406–10.

Lucas, A. (1991). Programming by early nutrition in man. In: Bock, G.R. & Whelan, J. (eds.) *The Childhood Environment and Adult Disease*, pp. 38–50. Ciba Foundation Symposium 156. Chichester: John Wiley.

Lucas, A., Brooke, O.G., Morley, R., Cole, T.J. & Bamford, M.F. (1990). Early diet of preterm infants and development of allergic or atopic disease: randomised prospective study. *Br Med J*, **300**, 837–40.

Lumey, L.H. (1992). Decreased birthweights in infants after maternal *in utero* exposure to the Dutch famine of 1944–1945. *Paediat Perinatal Epidemiol*, **6**, 240–53.

Martinez, F.D., Wright, A.L., Taussig, L.M., Holberg, C.J., Halonen, M. & Morgan, W.J. (1995). Asthma and wheezing in the first six years of life. *New Engl J Med*, **332**, 133–8.

Martyn, C.N., Barker, D.J.P., Jespersen, S. et al. (1995a). Growth in utero, adult blood pressure and arterial compliance. *Br Heart J*, **73**, 116–21.

Martyn, C.N., Meade, T.W., Stirling, Y. & Barker, D.J.P. (1995b). Plasma concentrations of fibrinogen and factor VII in adult life and their relation to intra-uterine growth. *Br J Haematol*, **89**, 142–6.

Martyn, C.N., Lever, A.F. & Morton, J.J. (1996). Plasma concentrations of inactive renin in adult life are related to indicators of foetal growth. *J Hypertension*, **14**, 881–6.

Merrett, T.G., Burr, M.L., Butland, B.K. et al. (1988). Infant feeding and allergy: 12-month prospective study of 500 babies born in allergic families. *Ann Allergy*, **61**, 13–24.

Michel, F.B., Bousquet, J., Greillier, P., Robinet-Leucy, M. & Coulomb, Y. (1980). Comparison of cord blood immunoglobulin E concentrations and maternal allergy for the prediction of atopic diseases in infancy. *J Allergy Clin Immunol*, **65**, 422–30.

Peters, T.J. & Golding, J. (1987). The epidemiology of childhood eczema: II. Statistical analyses to identify independent early predictors. *Paediatr Perinatal Epidemiol*, **1**, 80–94.

Phillips, D.I.W. (1993). Twin studies in medical research: can they tell us whether diseases are genetically determined? *Lancet*, **341**, 1008–9.

Phillips, D.I.W. (1996). Insulin resistance as a programmed response to fetal undernutrition. *Diabetologia*, **39**, 1119–22.

Phillips, D.I.W., Cooper, C., Fall, C., Prentice, L., Osmond, C., Barker, D.J.P. & Rees Smith, B. (1993). Fetal growth and autoimmune thyroid disease. *Q J Med*, **86**, 247–53.

Piccinni, M-P., Mecacci, F., Sampognaro, S. et al. (1993). Aeroallergen sensitization can occur during fetal life. *Int Arch Allergy Immunol*, **102**, 301–3.

Rantakallio, P. (1978). Relationship of maternal smoking to morbidity and mortality of the child up to the age of five. *Acta Paediat Scand*, **67**, 621–31.

Reed, C.E. & Corvallis, O. (1958). The failure of antepartum or neonatal exposure to grass pollen to influence the later development of grass sensitivity. *J Allergy*, **29**, 300–1.

Rich-Edwards, J., Stampfer, M., Manson, J., Rosner, B., Colditz, G., Willett, W., Speizer, F. & Hennekens, C. (1995). Birthweight, breastfeeding, and the risk of coronary heart disease in the Nurses' Health Study. *Am J Epidemiol*, **141**: S78.

Rona, R.J., Gulliford, M.C. & Chinn, S. (1993). Effects of prematurity and intrauterine growth on respiratory health and lung function in childhood. *Br Med J*, **306**, 817–20.

Ruiz, R.G.G., Richards, D., Kemeny, D.M. & Price, J.F. (1991). Neonatal IgE: a poor screen for atopic disease. *Clin Exp Allergy*, **21**, 467–72.

Ruiz, R.G.G., Kemeny, D.M. & Price, J.F. (1992). Higher risk of infantile atopic dermatitis from maternal atopy than from paternal atopy. *Clin Exp Allergy*, **22**, 762–6.

Saarinen, U.M. & Kajosaari, M. (1995). Breastfeeding as prophylaxis against atopic disease. *Lancet*, **346**, 1714.

Sauls, H.S. (1979). Potential effect of demographic and other variables in studies comparing morbidity of breast-fed and bottle-fed infants. *Pediatrics*, **64**, 523–7.

Schafer, T., Przybilla, B., Ring, J., Kunz, B., Greif, A. & Uberla, K. (1993). Manifestation of atopy is not related to patient's month of birth. *Allergy*, **48**, 291–4.

Schwartz, J., Gold, D., Dockery, D.W., Weiss, S.T. & Speizer, F.E. (1990). Predictors of asthma and persistent wheeze in a national sample of children in the United States. *Am Rev Resp Dis*, **142**, 555–62.

Seidman, D.S., Laor, A., Gale, R., Stevenson, D.K. & Danon, Y.L. (1991). Is low birth weight a risk factor for asthma during adolescence? *Br Med J*, **66**, 584–7.

Shaheen, S.O. & Barker, D.J.P. (1994). Early lung growth and chronic airflow obstruction. *Thorax*, **49**, 533–6.

Sibbald, B. & Rink, E. (1990). Birth month variation in atopic and non-atopic rhinitis. *Clin Exp Allergy*, **20**, 285–8.

Soothill, J.F., Stokes, C.R., Turner, M.W., Norman, A.P. & Taylor, B. (1976). Predisposing factors and the development of reaginic allergy in infancy. *Clin Allergy*, **6**, 305–19.

Stewart, R.J.C., Preece, R.F. & Sheppard, H.G. (1975). Twelve generations of marginal protein deficiency. *Br J Nutrit*, **33**, 233–53.

Strachan, D.P. (1994). Is allergic disease programmed in early life? *Clin Exp Allergy*, **24**, 603–5.

Strachan, D.P. (1995). Time trends in asthma and allergy: ten questions, fewer answers. *Clin Exp Allergy*, **25**, 791–4.

Strachan, D.P., Butland, B.K. & Anderson, H.R. (1996). Incidence and prognosis of asthma and wheezing illness from early childhood to age 33 in a national British cohort. *Br Med J*, **312**, 1195–9.

Strannegard, I-L., Svennerholm, L. & Strannegard, O. (1987). Essential fatty acids in serum lecithin of children with atopic dermatitis and in umbilical cord serum of infants with high or low IgE levels. *Int Arch Allergy Appl Immunol*, **82**, 422–3.

Tang, M.L.K., Kemp, A.S., Thorburn, J. & Hill, D.J. (1994). Reduced interferon-γ secretion in neonates and subsequent atopy. *Lancet*, **344**, 983–5.

Taylor, D.J., Thompson, C.H., Kemp, G.J., Barnes, P.R.J., Sanderson, A., Radda, G.K. & Phillips, D.I.W. (1995). A relationship between impaired fetal growth and reduced muscle glycolysis revealed by ^{31}P magnetic resonance spectroscopy. *Diabetologia*, **38**, 1205–12.

Vijayakumar, M., Fall, C.H.D., Osmond, C. & Barker, D.J.P. (1995). Birth weight, weight at one year, and left ventricular mass in adult life. *Br Heart J*, **73**, 363–7.

Warner, J.A., Miles, E.A., Jones, A.C. et al. (1994). Is deficiency of interferon gamma production by allergen triggered cord blood cells a predictor of atopic eczema? *Clin Exp Allergy*, **244**, 23–30.

Warner, J.A., Jones, A.C., Miles, E.A., Colwell, B.M. & Warner, J.O. (1996). Maternofetal interaction and allergy. *Allergy*, **51**, 447–51.

Watson, M., Lawrence, S., Collins, A. et al. (1995). Exclusion from proximal 11q of a common gene with megaphenic effect on atopy. *Ann Hum Genet*, **59**, 403–11.

Widdowson, E.M. & McCance, R.A. (1975). A review: new thought on growth. *Pediat Res*, **9**, 154–6.

Winick, M. & Noble, A. (1966). Cellular response in rats during malnutrition at various ages. *J Nutrit*, **89**, 300–6.

Zeiger, R.S., Heller, S., Mellon, M.H. & Halsey, J.F. (1992). Genetic and environmental factors affecting the development of atopy through age 4 in children of atopic parents: a prospective randomized study of food allergen avoidance. *Pediat Allergy Immunol*, **3**, 110–27.

10

Social factors and atopic dermatitis

Nicholas McNally and David Phillips

Socioeconomic status, health and epidemiology

The incidence of many diseases varies, sometimes considerably, according to social and economic conditions, culture and other environmental factors (Marmot, 1996). Socioeconomic status and social class have therefore become important concerns within epidemiology, and an increasing proportion of mortality and morbidity in developed and developing nations can now be explained by the growth in chronic disease with multifactorial aetiologies. Lifestyles and behaviour, heavily influenced by social factors, are now seen as crucial in health and disease.

There is a long tradition in Britain, perhaps less marked in some other countries, of public health interest in socioeconomic conditions and health (Macintyre, 1997). The well known Black Report, published in 1980 by the Department of Health and Social Services, concluded that marked differences in mortality rates existed between the occupational classes. In particular, the report confirmed the negative social class gradient for many diseases with a deterioration of the health experience and higher risk of premature death occurring in the unskilled and semi-skilled manual classes (class IV and V) relative to class I. These differences, the report suggested, could be understood largely in terms of specific features of the socioeconomic environment such as work accidents, overcrowding and cigarette smoking, all of which are class related in Britain and have clear causal significance in terms of health status (Townsend & Davidson, 1992).

In Britain, the occupation of the head of the family has traditionally been used as an approximate measure of socioeconomic status. There are two most commonly used measures of occupational class. First, the Registrar General's classification by occupational class is based on the level of skill, financial rewards and the status an individual confers within the community. This places people in groups ranging from social class I (professional and administrative occupations) to social class V (unskilled occupations). Secondly, the scale of socioeconomic groups (SEGs) categorizes people according to similar skills but perhaps puts greater emphasis on lifestyles (Cox et al., 1993). The advantage of using measures of socioeconomic status such as these is that they serve as useful surrogate measures of lifestyle. The classifications are taken as indicators of how ways of life and living standards differ between separate groups within the population (Townsend & Davidson, 1992). The two indices are summarized in Table 10.1.

Since the time of the Black Report, there have been extensive developments in the measurement of socioeconomic status, as it is increasingly recognized that social class is only a crude representation of social conditions and gives only an approximate index of the many factors that contribute to living standards (Power et al., 1996). Asset-based measures such as income, car ownership or housing have become increasingly used in Britain as indicators of social status, as have area-based indices of deprivation (Macintyre, 1997). Social class is clearly important in a geographical sense, since there is strong socioeconomic differentiation spatially. In Britain,

Table 10.1. Social class categorization in Britain (Robinson & Elkan, 1996)

RG's social class

I	Higher professional and administrative occupations.
II	Lesser professional occupations and employers in industry and retail trades.
III (N-M)	Skilled occupations (nonmanual).
III (M)	Skilled occupations (manual).
IV	Partly-skilled manual occupations.
V	Unskilled manual occupations.

Socioeconomic groups

1	Professional
2	Employers and managers
3	Intermediate junior nonmanual
4	Skilled manual
5	Semi-skilled manual and personal service
6	Unskilled manual

Table 10.2. Census variables used in the Townsend, Jarman and Carstairs indices (from Wilson, 1995)

Census variable	Townsend	Jarman	Carstairs
Unemployment	◆	◆	◆
Car ownership	◆		◆
Home ownership	◆		
Overcrowding	◆	◆	◆
Lone pensioners		◆	
Under 5		◆	
Social class		◆	◆
Changed address		◆	
Ethnic group		◆	
Lone parent		◆	

this often stems from and reflects the distribution of housing tenure and the effects of the housing market. Particularly marked in some locations is the earlier influence of social (public) housing, which was predominantly built in large estates. The private housing market has also been strongly spatially differentiated. This means that, as many diseases afflict different social groups at different rates, there are apparently geographically healthier and unhealthier areas and these spatial differences in apparent health status are sometimes quite spectacular. This has been made heavy use of previously and again more recently in territorial studies of deprivation and the development of deprivation indices which rank small areas rather than individuals on an index of deprivation. In British health studies, the most commonly used composite measures of deprivation include the Jarman index of underprivileged areas, the Carstairs index and the Townsend index (Robinson & Elkan, 1996). Table 10.2 illustrates the Census variables used to make up some of the most commonly used indices.

However, despite the increasingly recognized limitations of social class as an indicator of socioeconomic status, the use of occupational classifications has achieved considerable success in identifying

possible associated factors in the aetiology of many diseases. Moreover, Macintyre (1997) notes that observed inequalities in health are consistently found *whatever* the measure used. Attempts are now being made to review the existing measures of individual level occupational status and to supersede them with new classifications which employ a greater number (probably up to 20) of categories of occupational status as well as nonoccupational indicators from the Census which will be easily collapsed into smaller indices and allow comparison with the existing classifications (personal communication, Office of National Statistics).

As noted above and highlighted by the Black Report, negative social class gradients exist in Britain for most diseases (Townsend & Davidson, 1992) but there is growing contemporary evidence that for some diseases, notably certain cancers such as ovarian and melanoma, the reverse obtains and individuals of higher socioeconomic status are at greater risk of such diseases (Smith et al., 1996; Kelsey & Bernstein, 1996; Van den Eeden et al., 1991; Swerdlow et al., 1991). Some people in these groups may also be at greater risk from certain diseases related to stress and lifestyle (Blaxter, 1990).

Social class and atopy

As with many other forms of morbidity, rates of atopy appear to vary with social factors. However, in some cases this is a positive social class gradient, in which higher rates prevail amongst the highest social groups. Growing evidence suggests that a positive socioeconomic gradient exists for atopy as defined by positive results in skin prick tests (Shaheen et al., 1996; von Mutius et al., 1994; Gergen et al., 1987; Barbee et al., 1976; Freeman & Johnson, 1964; Smith, 1974), although this is not unequivocal, as other studies have not identified such trends (Astarita et al., 1988). There are also indications that a positive social class gradient may not exist for all allergic disease and, indeed, the reverse may be true for respiratory tract infections (Forster et al., 1990) and hospital admissions for asthma and wheezy bronchitis (Williams et al., 1994). In a national British cohort, dermatitis and hay fever have also been found to be associated with household size (Strachan, 1989), region of residence (Strachan, 1990) and county of residence (McNally et al., 1998), whereas asthma and wheezy bronchitis showed a different epidemiological pattern.

Atopic dermatitis: a social class gradient?

Early indications of a social class gradient in the prevalence of dermatitis in the United Kingdom were provided by analysis of the third British Cohort Study of 1970 (BCS70), a national sample of 11 920 children born in 1970. This showed the prevalence of reported dermatitis to be considerably higher in 'advantaged' socioeconomic groups, affecting 16.6% of children born from social class I (father's occupation a higher professional) compared with 8.9% from social class V (father's occupation unskilled), with a statistically significant trend over all social class groupings (Golding & Peters, 1987). Similar trends in prevalence of reported dermatitis were found with other indicators of socioeconomic status such as parental education, less overcrowding, and greater ownership of household possessions.

However, while these findings are interesting, the imprecise methods used to define atopic dermatitis (AD) means that it is difficult to determine whether children from higher social classes actually have a genuine higher risk of AD or whether the observed gradient is actually an artefact of different health-related behaviour and reporting among social class groups. A number of factors may be important. First, it seems likely that the terms *allergy* and *dermatitis* have become increasingly more fashionable in wealthier groups over recent decades and they might therefore be noted or reported more readily (Wüthrich, 1989; Taylor et al., 1984). Secondly, there is some evidence that the diagnosis of AD and hay fever, both by doctors and parents, is higher in constituent communities of higher socioeconomic status (Buser et al., 1993; Sibbald & Rink, 1991). Thirdly, wealthier families may be more likely than those in less advantaged social groups to consult their doctors and acquire the label AD for borderline conditions such as dry skin (Waters, 1971). Finally, recall of AD in the early years of life might be enhanced in wealthier families with fewer children on average, especially in the past.

Using data from the National Child Development Study (NCDS), the second of the British Cohort Studies, Williams et al. (1994) were able to test the hypothesis that the observed gradient in prevalence of AD by social class in Britain was actually due to the tendency, in more affluent families, to overreport the disease. The NCDS includes all those born in England, Wales and Scotland in one week in March 1958. The validation of parental-reported AD was possible because the NCDS included an examination of children by experienced school medical officers, for the presence of skin disease at the ages of 7, 11 and 16 (Shepherd, 1985). As with the BCS70 data, a striking social class gradient in the *reported* prevalence of AD was observed in the NCDS sample, with prevalence in social classes I and II being approximately twice as high as in classes IV and V. The strongest trend was observed when the children were aged 7 and under (see Figure 10.1).

Interestingly, similar social class trends were shown for the prevalence of *examined* AD at all ages in the follow-up study. The consistencies between the reported and examined gradients suggest that reporting bias was not the main reason for these trends. Moreover, the positive social class gradient was shown to persist after adjustment for region of residence, ethnic group, breast feeding, sex of child, parental smoking and family size. However, similar

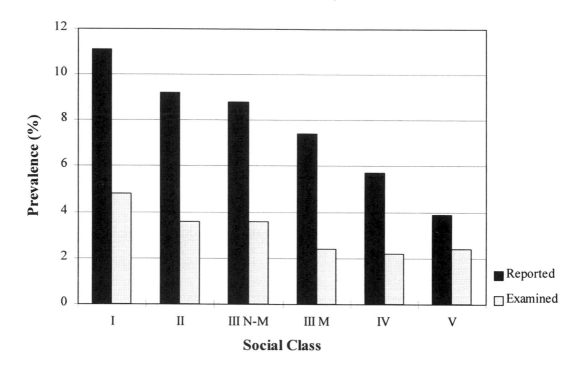

Fig. 10.1. Parent-reported and examined prevalence of eczema at seven years according to social class (Williams et al., 1994)

trends were not found for psoriasis and acne, the other inflammatory skin conditions recorded in the national cohort. This enhances the validity of the findings as it suggests that there was no general tendency for medical officers to overestimate visible skin disease in social classes I and II.

Indications of a positive social class gradient in the prevalence of AD are not just confined to British studies. The Swiss Scarpol study included 4465 children and identified a significant trend in reported lifetime prevalence of AD by social class with the highest prevalence found in social class I (15.9%) and the lowest in social class V (9.6%) (Wüthrich, 1996) (see Table 10.3). However, no significant trend in the point prevalence of AD was found.

Another study of atopic disease in schoolchildren in east and west Germany found that the risk of AD was increased (OR 1.83, 95% CI 0.83 to 4.02) amongst children whose parents were educated for ten years or more in school (Schäfer et al., 1996). A marked

social class gradient in the incidence of AD was also found among Chinese migrants living in San Francisco, using three categories of paternal occupation (Worth, 1962). The incidence of AD was 32%, 23% and 16% among white collar, blue collar and 'labourers', respectively. This study is discussed in greater detail in Chapter 13 where migrant studies are considered.

Why a positive social class gradient in dermatitis?

The effects of social class on the incidence and prevalence of AD could be manifested in a number of different ways. Dermatitis could be a disease of 'affluence'. Higher maternal education status among social class I and II families may have an influence. Of particular importance might be factors related to positive health-related behaviour such as the intake of mineral and vitamin supplements and an increased tendency to visit the doctor and be prescribed medicines. It is possible that increased exposure to topical corticosteroids (the principal treatment for AD in Britain) among social classes I

Table 10.3. Lifetime prevalence (parental report) of atopic dermatitis among Swiss schoolchildren (Wüthrich, 1996)

Social class	Lifetime reported prevalence (%)
I	15.9
II	12.5
III	12.9
IV	11.3
V	9.6

Note: χ^2 Linear trend $p<0.006$.

Table 10.4. Point prevalence of eczema at 7, 11 or 16 years by housing tenure (data from the NCDS) (Williams et al., 1994)

Housing tenure	Point prevalence of examined eczema (at 7, 11 or 16 years) (%)
Privately owned	6.1 (222/3622)
Privately rented	5.7 (52/907)
Council rented	4.5 (146/3254)
Rent free	2.0 (4/201)
χ^2 (for owned versus council rented property)	8.8 ($p=0.003$)

and II, resulting from increased consultation rates and demand for prescribed medicines, may also lead, in the long term, to an increase in disease chronicity or recurrence (Williams, 1992).

Increased uptake, at least historically, of immunization might also be an important risk factor for the expression of dermatitis which is characteristic of wealthier families. A study of the development of atopy in a population of Guinea-Bissau, West Africa, found that young adults who had experienced measles in childhood during a severe epidemic were significantly less likely to be atopic than those who had been vaccinated and had not had measles (Shaheen et al., 1996).

Perhaps more basic differences in the home environment of families in social classes I and II from those in social class IV and V, may be influential. These include (especially in the past) factors such as central heating, type of bedding, use of carpets and decreased air circulation due to better insulation, all of which may increase the risk of disease by influencing house dust mite populations. Beck et al. (1989) have shown that the movement of AD patients to houses with better indoor climates, particularly with high air exchange and low humidity, may be associated with an improvement in symptoms. Clearly, more refined studies are needed to determine whether specific factors in the home environment are important or whether residual confounding by other factors correlated with social class explain the findings.

Other potential exposures associated with the life-

styles of people in social classes I and II may also be important. For example, the differential use of showers or soaps may increase the vulnerability to sensitization by drying the skin. Increased close contact with pets, greater use of synthetic clothing fabrics and variations in exposure to ultraviolet light are also factors that need to be considered. Lifestyle differences between socioeconomic groups could also influence prenatal exposures. For example, higher maternal age and different maternal diet have been implicated with higher social status in the UK and other developed countries (Peters & Golding, 1987; Arshad et al., 1992; Williams, 1995).

Dermatitis and other socioeconomic indicators

Analysis of the effects of socioeconomic status on the prevalence of AD has not been restricted to the use of the Registrar General's classification of social class. Indeed, support for a positive socioeconomic gradient in the prevalence of AD has been provided by the investigation of other socioeconomic correlates. Further analysis of the NCDS data used household tenure as an indicator of socioeconomic status and found a significant difference in the prevalence of AD between types of housing tenure (Williams et al., 1994). Table 10.4 illustrates the results in detail.

The secular trends in the prevalence of AD, discussed in detail in Chapter 7, also provide some support for an association between AD and socioeconomic factors. If what is indeed being witnessed is a *real* increase in the prevalence of AD, it seems unlikely that genetic factors could account for such a rapid increase in reports. It is more likely that factors closely aligned with changing lifestyles and microenvironments, particularly those associated with affluence and development resulting in increased exposure to allergens, are one possible explanation.

Family size and atopic dermatitis

Family size is another useful correlate of socioeconomic status and has been the focus of a number of studies. Using data from the National Child Development Study, Strachan (1989) found the prevalence of parental-reported AD to be inversely related to family size, even when adjusted for other determinants of disease. Similar associations between smaller families and examined AD were later shown (Williams et al., 1992). These findings are supported by a German study which identified a linear decrease in the prevalence of atopic sensitization with the number of siblings (von Mutius et al., 1994). It would therefore seem that factors directly or indirectly related to the number of siblings may decrease the susceptibility of children to becoming atopic.

A possible explanation of this effect is that the higher chances of cross infection from siblings in large families may have a protective role in atopic disease expression. Indeed, the prevalence of atopy was found to be lower among subjects who were seropositive for hepatitis A than those who were seronegative, in a study of Italian military students (Matricardi et al., 1997). The age at infection could also be crucial, as analysis of the NCDS data also found that AD in the first year of life is independently related to the number of older children in the household (Strachan, 1989). Recent trends towards decreasing family size across all social class groups, but especially recently noticeable in the lower social classes, improvements in household amenities, the prevention of viral infectious diseases and higher standards of domestic hygiene, may all have reduced the opportunity for cross infection. Collectively, they may therefore go some way towards explaining the increasing prevalence of atopic disease documented in Chapter 7.

It has also been suggested that viral infection may trigger atopic sensitization, especially in asthma (Frick et al., 1979). There may well be links with the changes in sibship structure discussed above, particularly with regard to patterns in the exposure to common viruses, most notably the age at infection. It may be that the later exposure of children to certain viruses, perhaps a result of declining family size, may well therefore be important. It is also true in the United Kingdom and among other countries, however, that government policy is moving towards greater access to preschooling. This would again lead to earlier exposure to viruses among children attending nursery groups. Clearly, more studies are needed which test hypotheses as to whether childhood infections protect against or trigger AD and whether such infections can have different effects depending on the timing of exposure.

A further possible explanation for these findings relates to increased demands and stresses that are placed on the smaller modern family. Reductions in family support, reduced time spent as a family unit due to the employment of both parents, reduced contact with the extended family, as well as heightened anxiety over trivial skin complaints and pressure to succeed in schools, and peer group pressure for a blemishless skin, can all lead to a more stressful environment for the child. Stressful life events have been known to precede exacerbations of AD but it is still unclear whether there is a cause or effect relationship (Morren et al., 1994). The link between AD and psychological factors clearly warrants further investigation in a way which separates the preceding events from the psychosocial consequences of disease.

Implications and future directions

Atopic dermatitis, in the developed world in particular, does appear to have marked social status relationships in its incidence and prevalence. Contrary to many conditions, AD expression in developed world countries seems to be much higher among higher social class groups. The identification of patterns of AD prevalence by socioeconomic status represents important additions to knowledge of the epidemiology of the disease. The strength of these findings is enhanced by the consistencies in the trend observed using various indicators of socioeconomic status. Clearly, more detailed investigation of the link between the social and biological pathways that underlie the social patterning of AD is needed, in order to uncover more specific risk factors.

The studies reviewed here suggest the importance of environmental and lifestyle factors in the expression of AD and this has important implications for possible public health interventions aimed at reducing the burden of the disease. Particularly important among these would perhaps be the development of housing design and advice on maternal diet to reduce disease risk. Indeed, the socioeconomic environment can have a key influence on population health and the burden of disease, often more significant than the discovery of any cause or medical cure. Improvements in social status have been argued to have had a larger role in the decline of childhood infectious diseases in Europe than the introduction of specific therapies such as vaccination and antibiotics (McKeown, 1976), although advances in medicine have clearly also made a significant contribution to these trends.

The strongest evidence for a socioeconomic patterning of AD prevalence is derived from the major British cohort studies which relate to British children in the 1960s and 1970s. Social class differences may have altered subsequently although there are clearly other bases for concluding that factors correlated with socioeconomic status are important in the epidemiology of AD in developed nations. It should not be assumed, however, that such a social class gradient will remain constant over time. Heart disease and cirrhosis of the liver, for example, were once more common among the affluent, but are now more common among the poorer social classes (Marmot et al., 1978; Blaxter, 1981).

It is perhaps also unlikely that such a clear positive

social class gradient exists in many rural settings within developing nations. It has been suggested that increased secondary infections, increased exposure to primary irritants through childhood, crowding and reduced access and provision of medical care, may in fact give rise to a negative social class gradient for the prevalence of AD in such settings (Rajka, 1986). However, to date, studies of AD which include explicit social and socioeconomic measures in developing countries are virtually nonexistent. If it can be assumed that the trends in prevalence observed in some developed countries over the last three decades are linked to changes in lifestyle and increasing affluence, then this suggests that the burden of AD on developing nations is likely to increase as the forces of development gather impetus. In rapidly modernizing countries, there is growing evidence that AD already represents a considerable burden on the populations, for example in the industrializing countries of south-east Asia (Leung & Ho, 1994). Similar increases may well be imminent in many other highly populated developing countries (Paajanen, 1994). In fact, some of the highest prevalence estimates in the ISAAC data were found in Ibadan, Nigeria and Addis Ababa, Ethiopia (Asher et al., 1995).

In future research in the developed and developing world it seems sensible, at the very least, to consider social class and family size as potential confounders in epidemiological studies of AD. Moreover, if correlates of socioeconomic status associated with AD can be identified then this could have important public health policy implications. It may help reduce the burden of the disease in developed countries and help check the increasing potential burden of the disease in developing countries.

Summary of key points

- The incidence of many diseases varies, sometimes considerably, according to social and economic conditions.
- Growing evidence suggests that a positive socioeconomic gradient in the rates of atopy exists as defined by positive results in skin prick tests,

although this is not unequivocal as some studies have not identified such trends.

- Studies of children in the United Kingdom have found that the prevalence of reported and examined AD is higher among families in social class groups I and II than social class groups III and IV.

- The positive social class gradient in the prevalence of AD was found to persist even after adjustment for other determinants of disease.

- Indications of a positive social class gradient in the prevalence of AD were supported by studies from other developed nations.

- Differences in the behaviours, lifestyles and home environments may help to explain the difference in the prevalence of AD between different social class groups.

- Studies which use other socioeconomic correlates, such as housing tenure, support the hypothesis that AD is more common in families of higher socioeconomic status.

- The prevalence of parental-reported and examined AD has been found to be inversely related to family size, even when adjusted for other determinants of disease.

- Societal trends towards smaller families and higher standards of domestic hygiene may have reduced the opportunity for cross infection, possibly contributing to the increasing prevalence of AD which has been observed over the last four decades.

- The positive social class gradient in the prevalence of AD suggests the importance of environmental and lifestyle factors in the expression of AD, and this has important implications for possible public health interventions aimed at reducing the burden of disease.

References

Arshad, S.H., Matthews, S., Gant, C. & Hide, D. (1992). Effect of allergen avoidance on development of allergic disorders in infancy. *Lancet*, **339**, 1493–7.

Asher, M.I., Keil, U., Anderson, H.R., Beasley, R., Crane, J., Martinez, F., Mitchell, E.A. Pearce, N., Sibbald, B., Stewart, A.W., Strachan, D., Weiland, S.K. & Williams, H.C. (1995). International Study of Asthma and Allergies in Childhood (ISAAC): rationale and methods. *Europ Resp J*, **8**, 483–91.

Astarita, C., Harris, R.I., de Fusco, R., Franzese, A., Biscardi, D., Mazzacca, F.R. & Altucci, P. (1988). An epidemiological study of atopy in children. *Clin Allergy*, **18**, 341–50.

Barbee, R.A., Lebowitz, M.D., Thompson, H.C. & Burrows, B. (1976). Immediate skin test reactivity in a general population sample. *Ann Intern Med*, **84**, 129–33.

Beck, H-I., Bjerring, P.G. & Harving, H. (1989). Atopic dermatitis and the indoor climate. *Acta Dermatol Venereol*, Suppl. 144, 131–2.

Blaxter, M. (1981). *The Health of Children*. London: Heinemann.

Blaxter, M. (1990). *Health and Lifestyles*. London: Routledge.

Buser, K., Bohlen, F.V., Werner, P. Gernhuber, F. & Robra, B-P. (1993). Neurodermatitis-prävalenz bei schulkindern im landkreis Hannover. *Dtsch Med Wschr*, **118**, 1141–5.

Cox, B., Huppert, F.A. & Whichelow, M.J. (eds.) (1993). *The Health and Lifestyle Survey: Seven Years On*. Aldershot: Dartmouth.

Forster, J., Dungs, M., Wais, U. & Urbanek, R. (1990). Atopie-verdächtige symptome in den ersten zwei Lebensjahren. *Klin Pädiatr*, **202**, 136–40.

Freeman, C.L. & Johnson, S. (1964). Allergic diseases in adolescents. *Am J Dis Childh*, **107**, 459–66.

Frick, O.S., German, D.F. & Mill, J. (1979). Development of allergy in children. 1. Association with virus infection. *J Allergy Clin Immunol*, **63**, 228–41.

Gergen, P.J., Turkeltaub, P.C. & Kovar, M.G. (1987). The prevalence of allergic skin test reactivity to eight common aeroallergens in the US population: results from the second national health and nutrition examination survey. *J Allergy Clin Immunol*, **80**, 669–79.

Golding, J. & Peters, T.J. (1987). The epidemiology of childhood eczema. I. A population based study of associations. *Paediat Perinatal Epidemiol*, **1**, 67–79.

Kelsey, J.L. & Bernstein, L. (1996). Epidemiology and prevention of breast cancer. *Ann Rev Publ Hlth*, **17**, 47–67.

Leung, R. & Ho, P. (1994). Asthma, allergy and atopy in three South East Asian populations. *Thorax*, **49**, 1205–10.

Macintyre, S. (1997). The Black Report and beyond: what are the issues? *Soc Sci Med*, **44**, 723–45.

McKeown, T. (1976). *The Modern Rise of Population*. London: Edward Arnold.

McNally, N.J., Phillips, D.R. & Williams, H.C. (1998). The problem of atopic eczema: aetiological clues from the environment and lifestyles. *Soc Sci Med*, **46**, 729–41.

Marmot, M. (1996). The social pattern of health and disease. In: Blane, D., Brunner, E. & Wilkinson, R. (eds.) *Health and Social*

Organization: Towards a Health Policy for the 21st Century, pp. 42–67. London: Routledge.

Marmot, M.G., Adelstein, A.M., Robinson, N. & Rose, G.A. (1978). Changing social class distribution of ischaemic heart disease. *Br Med J,* **ii**, 1109–12.

Matricardi, P.M., Rosimini, F., Ferrigno, L., Nisini, R., Rapicetta, M., Chionne, P., Stroffolini, T., Paquini, P. & D'Amelio, R. (1997). Cross sectional retrospective study of prevalence of atopy among Italian military students with antibodies against hepatitis A virus. *Br Med J,* **314**, 999–1003.

Morren, M-A., Przybilla, B., Bamelis, M., Heykants, B., Reynaers, A. & Degreef, H. (1994). Atopic dermatitis: triggering factors. *J Am Acad Dermatol,* **31**, 467–73.

von Mutius, E., Martinez, F.D., Fritzsch, C., Nicolai, T., Reitmeir, P. & Thiemann, H-H. (1994). Skin test reactivity and number of siblings. *Br Med J,* **308**, 692–5.

Paajanen, H. (1994). Common skin diseases. In: Lankinen, K.S., Bergström, S., Mäkelä, P.H. & Peltomaa, M. (eds.) *Health and Disease in Developing Countries,* pp. 271–80. London: Macmillan.

Peters, T.J. & Golding, J. (1987). The epidemiology of childhood eczema. II. Statistical analyses to identify independent early predictors. *Paediat Perinatal Epidemiol,* **1**, 80–94.

Power, C., Bartley, M., Davey Smith, G. & Blane, D. (1996). Transmission of social and biological risk across the life course. In: Blane, D., Brunner, E. & Wilkinson, R. (eds.) *Health and Social Organization: Towards a Health Policy for the 21st Century,* pp. 188–203. London: Routledge.

Rajka, G. (1986). Atopic dermatitis: correlation of environmental factors with frequency. *Int J Dermatol,* **25**, 301–4.

Robinson, J. & Elkan, R. (1996). *Health Needs Assessment: Theory and Practice.* London: Churchill Livingstone.

Schäfer, T., Vieluf, D., Behrendt, H., Krämer, U. & Ring, J. (1996). Atopic eczema and other manifestations of atopy: results of a study in East and West Germany. *Allergy,* **51**, 532–9.

Shaheen, S.O., Aaby, P., Hall, A.J., Barker, D.J.P., Heyes, C.B., Shiell, A.W. & Goudiaby, A. (1996). Measles and atopy in Guinea-Bissau. *Lancet,* **347**, 1792–6.

Shepherd, P.M. (1985). *The National Child Development Study: an Introduction to the Origins of the Study and the Methods of Data Collection.* London: NCDS User Support Group, City University.

Sibbald, B. & Rink, E. (1991). Labelling of rhinitis and hayfever by doctors. *Thorax,* **46**, 378–81.

Smith, D., Taylor, R. & Coates, M. (1996). Socioeconomic differentials in cancer incidence and mortality in urban New South Wales 1987–1991. *Aust N Z J Publ Hlth,* **20**, 129–37.

Smith, J.M. (1974). Incidence of atopic disease. *Med Clin N Am,* **58**, 3–24.

Strachan, D.P. (1989). Hay fever, hygiene and household size. *Br Med J,* **299**, 1259–60.

Strachan, D.P. (1990). Regional variations in wheezing illness in British children: the effect of migration during early childhood. *J Epidemiol Commun Hlth,* **44**, 231–6.

Swerdlow, A.J., Douglas, A.J., Huttly, S.R. & Smith, P.G. (1991). Cancer of the testis, socioeconomic status, and occupation. *Br J Industr Med,* **48**, 670–4.

Taylor, B., Wadsworth, J., Wadsworth, M. & Peckham, C. (1984). Changes in the reported prevalence of childhood eczema since the 1938–45 war. *Lancet,* 1255–7.

Townsend, P. & Davidson, N. (eds.) (1992). *Inequalities in Health: the Black Report and the Health Divide.* London: Penguin.

Van den Eeden, S.K., Weiss, N.S., Strader, C.H. & Daling, J.R. (1991). Occupation and the occurrence of testicular cancer. *Am J Industr Med,* **19**, 327–37.

Waite, D.A., Eyles, E.F., Tonkin, S.L. & O'Donnell, T.V. (1980). Asthma prevalence in Tokelauan children in two environments. *Clin Allergy,* **10**, 71–5.

Waters, W.E. (1971). Migraine, social class, and familial prevalence. *Br Med J,* 71–81.

Williams, H.C. (1992). Is the prevalence of atopic dermatitis increasing? *Clin Exp Dermatol,* **17**, 385–91.

Williams, H.C. (1995). Atopic eczema: we should look to the environment. *Br Med J,* **311**, 1241–2.

Williams, H.C., Strachan, D. & Hay, R.J. (1992). Eczema and family size. *J Invest Dermatol,* **98**, 601.

Williams, H.C., Strachan, D.P. & Hay, R.J. (1994). Childhood eczema: disease of the advantaged? *Br Med J,* **308**, 1132–5.

Wilson, S. (1995). *Aiming for Health in the Year 2000: Annual Report of the Director of Public Health.* Nottingham Health District.

Worth, R.M. (1962). Atopic dermatitis among Chinese infants in Honolulu and San Francisco. *Hawaii Med J,* **22**, 31–4.

Wüthrich, B. (1989). Epidemiology of the allergic diseases: are they really on the increase? *Int Arch Allergy Appl Immunol,* **90**, 3–10.

Wüthrich, B. (1996). Epidemiology and natural history of atopic dermatitis. *Allergy Clin Immunol Int,* **8**, 77–82.

11

The 'old mother' hypothesis

Anne Braae Olesen and Kristian Thestrup-Pedersen

Introduction

Industrialized countries have changed markedly in many ways during recent decades. This has led to changes and concerns regarding pollution, ozone depletion, change in food habits and indoor climate.

There are also significant changes for children in their increased education and later arrival at the job market. The changes starting in the 1960s have been quite remarkable, especially for women's social and organizational conditions. This has enabled women to achieve education and academic degrees quite comparable to what men have had for many years. Thus, the percentage of female doctors graduating from the University of Aarhus, Denmark, was 15% in 1965 and 52% in 1994.

A result of these changes has been that the age of first-time mothers has increased year by year. One reason for this, in many countries, has been the introduction of new kinds of birth control such as the contraceptive pill or access to legalized abortion. The use of such procedures reflects many underlying reasons such as women's desire for liberation and independence in otherwise male-dominated societies. This chapter looks at the relationship between maternal factors such as age of first-time mothers and gestational age, and the later development of atopic dermatitis.

Maternal factors and the increased prevalence of atopic dermatitis

Chapter 7 in this book, and many articles as reviewed elsewhere (Williams, 1992), describes how the prevalence of atopic dermatitis (AD) has increased significantly during recent decades in several European countries. Chapter 8 describes how AD is, to a major extent, a genetically determined disorder.

How can the prevalence of a genetically determined disorder increase in such a short time? The most obvious explanation is that the diagnosis is used more frequently by doctors than previously. If this is not the only explanation, then a genetically determined trait must somehow be more easily revealed – in other words, the disease has become clinically manifest and not latent.

Many environmental factors have been studied such as pollution, smoking, change in indoor climate and allergen exposure, but these exposures have not convincingly correlated with expression of AD. Breast feeding and allergen avoidance was found to delay the expression of AD (Arshad et al., 1992), and socioeconomic class was also found to be correlated with an increased prevalence of AD (Golding & Peters 1987; Williams et al., 1994).

Atopic dermatitis is largely a disease of 'children', i.e. a disease expressed early in life. Its major symptoms relate to the 'immune system'. It has been shown that it is possible to establish cytokine and not antigen-driven T-lymphocyte cell lines from skin biopsies of adults with AD (Kaltoft et al., 1994, 1995). These cells are not present in peripheral blood. This has led us to suggest that the immune deviations in AD may be related to a faulty maturation of the T-lymphocyte immune system (Thestrup-Pedersen et al., 1997) – a system that is very active early in life and which during the

Table 11.1. Factors associated with age of the mother

Biological conditions
Fecundity
Contraception
Abortion – spontaneous or provoked
Parity
Birth weight
Gestational age

Social and organizational conditions
Socioeconomic status
Educational qualifications
Working conditions, i.e. certain circumstances in paid work
Physical environment
Maternal health behaviour, i.e. easy access to doctors, compliance with prophylactic investigations of children's health, vaccinations

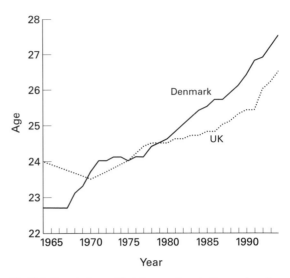

Fig. 11.1. Reported age of first-time mothers in Denmark and the United Kingdom

teenage years is reduced in activity (Mackall et al., 1995).

We have therefore speculated that there may be factors related to gestation and fetal maturation, which would associate with later clinical expression of a genetically inherited trait such as AD. If such factors were evident, then the age of the mother could be important as well.

The 'old mother hypothesis'

The 'old mother hypothesis' is forwarded as a possible contributing factor to explain the increasing prevalence of AD. It is based upon the following lines of evidence:

(a) the age of first-time mothers has changed quite significantly during the last three decades;
(b) a relationship between increasing prevalence of AD and increasing parity;
(c) studies which have examined the link between AD and birth factors.

It is biologically plausible that older mothers could give birth to children with changed health risks for conditions such as AD. A relevant example is Down's syndrome, where advancing maternal age results in increased error of meiosis and declining rates of spontaneous abortion above normal fetuses. Table 11.1 lists factors which associate with age of the mother.

Age of first-time mothers in European countries

Figure 11.1 depicts the age of first-time mothers in Denmark and the UK from the 1960s until today. It is seen clearly that a steady and significant increase in age at first birth has taken place. Figure 11.2 illustrates how the percentage of first-time mothers aged 20 and below has dropped in the UK over the last three decades. Table 11.2 shows that many countries in Europe have experienced a significant increase in the age of first-time mothers over the last 25 years. The increase in maternal age for the countries in western Europe ranges from 16.5% in Holland to 4.1% in Portugal. Such changes are remarkable when one considers that it covers the whole female population. A few eastern European countries such as Bulgaria, Poland, the Czech Republic and Slovak Republic have not experienced similar changes. However, the authors are not aware of any epidemiological studies in these countries which have focused on the incidence or prevalence of AD over the last three decades. Many other factors, however,

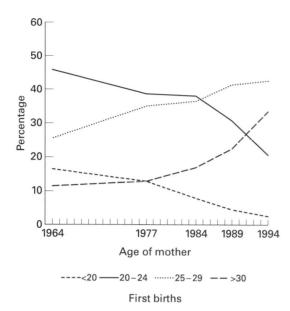

----<20 ——20–24 ·······25–29 —— >30

First births

Fig. 11.2. British statistics demonstrating how first-born children are now born to older mothers in the UK. Thus, 18% of first-time mothers were younger than 20 years in 1964 compared with 3% in 1994

could also play a significant role in the expression of AD in those countries.

Germany is quite interesting given the fact that the prevalence of positive prick tests was significantly higher in western compared with eastern Germany (von Mutius et al., 1994). However, the prevalence of respiratory atopic disease did not seem to differ (von Mutius et al., 1992). It is evident how the age of first-time mothers in eastern Germany did not change until after 1989, when Germany was unified (Figure 11.3). The relationship between AD and these different cohorts of older mothers over time warrants further investigation, although many factors such as different socioeconomic conditions are also occurring simultaneously.

Atopic dermatitis and parity

A possible method for looking at the influence of maternal age on AD could be to observe whether a woman has her AD child 'later in life', i.e. if child number two or three has an increased frequency of

Table 11.2. Age of first-time mothers in various European countries. The right-hand column shows the increase between most recent year compared to earliest year of recording

Country	1970	1975	1980	1985	1990	1991	1992	1993	1994	Increase (%)
Netherlands	24.3	25.0	25.6	26.5	27.6	27.7	28.0	28.3		16.5
East Germany	22.5	22.5	22.3	22.3		24.9	25.4	26.2		16.4
Finland	23.7	24.7	25.7	26.1	26.8	26.9	27.0	27.2	27.4	15.6
France	23.8	24.2	24.9	25.9	27.0	27.2	27.4			15.1
Denmark	23.7	24.0	24.6	25.5	26.4	26.8	26.9	27.2		14.8
West Germany	24.3	24.8	25.2	26.2	26.9	27.1	27.3	27.6		13.6
Switzerland	25.1	25.7	26.4	27.0	27.6	27.8	28.0	28.1	28.3	12.7
UK	23.5	24.0	24.4	24.8	25.5	25.7	26.0	26.2		11.5
Norway	23.6	24.2	25.2	26.1	25.5	25.7	25.9	26.0	26.3	11.4
Sweden		24.5	25.5	26.1	26.3	26.5	26.7	27.0		10.2
Austria	23.7	24.0	24.3	25.1	26.1	26.1	26.0	25.5	25.9	9.2
Portugal	24.4	24.0	23.6	23.8	24.7	24.9	25.0	25.2	25.4	4.1
Slovak	21.7	22.0	22.4	22.3	22.1	21.3	21.9	22.0	22.1	1.8
Czech	22.5	22.5	22.4	22.4	22.5	22.4	22.5	22.6	22.9	1.8
Poland	22.5	22.7	23.0	23.3	23.0	22.9	22.6	22.6	22.7	0.9
Bulgaria	21.9	22.0	21.9	21.9	22.0	21.8	21.8	21.3		−2.7

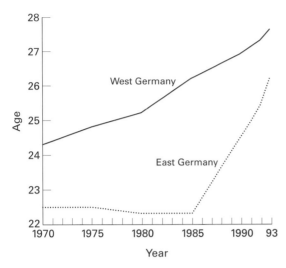

Fig. 11.3. Age of first-time mothers in the former west Germany compared with the former east Germany

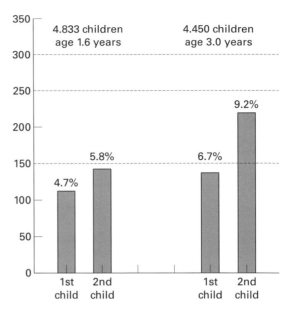

Fig. 11.4. In Japan all children must be examined by a medical doctor after 1½ years of life (1.6 years) and after 3 years. A national study of the prevalence of eczema was performed in the early 1990s (Japanese Government Report, 1993). The diagram shows how many children were found to have AD and their rank in the family. The difference between the prevalence of AD in three-year-old children was statistically significant

AD. Such an investigation may be confounded by the fact that parity itself has an influence on the expression of AD, or that factors such as a previous child will change the microbiological impact on the second or third child. We have shown that AD is seen more frequently in child number two than in child number one (Olesen et al., 1996). This is supported by similar observations in Japan during a national investigation for AD (Figure 11.4) (Japanese Ministry of Health and Welfare, 1993). This finding could indirectly support the view that the age of the mother may influence disease expression.

Direct studies of maternal age and atopic dermatitis

A British epidemiological study of childhood eczema was performed among 12 555 children born in 1970 (Golding & Peters, 1987). A large proportion of associations was statistically significant at the 1% level, among them social class, maternal age and birth weight. However, when adjusted for confounding factors, the maternal age association became statistically insignificant.

We studied a cohort of 7862 children who at the time of investigation were between five and eight years old. We analysed two groups within this population. In the first study we made a follow-up of all 'single born' children using information from all dermatologists in the city of Åarhus, and the Danish Birth Register. In this cohort 403 children out of 7862 had a definitive diagnosis of AD made by specialists in dermatology.

In the second study we made a stratified subsample of the same population based on gestational age strata. This follow-up was based on parental information and statistics from the Danish Birth Register, and included 985 single born children. We found among these children 184 with AD.

We did not see a statistically significant correlation with the age of the mothers and AD. In the first study of a birth cohort of 7862 children we saw an increasing relative risk from 25 to 34 years of age. However, mothers older than 34 years of age seem to have a rapidly falling risk for having an atopic

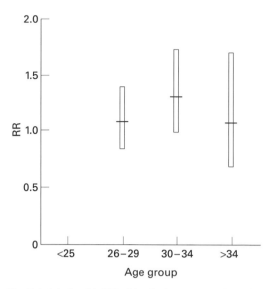

Fig. 11.5. Relative risk (RR) of developing AD in mothers of different age groups (Olesen et al., 1996). There was a trend towards a correlation in the age group 30–34 years, but it was statistically insignificant

eczema child (Figure 11.5). A similar trend was found in our second questionnaire study. The finding illustrates that there was a trend of increased mother age in the age group 30–34 years, but not in older age groups. Future studies must be performed in order to elucidate this finding further. However, the reason for 'mothers' to have children is probably not related to its risk of developing AD, and therefore it may be impossible to show directly any age difference between 'atopic' and 'nonatopic' mothers.

Atopic dermatitis and other birth factors

Prematurity and atopic dermatitis

Recent epidemiological studies have looked at parameters occurring during gestation and at birth which statistically relate to later expression of AD. It has been quite clearly shown that there is no relation between 'prematurity' and AD (David & Ewing, 1988; Olesen et al., 1997). Thus, a child born premature will not have an increased risk of developing AD.

Postmaturity and atopic dermatitis

In the cohort study described on page 151, we found a significant correlation between children born later than 40 weeks' gestation and development of AD. Among postterm children 151 of 2410 had developed the skin disease, i.e. relative risk = 1.32; 95% confidence intervals CI = 1.06–1.63, when adjusted for the following confounding factors: birth weight, parity, age of mother and gender. In the second questionnaire-based study, among 271 postterm children, 62 had developed AD, giving a relative risk of 1.35; 95% confidence interval 0.96–1.89, when adjusted for the confounders mentioned above.

Oral contraceptive use

The increase in the age of first-time mothers must be related to many factors affecting society. It has been shown in one report that there is a correlation between expression of AD and previous use of contraceptive hormones during the last 18 months prior to conception (Peters & Golding, 1987). The increase of AD cannot, however, be solely a consequence of the contraceptive pill, because this contraceptive method has never been introduced in Japan – a country where an increase has been observed both of the age of first-time mothers and also of an increased expression of AD. Given our hypothesis that AD is a manifestation of a dysmatured T-lymphocyte system, it would still be important to study how hormonal contraception may influence immune maturation (Chapter 9). It is known in rats that growth hormone can promote the maturation of T-lymphocytes under experimental in vitro conditions (Murphy, Durum & Longo, 1992). The authors are not aware of human studies in this area.

Conclusion

Maternal age has changed quite significantly within the industrialized world. We have shown how the length of a child's gestation may relate to later expression of AD. We also have evidence to show that the immune system is not properly matured in AD patients. The prolonged gestation in children who later develop AD could reflect a dysmaturation step of the immune system. Older mothers could be relatively insufficient in supporting the immune maturation process. Therefore, children with latent AD will more easily express clinical eczema if their mother is older. So far, the evidence linking AD to increased maternal age is conflicting and could be due to other confounding factors.

There are other factors in early infancy which need to be investigated more thoroughly in relation to dysmaturation of the immune system. One concerns the introduction of measles vaccination which may have changed the immune system's maturation early in life (Shaheen, 1995; Starr, 1996). Both measles and AD typically occur between the ages of two and four years and it is possible that measles vaccination has altered the immune balance and previous 'protective role' of measles infection in early life. The use of hormonal contraception has also been found to correlate with later expression of AD and this needs to be looked into further. Future investigations should focus on prospective studies where one of the factors being investigated is the age of the mother.

Summary of key points

- The prevalence of atopic dermatitis (AD) has probably increased substantially in Europe over the last three decades.
- Genetic factors are unlikely to account for these changes.
- Over the last 20 years maternal age of first-time mothers has increased by around 10% in Europe.
- Some evidence exists to suggest that AD is associated with dysmaturity of the T-lymphocyte immune system.
- The risk of AD is increased in second and third born children compared with first born children.
- One possible explanation for increased risk of AD with increasing parity is increasing maternal age.
- One UK birth cohort study has found a relationship between atopic prevalence and increasing maternal age. This association was abolished after adjusting for potential confounders.
- A study cohort of Danish children found no overall association between maternal age and atopic prevalence, although a higher risk of AD was noted in the 30–34-year age group of mothers.
- This same study showed a relationship between increased gestational age and later expression of AD.
- Maternal age may be a marker of other possible risk factors for AD rather than a direct cause of error in meiosis, as in Down's syndrome.
- Factors occurring in early life, such as use of oral contraceptives and use of vaccinations, require more study as they may provide one possible key to the increasing prevalence of AD.

References

Arshad, S.H., Matthews, S., Gant, D. & Hide, D. (1992). Effect of allergen avoidance on allergic disorders in infancy. *Lancet*, **339**, 1493–7.

David, T.J. & Ewing, C.I. (1988). Atopic eczema and preterm birth. *Arch Dis Childh*, **63**, 435–6.

Golding, J. & Peters, T.J. (1987). The epidemiology of childhood eczema. I. A population based study of associations. *Paediat Perinatal Epidemiol*, **1**, 67–79.

Japanese Ministry of Health and Welfare (1993). National Investigation for Atopic Dermatitis. Government Report.

Kaltoft, K., Pedersen, C.B., Hansen, B.H., Lemonidis, A.S., Frydenberg, J. & Therstrup-Pedersen, K. (1994). Atopic dermatitis is associated with a subset of skin homing genetically aberrant T-cell clones with continuous growth in vitro. *Arch Dermatol Res*, **287**, 42–7.

Kaltoft, K., Hansen, B.H., Pederson, C.B., Pedersen, S. & Thestrup-Pederson, K. (1995). Continuous human T lymphocyte cell lines with solitary cytokine dependent growth and with common clonal chromosome aberrations. *Cancer Genet Cytogenet*, **85**, 68–71.

Mackall, C.L., Fleisher, T.A., Brown, M.R., Andrich, M.P., Chen, C.C., Feuerstein, I.M., Horowitz, M.E., Magrath, I.T., Shad, A.T., Steinberg, S.M., Wexler, L.H. & Gress, R.E. (1995). Age, thymopoiesis, and CD4+ T-lymphocyte regeneration after intensive chemotherapy. *N Engl J Med*, **332**, 143–9.

Murphy, W.J., Durum, S.K. & Longo, D.L. (1992). Human growth hormone promotes engraftment of murine or human T cells in severe combined immunodeficient mice. *Proc Natl Acad Sci USA*, **89**, 4481–5.

Olesen, A.B., Ellingsen, A.R., Larsen, F.S., Larsen, P.Ø., Veien, N.K. & Thestrup-Pedersen, K. (1996). Atopic dermatitis may be linked to whether a child is first or second born and/or the age of the mother. *Acta Dermatol Venereol (Stockh.)*, **76**, 457–60.

Olesen, A.B., Ellingsen, A.R., Olesen, H., Juul, S. & Thestrup-Pedersen, K. (1997). Atopic dermatitis and birth factors: historical follow up by record linkage. *Br Med J*, **314**, 1003–8.

Peters, T.J. & Golding, J. (1987). The epidemiology of childhood eczema: II. Statistical analyses to identify independent early predictors. *Paediat Perinatal Epidemiol*, **1**, 80–94.

Shaheen, S.O. (1995). Changing patterns of childhood infection and rise in allergic disease. (Review.) *Clin Exp Allergy*, **25**, 1034–7.

Starr, S.E. (1996). Novel mechanism of immunosuppression after measles. *Lancet*, **348**, 1257–8 (editorial).

Thestrup-Pedersen, K., Ellingsen, A.R., Olesen, A.B., Lund, M. & Kaltoft, K. (1997). Atopic dermatitis may be a genetically determined dysmaturation of ectodermal tissue, resulting in disturbed T lymphocyte maturation. *Acta Dermatol Venereol (Stockh.)*, **77**, 20–21.

von Mutius, E., Fritzsch, C., Weiland, S.K., Röll, G. & Magnussen, H. (1992). Prevalence of asthma and allergic disorders among children in united Germany: a descriptive comparison. *Br Med J*, **305**, 1395–9.

von Mutius, E., Martinez, F.D., Fritzsch, C., Nicolai, T., Reitmeir, P. & Thiemann, H-H. (1994). Skin test reactivity and number of siblings. *Br Med J*, **308**, 692–5.

Williams, H.C. (1992). Is the prevalence of atopic dermatitis increasing? *Clin Exp Dermatol*, **17**, 385–91.

Williams, H.C., Strachan, D.P. & Hay, R.J. (1994). Childhood eczema: disease of the advantaged? *Br Med J*, **308**, 1132–5.

12

The possible role of environmental pollution in the development of atopic dermatitis

Torsten Schäfer and Johannes Ring

Introduction

Atopic dermatitis (AD) occurs in individuals who have a genetic predisposition and have been exposed to certain environmental influences. It is the most prevalent chronic inflammatory skin disease in childhood (Ruzicka et al., 1991). As pointed out in earlier chapters there is good evidence that this condition has significantly increased over recent decades. However, it is still unclear which factors are responsible for the increase. For AD the role of genetic predisposition to the disease is well established (Niermann, 1964; Schultz Larsen et al., 1986; Küster et al., 1990). Within the multifactorial pathogenesis several contributing external factors have been described. In addition to sex (Engbak, 1982; Erisson-Lihr, 1955; Larsson & Liden, 1980) and age (Rajka, 1989), psychosomatic influences (Young et al., 1986), exposure to aeroallergens (Vieluf et al., 1993) and food allergens (Przybilla & Ring, 1990), climatic stimuli (Young, 1980), and socioeconomic status (Williams et al., 1994) have been linked to AD. However, the postulated increase cannot be explained totally by these risk factors. Environmental contaminants and, in particular, air pollutants have been suspected as factors which possibly aggravate AD (Ring, 1991; Ring et al., 1995). The biological plausibility of this suggestion arises from the fact that most air pollutants act as nonspecific irritants as well as immunomodulators, e.g. enhancing IgE formation in animals (Behrendt et al., 1991; Suzuki et al., 1989; Takafuji et al., 1989). Exposure to air pollutants and,

in particular, to tobacco smoke has been linked to chronic inflammation of the upper respiratory tract, impaired lung function in children, and asthma (Burr et al., 1989; Fergusson et al., 1985; Martinez et al., 1988). Although biologically plausible, there is still very little evidence from experimental or epidemiological studies for an association between exposure to (air) pollutants and AD. Eberlein-König et al. (1995), in a preliminary experimental investigation, showed that some parameters of skin function such as transepidermal water loss can be affected by air pollutants in patients with AD. Some results of our own epidemiological studies are described in this chapter.

Pollutants

Ingested pollutants

Arsenic and heavy metals

An association between exposure to arsenic and heavy metals and AD has not been investigated so far, although some effects on the immune system and a high affinity to the skin have been described for some components of these materials.

Arsenic is more toxic in its inorganic form and exposure is mostly due to food (seafood), water and pesticide uptake, as well as several occupational sources. Arsenic is mainly taken up by the gastrointestinal tract and is also able to cross the placenta. From the dermatological point of view it is of special interest that arsenic binds favourably to sulfhydryl groups of keratin. Therefore, the highest concentrations are found in hair and nails as well as the epidermis. It is well known that arsenic causes keratosis and melanosis and also acts as a carcinogen. In addition, irritant effects leading to dermatitis have been described (Peters et al., 1984). Arsenic is rapidly cleared from the blood ($t_{1/2}$<12 h) and excreted mainly by the kidneys. Blood measurements therefore tend to reflect the acute exposure, whereas urine concentrations allow for a better assessment of chronic exposure (Amdur et al., 1993).

Cadmium is a toxic metal which is taken up by food (seafood, organs), air and water, and accumulates mainly in kidney and liver tissue. Cigarettes which contain 1–2 μg cadmium are also a major source of exposure. Cadmium is excreted slowly by the kidneys and blood cadmium levels are usually lower than 1 μg/dl. Little is known about the effect of cadmium on the human immune system (Descotes, 1992). Experimental data from rodents indicate that, overall, cadmium enhances the humoral immune response at low exposure levels (Malave & de Ruffino, 1984), whereas higher exposure leads to a decrease in antibody production or no effect at all (Koller & Roan, 1975; Daum et al., 1993). The cell-mediated immunity, in contrast, was more consistently shown to be depressed (Müller et al., 1979). There are practically no clinical reports of the effect of cadmium exposure on allergic reactions in humans. A few experimental data exist, however. Kastelan et al. (1981) showed a dose-dependent inhibition of phytohaemagglutinin-induced lymphocyte proliferation in vitro. Furthermore, it was reported that cadmium affects the mediator release (Behrendt et al., 1988; Wieczorek & Behrendt, 1989; Behrendt, 1992) and might therefore also be an interesting candidate for the analysis of an association with AD.

Mercury is important from a toxicological standpoint, both in its organic as well as its inorganic form. It can be found in preservatives, dental amalgam, pharmaceutical and cosmetic products, and food, as well as in several occupational sources. Organic mercurials are highly absorbed by the gastrointestinal tract, and also in a considerable amount by the dermis. Both mercury forms are able to cross the placental barrier but show different toxicological profiles. Inorganic mercurials are excreted primarily, and organic compounds secondarily, by the kidneys. The effects of mercuric chloride have been intensively investigated in rodents. It was shown that mercury can induce the production of clinically relevant autoantibodies. The origin of this effect is the CD4+ T-cell-dependent polyclonal activation of B cells (Druet, 1995). The manifestations observed include a lymphoproliferation of B and T helper cells, hyperimmunoglobulinaemia and the production of autoantibodies (Pelletier et al., 1988; Kubicka-Muranyi et al., 1996; Hultmann & Enestroem, 1988). In strains of susceptible mice, immune complex nephritis and IgG deposits in blood vessel walls were observed after administration of $HgCl_2$ (Hultmann & Enestroem, 1987; Druet, 1995). Similar effects may also play a role in humans. Schrallhammer-Benkler et al. (1992) reported a case of 'acute mercury intoxication with lichenoid drug eruption followed by mercury contact allergy and development of antinuclear antibodies'. Organic mercury compounds are well known contact allergens (Mayenburg, 1989) and, within these, thimerosal may be the most common representative (Schäfer et al., 1995). An association between mercury exposure and other inflammatory skin diseases remains to be investigated.

Water pipes, paints, ceramic dishes and, in the past, gasoline (petrol) are major general sources of lead exposure. Up to 20% of the ingested lead is absorbed but inhalation is also a major pathway. Lead is stored in soft tissues (liver, kidney, central nervous system) and the skeletal system, and mainly excreted by the kidneys. Nails, sweat and hair constitute minor excretory paths. Since lead interferes with the biosynthesis of heme (ALA-dehydratase, ferrochelatase), the most prominent disease involving the skin which can be provoked by lead is porphyria. Inflammatory skin diseases have not been connected with lead exposure so far, but there is experimental evidence that triethyl lead can

increase the histamine release from human basophils (Juergensen & Behrendt, 1989).

Other compounds

Several other important environmental pollutants
need further attention with regard to their association with allergic diseases in general, and AD in particular. A 'marker' skin disease of exposure to
halogenated hydrocarbons such as dibenzodioxines
and dibenzofuranes is chloracne (Kimmig & Schulz,
1957). The immunosuppressive effects of these substances have been described in vitro (Vos & Moore,
1974; Birnbaum, 1994; Neubert et al., 1991) and in
vivo (Evans et al., 1988; Hoffman et al., 1986). The
most pronounced effect is thymus atrophy which
was observed in rodents treated with rather high
doses of 2,3,7,8-tetrachlorodibenzo-p-dioxin (Buu-
Hor et al., 1972). For lower doses immunosuppressive effects have been reported concerning certain
subsets of T-lymphocytes such as CD4+ and
Cdw29+ cells in rodents and marmosets (Buu-Hor et
al., 1972). A reduction of human CD4+ cells was
observed after incubation with TCDD and poke weed
mitogen (Neubert et al., 1991). Little is known of the
immunosuppressive effect of dioxines from human
in vivo studies and the results are still conflicting.
Earlier findings reported significant increased frequencies of anergy, determined by common recall
antigens in skin tests, and abnormal T-cell subsets in
a group of TCDD exposed people (Hoffman et al.,
1986). However, these findings were no longer
present in a follow-up study (Evans et al., 1988).

Other organic compounds from different sources,
such as benzene, toluene, xylene, PCB, solvents and
pesticides, might also be worth further investigation
with respect to allergies. Pyrethrum, for example, is
known to cause contact dermatitis and burning,
itching and tingling skin sensations possibly
induced by the depolarizing effect of this agent (He
et al., 1989; Tucker & Flannigan, 1983). Other pesticides, e.g. pentachlorphenol, also have an irritative
capacity which might aggravate an atopic skin condition.

Air pollutants

When discussing air pollutants, it has become clear
from data comparing east and west European countries available in the last few years that at least two
types of air pollution have to be distinguished
(Behrendt et al., 1995). Type I is characterized as the
reducing type mainly resulting from incomplete
combustion of coal (with a high content of sulphur)
and conditions of fog and cool temperatures. Typical
components of this air pollutant pattern, also known
as the classical 'London type' smog, are sulphur
dioxide and large dust particles.

Type II air pollution is characterized by components such as oxides of nitrogen, hydrocarbons and
such photochemical oxidants as ozone. Most of this
so-called oxidizing or photochemical type is the
result of atmospheric reaction products of automobile exhaust. The development of this type of air pollution is promoted by a combination of high traffic
intensity and sunlight, which occurs in particular in
peripheral zones of bigger cities. These circumstances are further aggravated when the pollutants
are trapped by meteorological inversion layers,
which is the case in Los Angeles (Amdur et al., 1993).
Type II air pollution is also predominant in major
western European cities.

Indoor and outdoor pollution – measurement

The measurement of pollutants in the appropriate
body compartments can be considered as the most
informative biologically relevant exposure assessment. This method of measurement, however, is not
available for all pollutants (e.g. air pollutants) and
usually is expensive as well as time-consuming, and
usually requires an uncomfortable invasive proce-
dure in order to obtain specimens. Valid assessments can be obtained by monitoring the person's
exposure (personal samplers) or by directly sampling exposures in the individual's home environment. These measures, however, are relatively
expensive and therefore only limited data are available. Sequential exposure measurements may

reduce some of the limitations of measuring highly variable factors such as air pollution at one point in time. Relevant information on specific exposures can also be obtained by questionnaire or interview. The adaptation of job categories can provide a simple but crude means of roughly categorizing exposure. More detailed questions on particular sources of pollutants (e.g. gas stove, chemical laundry, petrol station, traffic) may contribute to a valid exposure assessment.

The exposure to air pollutants in particular may vary significantly between the indoor microenvironment and outdoor environment. The degree of this variation, of course, depends on the method and amount of ventilation or isolation and the presence of indoor sources including tobacco smoke. For an accurate exposure assessment the individual time spent in- or outdoors has to be taken into consideration.

Associations between atopic dermatitis and air pollution

Tobacco smoke

Experimental data have provided evidence that tobacco smoke (Zetterström et al., 1981) increases IgE synthesis and thereby may contribute to the immunological sensitization. Additionally, these adjuvant effects may enhance chronic inflammation, damage the mucosal barrier and increase the allergenicity of certain allergens (Behrendt et al., 1991; Ring & Behrendt, 1993). Total serum IgE levels of active tobacco smokers are higher than those of nonsmokers (Bahna et al., 1983; Warren et al., 1982). The exposure to maternal environmental tobacco smoke also leads to immunological changes in the children (Kjellman, 1981). These effects are followed by clinical symptoms: children of households in which the mother is a smoker suffer from significantly more upper respiratory tract infections and impaired lung function when compared with children of nonsmokers (Burr et al., 1989; Fergusson et al., 1985). Maternal smoking during pregnancy, however, is associated with a number of

Table 12.1. Mean levels of indoor and outdoor measures of NOx and SO_2 in different Bavarian study sites (1989, 1990) (adapted Schäfer et al., 1997)

Mean ($\mu g/m^3$)	I	II	Region III	IV (control)
Indoor SO_2	5.0	5.2	7.2	4.4
Indoor NOx	6.2	7.4	5.3	5.6
Outdoor SO_2	21.9	37.1	5.2	8.2
Outdoor NOx	4.9	17.4	6.7	7.9

serious health effects in the offspring. These effects include premature birth, intra-uterine growth retardation and impaired behavioural capabilities (Abel, 1980). It has been demonstrated that nicotine crosses the placenta (Larsson & Silvette, 1969) and is excreted into breast milk (Hatcher & Crosby, 1927). The nicotine metabolite cotinine is elevated in the amniotic fluid of pregnant women exposed to environmental tobacco smoke (Jordanov, 1990). Certain immunological changes have been reported as an effect of smoking. Children of mothers who had smoked during pregnancy showed elevated levels of IgE, IgA and IgG3 (Magnusson, 1986; Magnusson & Johansson, 1986) in their cord blood and other altered immune functions (Paganelli et al., 1979). Elevated levels of cord blood IgE have been linked to a higher risk of atopy (Magnusson, 1988). In contrast to the demonstration of immunological changes by maternal smoking during pregnancy, little is known regarding the influence of maternal smoking during pregnancy on atopic manifestations. To address this question we conducted a multicentre cross-sectional study in different regions of Bavaria, southern Germany (Überla et al., 1991; Kunz et al., 1991). A total number of 950 five- to six-year-old preschool-children who were scheduled for the compulsory school entrance medical examination were invited to participate. A written formal consent was obtained from 678 (71.4%) parents. Three regions (I–III) with rather high outdoor exposure, especially to SO_2 and NOx, and a control region (IV) with lower

Table 12.2. Cumulative incidence of atopic diseases in different Bavarian study sites (1988–90) (adapted from Schäfer et al., 1997)

Parameter (%)	I	II	Region III	IV (control)
Atopic dermatitis	14.6	14.8	15.5	7.9
Hay fever	4.1	10.9	25.6	6.3
Asthma	8.1	5.1	3.0	4.8

degrees of air pollution, were chosen. We used a standardized questionnaire to obtain data on the personal and family history of atopic diseases as well as other relevant sociodemographic parameters. A skin prick test was performed with common aeroallergens using a multipuncture device.

The mean values for measures of the indoor and outdoor exposure to SO_2 and NOx in 1989 and 1990 are listed for the different study sites in Table 12.1. The most polluted areas with respect to outdoor SO_2 were regions I and II. A comparison between indoor and outdoor exposure measures makes clear that both reflect different situations.

The cumulative incidences obtained by questionnaire of the three major atopic diseases are displayed in Table 12.2 for the different study regions. We observed a trend towards higher frequencies of atopic diseases in more polluted areas, which was most pronounced for AD and hay fever.

Within the questionnaire we also obtained data on previous maternal smoking habits: 12.6% of the mothers (84 out of 666) reported that they had smoked during pregnancy (62, or 73.2%) or while breast feeding (22, or 26.8%) the examined child. All but 10 of these mothers still smoked at the time of the study and no woman had started smoking after pregnancy. Current smoking was highly associated with former smoking and with actual indoor NOx levels ($p<0.0001$). Indoor NOx exposure in households of women who were reported to have smoked during pregnancy was significantly higher than in households of women who denied smoking (8.0

versus 5.5 μg/m³, $p<0.0001$). Information on the quantity of consumed cigarettes during pregnancy was probably not recalled precisely, so no quantitative analysis was done. At the time of investigation 33.5% of the mothers smoked and within this group those who smoked during pregnancy tended to smoke more heavily (38.8% versus 9.8%>11 cigarettes/day, OR 5.8; CI 2.9–11.8). The current smoking habits or the exposure to NOx and SO_2, however, were not positively associated with any manifestation of atopy in the children. Furthermore, the family history of atopic diseases did not differ significantly within the groups of smoking and non-smoking mothers.

We primarily analysed risk factors for the manifestation of atopy. Therefore, the outcome variable 'manifestation of atopy' was defined as a positive individual history for AD, hay fever or asthma or a positive skin prick test to grass pollen, house dust mite or cat. Gender, location, exposure to SO_2 and NOx, and maternal smoking during pregnancy and lactation were included as risk factors. The analysis was done using the technique of 'classification and regression trees' (CARTs) which shows graphically in a hierarchical fashion the influence of the covariates on the selected variable (Dirschedl, 1991). For a total of 421 children complete data were available for this analysis: 158 of these children (37.5%) showed manifestations of atopy. The variable 'manifestation of atopy' was primarily influenced by two parameters, 'maternal smoking during pregnancy or lactation' and the indoor NOx exposure. The parameter with the strongest influence led to the first split in the CART: this was maternal smoking during pregnancy or lactation. Out of 46 children whose mothers smoked during pregnancy 24 (52.2%) showed manifestations of atopy versus 134 of 375 (35.7%) for non-smoking mothers ($p<0.044$). The definite p-value for the influence of NOx (Q1 versus Q2–4) on the depending variable was 0.052, which was not significant but demonstrated a possible influence. In the final CART analysis the NOx exposure led to the second split, a separation within the group of mothers who did not smoke during pregnancy or lactation. In contrast to the a priori hypothesis more

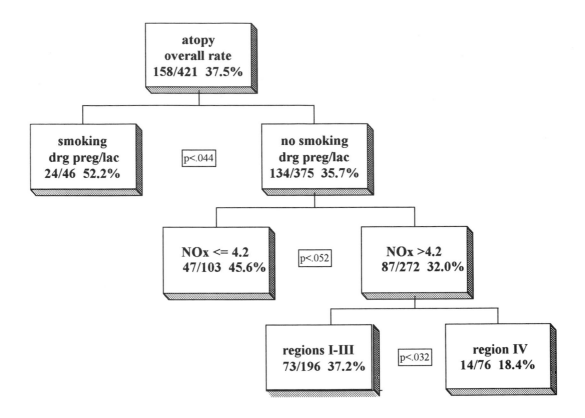

Fig. 12.1. Classification and regression tree (CART) for manifestations of atopy in 421 Bavarian preschoolchildren (adapted from Schäfer et al., 1997)

children with manifestations of atopy were found in the lowest category of indoor NOx exposure (45.6% Q1 versus 32% Q2–4). The quartiles 2–4 of the NOx exposure were separated in a third split by the influence of the investigation site. In this group the children of the so-called clean air areas (group IV) had significantly less manifestations of atopy (14 of 76, 18.4%) compared to all other groups (73 of 196, 37.2%; $p<0.032$) (Figure 12.1).

The influence of maternal smoking habits on the individual measures of atopy was further analysed bivariately. Smoking during pregnancy and/or lactation was neither associated with the child's skin prick test reactivity nor a history of respiratory atopic diseases, but only with a positive history of AD; 18.1% (98 of 541) of the children whose mothers did not smoke gave a history of AD, whereas in 33.8% (26 of 77) of the children whose mothers had smoked during pregnancy and/or lactation AD was reported (OR 2.30, 1.32–3.12) (Table 12.3).

In this study maternal smoking during pregnancy and/or lactation was found to be associated with an increased risk of 2.3 (1.3–3.1) for AD in the offspring (Schäfer et al., 1997). The degree to which the effects of prenatal exposure to components of tobacco smoke on the immune system are causally linked to the later outcome cannot yet be answered. Earlier studies by Rantakallio (1978) had associated smoking during pregnancy with alterations of the child's skin. There the cumulative incidence during the first five years of life, according to hospital admissions for diseases of the skin and the subcutaneous tissue, was found to be 22.5 per 1000 live births in the group of mothers who smoked during pregnancy ($n = 1821$) compared with 8.2 per 1000 in

Table 12.3. Associations between maternal smoking during pregnancy and lactation and atopic diseases in the offspring (adapted from Schäfer et al., 1997)

Atopic disease	OR	95% CI
Hay fever	n.s.	
Asthma	n.s.	
Atopic dermatitis	2.30	1.32–3.12

the nonsmoker group ($n = 1823$) ($p < 0.0001$). Among these diseases AD and urticaria were observed 4.7 times more often in the smoker group. Other factors, such as socioeconomic status, may in part also account for these differences. It has also been shown that children with AD whose mothers smoke are more likely to develop asthma later on (Murray & Morrison, 1990).

The unexpected inverse correlation between indoor NOx exposure and manifestation of atopy within the group of mothers who did not smoke during pregnancy or lactation cannot be fully explained. It was suspected that parents of obviously atopic children refrained from smoking (the major indoor NOx source) as a preventive measure, but data confirming that hypothesis are not available. Family history of atopic diseases, which was not included in the model, might have confounded the relationship. There was, however, no statistically significant difference in the various exposure groups with regard to this parameter. The third split in the CART confirms the original expectations in so far that, for the remaining subgroup, significantly fewer manifestations of atopy were found in the so-called clean air regions. This evidence on the incidence of AD confirms the current preventive recommendations to avoid smoking, especially during pregnancy and lactation.

Industrial and traffic pollution in east versus west Germany

The fall of the Berlin Wall in 1989 offered the unique opportunity to compare cohorts which had been exposed to different degrees and kinds of (air) pollutants over a long time period. It can be assumed that there is no substantial genetic heterogeneity between subjects in east and west Germany. With respect to air pollutant patterns east Germany showed, in part significantly, higher degrees of exposure to the reducing type of air pollution, including SO_2, dust fall and suspended particles. This was mainly a consequence of combustion of coal with a high content of sulphur and the lack of modern filter techniques. In contrast, the inner city areas of west German communities were mainly exposed to NOx, in some cases to higher degrees than in east Germany. This exposure can be considered as a consequence of the intensity of automobile traffic and reflects the oxidative type of air pollution. Figure 12.2 summarizes the mean outdoor exposures of SO_2, NOx, dust fall and suspended particles for selected study regions in east (Halle an der Saale) and west (Duisburg North and South, Essen) Germany including a countryside control region (Borken).

In 1991 all 1930 preschoolchildren living in predefined areas (according to exposure criteria) in these regions were contacted about this cross-sectional study (Schäfer et al., 1996). These 5–7-year-old children were invited to participate as volunteers in further investigations additional to the local compulsory preschool examination. Informed consent was given by the children and their parents. Completed questionnaires were obtained from 1470 children (76.2%). The dermatological examination was completed in 1273 (66.0%). Since in 1991 almost no children of foreign nationality lived in Halle, so the results are given for children of white German nationality only.

Detailed numbers on response rates, sex distribution and percentage of German children are given in Table 12.4.

Again, we used a questionnaire to assess the personal and family history of atopic diseases as well as numerous other possible risk factors for the development of atopic diseases, e.g. parameters of the socioeconomic status and relevant allergen and air pollutant exposure. Translations of standardized

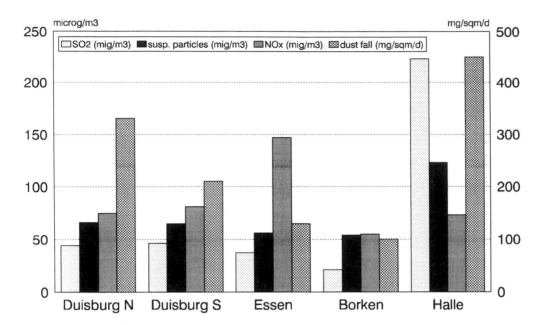

Fig. 12.2. Patterns of air pollutants in selected study regions in an epidemiological study in east and west Germany (mean values for Duisburg and Essen 1986–1990, Borken 1990, Halle 1989) (adapted from Schäfer et al., 1996)

questions, which are used in the International Study on Allergy and Asthma in Childhood (ISAAC), and in another German comparison study (von Mutius et al., 1992), were used to obtain the history of atopic diseases. A total number of 19 physicians from the Department of Dermatology of Hamburg University examined the entire skin surface of the children. With the help of a recently developed instrument, skin manifestations of AD were registered qualitatively and quantitatively. In addition to the extent of the disease, the characteristic items (erythema, oozing, crusts, excoriation and lichenification) were documented using a grading score from 0 to 3 (0 = absent, 1 = mild, 2 = moderate, 3 = severe). The extent was assessed using the 9% rule of burn injuries. To assure a high degree of standardization all investigators were trained in the use of the instrument.

The dependent variable 'present AD' was tested in a logistic regression model for the influence of direct

and indirect parameters of air pollutant exposure, which were the distance of the homes to a heavy traffic road, the exposure to automobile exhaust >1 h/day, indoor use of gas, exposure to environmental tobacco smoke, and the living place (four dummy variables with Borken as reference). Gender, age, genetic predisposition, bedroom sharing, education level of the parents and the month of investigation were included as confounding variables. In this basic model only variables described as risk factors in earlier studies were included. Finally, an exploratory analysis was added to determine the effect of three other possibly influencing factors (contact to animals, presence of furs in bedrooms, previous helminthic infection) which were not included in the basic model. The overall prevalence of AD in the preschoolchildren was 12.9%. Within the different study regions the prevalence ranged from 5.7% (Duisburg North) to 17.5% (Halle an der Saale) (Figure 12.3).

The highest prevalence of AD was found in east Germany (Halle an der Saale). This was not significantly different from the control region, Borken. However, this prevalence was significantly higher than that from the west German city of

Table 12.4. Population sizes and response in an epidemiological study with preschoolchildren in east and west Germany (adapted from Schäfer et al., 1996)

	Duisburg N	Duisburg S	Essen	Borken	Halle	Total
Families contacted	440	380	418	292	400	1930
Questionnaire answered	295	321	265	273	316	1470
Response rate (%)	67.1	84.5	63.4	93.5	79	76.2
Dermatological examination	187	304	228	267	287	1273
Response rate (%)	42.5	80	54.6	91.4	71.8	66
German children (%)	56.7	85.2	80.1	94.8	99.3	85.3
Performed skin prick tests	147	249	179	238	282	1095
Valid skin prick tests	129	211	162	224	279	1005

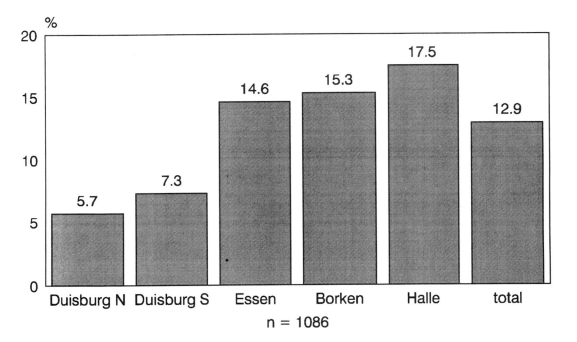

Fig. 12.3. Prevalence of AD (examination) in preschoolchildren in an epidemiological study in east and west Germany (adapted from Schäfer et al., 1996)

Duisburg (Halle versus Duisburg N + S: OR 2.93, CI 1.79–4.79).

A multivariate logistic regression analysis was done according to the model which was described above. As a result girls were found to be more susceptible to AD than boys (OR 0.63, CI 0.43–0.92 boys versus girls) with differences being most impressive in Borken (8.9% in boys, 20.2% in girls) and Duisburg South (3.7% in boys, 11.3% in girls). A positive family history of allergic diseases was also associated with AD (OR 1.52, CI 1.03–2.25.

In all study sites, except Essen, AD was more frequent in children whose parents had graduated after ten or more years of school. This difference was significant for Duisburg South ($p = 0.039$), but not for the total study population (OR 1.83, CI 0.83–4.02).

The clinical manifestation of AD may fluctuate

during the course of the year. We found a significantly lower rate of AD in the second of two subsequent months during the examination period February through May (OR 0.55; CI 0.37–0.81 May versus April and March versus February in Halle, respectively).

As an indirect parameter for NOx exposure, use of indoor gas for cooking without an extractor hood was associated with AD (OR 1.68; CI 1.11–2.56). That is to say about 70% more cases of AD were observed in households with this indoor NOx source. Higher rates of AD were also found in children whose homes were located closer than 50 m to a high traffic volume road (OR 1.71; CI 1.07–2.73). This may substitute as an indicator for automobile exhaust as a risk factor for AD.

After controlling for confounders the prevalence of AD was still markedly lower in Duisburg when compared with the control region, Borken. The difference turned out to be significant for Duisburg South (OR 0.52; CI 0.30–0.96). The other tested parameters yielded no statistically relevant results.

With respect to allergen exposure AD was found to be associated with contact to rabbits (OR 1.81, CI 0.96–3.41; for girls only: OR 2.90, CI 1.36–6.19) and the presence of animal furs in the bedroom (OR 2.17, CI 1.00–4.67). There was also an association between AD and previous intestinal parasitic infections (OR 1.61, CI 0.98–2.64). Additional inclusion of these factors in the basic logistic regression model changed the adjusted odds ratios only marginally.

Results of these analyses are summarized in Table 12.5.

This first comparative epidemiological study on the prevalence of AE in east and west Germany, including an actual dermatological examination, yielded on average high prevalence rates with a great variation between different study sites. The prevalence of AD in east Germany was higher (17.5%; adj. OR 1.39, CI 0.77–2.52 compared to Borken) than in all other study regions. Although the degree of air pollution is not fully reflected by these numbers the prevalence in east Germany is higher than that found by others (Schultz Larsen, 1993; Taylor et al.,

Table 12.5. Risk factors for atopic dermatitis in an epidemiological study in east and west Germany (adapted from Schäfer et al., 1996)

Parameter	OR	CI (95%)
Male gender	0.63	0.43–0.92*
Location (reference Borken)		
Duisburg south	0.52	0.30–0.96*
Duisburg north	0.42	0.15–1.16
Essen	0.85	0.46–1.54
Halle	1.39	0.77–2.52*
Positive family history of atopic diseases	1.52	1.03–2.25*
Month of investigation	0.55	0.37–0.81*
(May vs. April/March vs. February)		
High parental educational level	1.83	0.83–4.02[a]
Contact to rabbits	1.81	0.96–3.41
	2.90	1.36–6.19*[b]
Animal furs in bedroom	2.17	1.01–4.67*
Indoor use of gas without hood	1.68	1.11–2.56*
Homes close to high traffic road (<50 m)	1.71	1.07–2.73*
Previous helminthic infection	1.61	0.98–2.64

Adjusted for:
age, bedroom sharing, ETS, exposure to automobile exhaust (>1 h/day)
a: significant in Duisburg-South ($p = 0.039$)
b: results for girls

1984). The markedly lower frequency of AD in Duisburg could not be explained by testing for known confounders.

Anamnestic parameters of exposure to air pollutants, which may also increase the total IgE level, were associated with the manifestation of AD (use of gas without an extractor hood, living near a high traffic volume road). Similar results connecting automobile exhaust and pollinosis had been published by Ishizaki et al. (1987). This east–west German comparison yielded some unexpected results. As reported earlier (Behrendt et al., 1993; Schlipköter et al., 1992; Krämer et al., 1991) the frequencies of respiratory allergies and specific IgE levels were not elevated in east Germany in contrast to the total IgE levels, which were significantly higher compared with west German regions. Similar results were obtained in another east–west German study (von Mutius et al., 1992). Atopic dermatitis seems to follow a different course from respiratory atopic diseases. The complex subject of the influence of air pollutants on allergic sensitization and disease (Holt, 1989; Rajka, 1986; Ring et al., 1995) needs further research in experimental, epidemiological and clinical studies.

Conclusion

There is preliminary evidence that environmental pollutants can contribute to the manifestation of AD. Future epidemiological studies should utilize the best measures of outcome (actual dermatological examination) and exposure (personal sampling) achievable. Modern techniques in biostatistics should be used to control for known confounders.

Summary of key points

- The prevalence of atopic dermatitis (AD) has increased.
- Environmental influences may play a role in the manifestation of AD.
- For several pollutants an irritative as well as an immunomodulatory effect have been described.
- Certain air pollutants can aggravate asthma-related symptoms.
- Although biologically plausible, information linking AD with air pollutants is still small.
- Ingested pollutants have never been investigated as risk factors for AD.
- In a study of 678 preschoolchildren in Bavaria maternal smoking during pregnancy and/or lactation was found to be an important risk factor for AD.
- In a study of 1470 children in one east and four west German communities AD was found to be higher in east Germany.
- This finding is in contrast to the results for respiratory atopic diseases.
- The use of indoor gas without hood for cooking purposes and proximity to automobile traffic were found to be independent risk factors for AD in children.
- Future studies on pollution and AD should specify the type of pollution and utilize the best measures of exposure and outcome possible.

References

Abel, E. (1980). Smoking during pregnancy: a review of effects on growth and development of offsprings. *Human Biol*, **52**, 593–625.

Amdur, M., Doull, J. & Klaassen, C. (1993). *Casarett and Doull's Toxicology*. New York: McGraw-Hill.

Bahna, S., Heiner, D. & Myhre, B. (1983). Immunoglobulin E pattern in cigarette smokers. *Allergy*, **38**, 57–64.

Behrendt, H. (1992). Allergotoxikologie: Ein Forschungskonzept zur Untersuchung des Einflusses von Umweltschadstoffen auf die Allergieentstehung. In: Ring, J. (ed.) *Allergieforschung: Probleme, Strategien und klinische Relevanz*, pp. 123–30. Muenchen: MMV.

Behrendt, H., Wieczorek, M., Wellner, S. & Winzer, A. (1988). Effect of some metal ions (Cd++, Pb++, Mn++) on mediator release from mast cells in vivo and in vitro. In: Seemayer, N. & Hadnagy, W. (eds.) *Environmental Hygiene*, pp. 105–10. Berlin: Springer-Verlag.

Behrendt, H., Friedrichs, K., Kainka-Staenicke, E., Darsow, U. et al. (1991). Allergens and pollutants in the air – a complex interaction. In: Ring, J. & Przybilla, B. (eds.) *New Trends in Allergy III*. pp. 467–78. Berlin: Springer-Verlag.

Behrendt, H., Krämer, U., Dolgner, R., Hinrichs, J. et al. (1993). Elevated levels of total serum IgE in East German children: atopy, parasites or pollutants? *Allergy J*, **3**, 31–40.

Behrendt, H., Friedrichs, K., Krämer, U. Hitzfeld, B. et al. (1995). The role of indoor and outdoor air pollution in allergic diseases. In: Johansson, S. (ed.) *Progress in Allergy and Clinical Immunology*, Vol. 3, pp. 83–9. Seattle: Hogrefe & Huber.

Birnbaum, L. (1994). The mechanism of dioxin toxicity: relationship to risk assessment. *Env Hlth Perspect*, **102**, Suppl. 9, 157–67.

Burr, M., Miskelly, F., Butland, B., Merrett, T. et al. (1989). Environmental factors and symptoms in infants at high risk of allergy. *J Epidemiol Comm Hlth*, **43**, 125–32.

Buu-Hor, N., Chanh, P., Sesque, G., Azum-Gelade, M. et al. (1972). Organs as targets of dioxin (2,3,7,8-tetra-chlorodibenzo-p-dioxin) intoxication. *Naturwissenschaften*, **59**, 174–5.

Daum, J., Shepherd, D. & Noelle, R. (1993). Immunotoxicology of cadmium and mercury on B-lymphocytes I. Effects on lymphocyte function. *Int J Immunopharmacol*, **15**, 383–94.

Descotes, J. (1992). Immunotoxicology of cadmium. In: Nordberg, G., Herber, R. & Alessio, L. (eds.) *Cadmium in the Human Environment: Toxicity and Carcinogenicity* No. 118, pp. 385–90. Lyon: International Agency for Research on Cancer (WHO) Scientific Publications.

Dirschedl, P. (1991). Exploration von Risikofaktoren mit Klassifikationsbäumen. In: Ring, J. (ed.) *Epidemiologie allergischer Erkrankungen*, pp. 21–34. Muenchen: MMV.

Druet, P. (1995). Metal-induced autoimmunity. *Hum Exp Toxicol*, **14**, 120–1.

Eberlein-König, B., Pechak, J., Gebefuegi, I., Kuehnl, P. et al. (1995). Airborne nitrogen dioxide or formaldehyde influence parameters of skin function and of cellular activation in atopic eczema patients and controls. *J Allergy Clin Immunol*, **95**, 249.

Engbak, S. (1982). *The Morbidity of School Age*. Copenhagen: Lageforeningen.

Erisson-Lihr, Z. (1955). The incidence of allergic disease in childhood. *Acta Allergol*, **8**, 289–313.

Evans, R., Webb, K., Knutsen, A., Roodman, S. et al. (1988). A medical follow-up of the health effects of long-term exposure to 2,3,7,8-tetrachlorodibenzo-p-dioxin. *Arch Environ Hlth*, **43**, 273–8.

Fergusson, D., Hons, B. & Horwood, L. (1985). Parental smoking and respiratory illness during early childhood: a six-year longitudinal study. *Pediat Pulmonol*, **2**, 99–106.

Hatcher, R. & Crosby, K. (1927). The elimination of nicotine in the milk. *J Pharm Exp Ther*, **32**, 1–6.

He, F., Wang, S., Liu, L., Chen, S. et al. (1989). Clinical manifestations and diagnosis of acute pyrethroid poisoning. *Arch Toxicol*, **63**, 54–8.

Hoffman, R., Stehr-Green, P., Webb, K., Evans, G. et al. (1986). Health effects of long-term exposure to 2,3,7,8-tetrachlorodibenzo-p-dioxin. *J Am Med Ass*, **255**, 2031–8.

Holt, P. (1989). Environmental pollutants as co-factors in IgE production. *Curr Opinion Immunol*, **1**, 643–6.

Hultmann, P. & Enestroem, S. (1987). The induction of immune complex deposits in mice by peroral and parental administration of mercuric chloride: strain dependent susceptibility. *Clin Exp Immunol*, **67**, 283–92.

Hultmann, P. & Enestrom, S. (1988). Mercury induced antinuclear antibodies in mice: characterization and correlation with renal immune complex deposits. *Clin Exp Immunol*, **71**, 269–74.

Ishizaki, T., Koizumi, K., Ikemore, R., Ishiyama, Y. et al. (1987). Studies of prevalence of Japanese cedar pollinosis among residents in a highly cultivated area. *Ann Allergy*, **48**, 265–70.

Jordanov, J. (1990). Cotinine concentration in amniotic fluid and urine of smoking, passive smoking and non-smoking pregnant women at term and in the urine of their neonates on the 1st day of life. *Pediatrics* **149**, 734–7.

Juergensen, H. & Behrendt, H. (1989). The effect of organolead compound triethyllead on human basophils and rat mast cells. *Allergologie*, **12** (Suppl.), 65.

Kastelan, M., Gerencer, M., Kastelan, A. & Gamulin, S. (1981). Inhibition of mitogen and specific antigen-induced human lymphocyte proliferation by cadmium. *Exp Cell Biol*, **49**, 15–19.

Kimmig, J. & Schulz, K. (1957). Occupational acne (so called cloracne) due to the chlorinated aromatic cyclic esters. *Dermatologica*, **115**, 540–6.

Kjellman, N. (1981). Effect of parental smoking on IgE levels in children. *Lancet*, **5**, 993–4.

Koller, L. & Roan, J. (1975). Antibody suppression by cadmium. *Arch Environ Hlth*, **30**, 598–601.

Krämer, U., Behrendt, H., Dolgner, R., Kainka-Staenicke, E. et al. (1991). Auswirkungen der Umweltbelastungen auf allergologische Parameter bei 6jaehrigen Kindern. Ergebnisse einer Pilotstudie im Rahmen der Luftreinhalteplaene von Nordrheim-Westfalen. In: Ring, J. (ed.) *Epidemiologie allergischer Ekrankungen*. Muenchen: MMV.

Kubicka-Muranyi, M., Kremer, J., Rottmann, N. Lübben, B. et al. (1996). Murine systemic autoimmune disease induced by mercuric chloride: T helper cells reacting to self proteins. *Int Arch Allergy Immunol*, **109**, 11–20.

Kunz, B., Ring, J., Dirschedl, B., Przybilla, B. et al. (1991). Innenraumbelastung und atopische Erkrankungen bei Kindern. In: Ring, J. (ed.) *Epidemiologie allergischer Erkrankungen*, pp. 202–20. Muenchen: MMV.

Küster, W., Petersen, M., Christophers, E., Goos, M. et al. (1990). A family study of atopic dermatitis. *Arch Derm Res*, **282**, 98–102.

Larsson, P. & Silvette, H. (1969). *Tobacco: Experimental and Clinical Studies. A Comprehensive Account of World Literature Supplement*. Baltimore: Williams & Wilkins.

Larsson, P. & Liden, S. (1980). Prevalence of skin diseases among adolescents 12–16 years of age. *Acta Dermatol Venereol (Stockh.)*, **60**, 415–23.

Magnusson, C. (1986). Maternal smoking influences cord serum IgE and IgD levels and increases the risk for subsequent infant allergy. *J Allergy Clin Immunol*, **78**, 898–904.

Magnusson, C. (1988). Cord serum IgE in relation to family history and as a predictor of atopic disease in early childhood. *Allergy*, **43**, 241–51.

Magnusson, C. & Johansson, S. (1986). Maternal smoking leads to increased cord serum IgG3. *Allergy*, **41**, 302–7.

Malave, L. & de Ruffino, D. (1984). Altered immune response during cadmium administration in mice. *Toxicol Appl Pharmacol*, **74**, 46–56.

Martinez, F., Antognoni, G., Macri, F., Bonci, E. et al. (1988). Parental smoking enhances bronchial responsiveness in nine-year-old children. *Am Rev Resp Dis*, **138**, 518–23.

Mayenburg, J. (1989). Quecksilber als Allergen. *Allergologie*, **12**, 235–42.

Müller, S., Gillert, K., Krause, C., Jautzke, G. et al. (1979). Effects of cadmium on the immune system of mice. *Experientia*, **35**, 909–10.

Murray, A. & Morrison, B. (1990). It is children with atopic dermatitis who develop asthma more frequently if the mother smokes. *J Allergy Clin Immunol*, **86**, 732–9.

von Mutius, E., Fritzsch, F., Weiland, S., Roell, G. et al. (1992). Prevalence of asthma and allergic disorders among children in united Germany: a descriptive comparison. *Br Med J*, **305**, 1395–9.

Neubert, R., Jacob-Müller, U., Helge, H., Stahlmann, R. et al. (1991). Polyhalogenated dibenzo-p-dioxin (TCDD) on lymphocytes of venous blood from man and a non-human primate (Callithrix jacchus). *Arch Toxicol*, **65**, 213–9.

Niermann, H. (1964). *Zwillingsdermatologie*. Berlin: Springer-Verlag.

Paganelli, R., Ramadas, D., Layward, L., Harvey, B. et al. (1979). Maternal smoking and cord blood immunity function. *Clin Exp Immunol*, **36**, 256–9.

Pelletier, L., Pasquier, R. & Guvettier, C. (1988). HgCl$_2$ induces T and B cells to proliferate and differentiate in BN rats. *Clin Exp Immunol*, **71**, 336–42.

Peters, H., Croft, W., Woolson, E., Darcey, B. et al. (1984). Seasonal arsenic exposure from burning chromium-copper-arsenate-treated wood. *J Am Med, Ass*, **251**, 2393–6.

Przybilla, B. & Ring, J. (1990). Food allergy and atopic eczema. *Semin Dermatol*, **3**, 220–5.

Rajka, G. (1986). Atopic dermatitis. Correlation of environmental factors with frequency. *Int J Dermatol*, **25**, 301–4.

Rajka, G. (1989). *Essential Aspects of Atopic Dermatitis*. Berlin: Springer-Verlag.

Rantakallio, P. (1978). Relationship of maternal smoking to morbidity and mortality of the child up to the age of five. *Acta Paediat Scand*, **67**, 621–31.

Ring, J. (1991). *Epidemiolgie allergischer Erkrankungen*. Muenchen: MMV.

Ring, J. & Behrendt, H. (1993). Allergy and IgE production: role of infection and environmental pollution. *Allergy J*, **2**, 27–30.

Ring, J., Behrendt, H., Schäfer, T., Vieluf, D. et al. (1995). Impact of pollution in allergic diseases. Clinical and epidemiological studies. In: Johansson, S. (ed.) *Progress in Allergy and Clinical Immunology*, Vol. 3, pp. 174–82. Seattle: Hogrefe & Huber.

Ruzicka, T., Ring, J. & Przybilla, B. (1991). *Handbook of Atopic Eczema*. Berlin: Springer-Verlag.

Schäfer, T., Enders, F. & Przybilla, B. (1995). Sensitization to thimerosal and previous vaccination. *Cont Dermatitis*, **32**, 114–6.

Schäfer, T., Vieluf, D., Behrendt, H., Krämer, U. et al. (1996). Atopic eczema and other manifestations of atopy: results of a study in East and West Germany. *Allergy*, **51**, 532–9.

Schäfer, T., Dirschedl, P., Kunz, B., Ring, J. et al. (1997). Maternal smoking during pregnancy and lactation increases the risk for atopic eczema in the offspring. *J Am Acad Dermatol*, **36**, 550–6.

Schlipköter, H., Krämer, U., Behrendt, H., Dolgner, R. et al. (1992). Impact of air pollution on children's health. Results from Saxony-Anhalt and Saxony as compared to North-Rhine-Westphalia. Health and ecologic effects. *Critical Issues in the Global Environment*. Pittsburgh: A.W.M. Association.

Schrallhammer-Benkler, K., Ring, J., Przybilla, B., Meurer, M. et al. (1992). Acute mercury intoxication with lichenoid drug eruption followed by mercury contact allergy and development of antinuclear antibodies. *Acta Dermatol Venereol (Stockh.)*, **72**, 294–6.

Schultz Larsen, F. (1993). The epidemiology of atopic dermatitis. In: Burr, M. (ed.) *Epidemiology of Clinical Allergy*, pp. 9–28. Basel: Karger.

Schultz Larsen, F., Holm, N. & Henningsen, K. (1986). Atopic dermatitis: a genetic–epidemiology study in a population-based twin sample. *J Am Acad Dermatol*, **15**, 487–94.

Suzuki, S., Takafuji, S. & Miyamoto, T. (1989). Particle air pollutants as enhancers of IgE production. *Allergy Clin Immunol News*, **1**, 76.

Takafuji, S., Suzuki, S., Muranaka, M. & Miyamoto, T. (1989). Influence of environmental factors on IgE production. In: Metzger, H. (ed.) *IgE, Mast Cells and the Allergic Response*, pp. 188–204. London: John Wiley.

Taylor, B., Wadsworth, J., Wadsworth, M. & Peckham, C. (1984). Changes in the reported prevalence of childhood eczema since the 1939–45 war. *Lancet*, 1255–7.

Tucker, S. & Flannigan, S. (1983). Cutaneous effects from occupational exposure to Fenvalerate. *Arch Toxicol*, **54**, 195–202.

Überla, K., Dirschedl, P., Greif, A., Huber, H. et al. (1991). *Pilot-Untersuchungen auf gesundheitliche Indikatoren im Umfeld der Sondermüllverbrennungsanlage und Deponie Schwabach*. Muenchen: MMV.

Vieluf, D., Kunz, B., Bieber, T., Przybilla, B. et al. (1993). 'Atopy Patch Test' with aeroallergens in patients with atopic eczema. *Allergy J*, **2**, 9–12.

Vos, J. & Moore, J. (1974). Suppression of cellular immunity in rats and mice by maternal treatment with 2,3,7,8-tetra-chlorodibenzo-p-dioxin. *Int Arch Allergy Appl Immunol*, **47**, 777–94.

Warren, C., Holford-Strevens, V., Wong, C. & Manfreda, J. (1982). The relationship between smoking and total immunoglobu-lin E levels. *J Allergy Clin Immunol*, **69**, 370–5.

Wieczorek, M. & Behrendt, H. (1989). Wirkungen von Cadmium und Blei auf Mediatorzellen allergischer Reaktionen. *Allergologie*, **12**, 158–60.

Williams, H., Strachan, D. & Hay, R. (1994). Childhood eczema: disease of the advantaged? *Br J Dermatol*, **308**, 1132–5.

Young, E. (1980). Seasonal factors in atopic dermatitis and their relationship to allergy. *Acta Dermatol Venereol (Stockh.)*, **92**, (Suppl), 111–2.

Young, S., Rubin, J. & Daman, H. (1986). *Psychobiological Aspects of Allergic Disorders*. New York: Praeger.

Zetterström, O., Osterman, K., Machedo, L. & Johansson, S. (1981). Another smoking hazard: raised IgE concentration and increased risk of occupational allergy. *Br Med J*, **283**, 1215–7.

13

Atopic dermatitis in migrant populations

Carol Burrell-Morris and Hywel C. Williams

Introduction

Why study migrant groups?

Previous chapters in this book have suggested that the aetiology of atopic dermatitis (AD) is a complex interaction between genetic and environmental factors. The absence of any clear genetic markers for most cases of AD has meant that separating the effects of genetic versus environmental factors in cross-sectional, cohort or case-control studies has been extremely difficult to date. Some have used family history of atopic disease as a surrogate measure of the genetic influence of AD, but such a measure is far from adequate as close relatives, by definition, are likely to share a very similar environment. Twin studies have been useful in telling us something about the role of nature versus nurture (Schultz Larsen, 1986) but, as was pointed out in Chapter 8, these also have their limitations.

Another approach to separating the effects of genetics versus environmental factors is the study of genetically similar people who migrate from one country to another, where they might be exposed to a range of different environmental factors. The assumption underlying migrant studies is that, if genetically similar people who migrate from one country to another acquire a different risk of disease, the change in risk status might be attributable to environmental factors present in the adopted country. It seems very unlikely that genetic factors could account for changes in disease rates in migrant groups which occur over the span of a decade or one generation.

Before the 'it cannot be genetic' argument is dismissed in such migrant studies, it is important to consider the possibility of somatic mutations or, perhaps more plausibly, that previously dormant 'atopic' genes are activated on exposure to certain environmental triggers, such as higher antigen loads. Conversely, it is possible that previously active suppressor genes are inactivated, by loss of helminthic parasites for example. In such a situation, it becomes an academic argument as to whether the change in disease rate is 'genetic' or 'environmental'. Both could clearly be involved, either in the sense of increasing multiplicative risk or in terms of effect modification. Too much scientific energy has been wasted in arguing whether atopic dermatitis is predominantly a genetic disease or otherwise – what is important is discovering which environmental triggers increase the risk of disease, by how much, and whether disease risk can be reduced if those factors are removed or abolished.

In addition to making inferences about environmental risk factors based on changes in disease rates following migration, one could also postulate that migrant studies could be useful in suggesting that certain environmental factors may not be as important as previously suspected if disease rates fail to change substantially on exposure to such factors. For example, if AD rates remain unchanged in people who migrate from a country where there is low environmental exposure (e.g. to industrial pollution) to another where there is high exposure, this suggests that such exposures may be less important than previously suggested (Behrendt et al., 1993; Bobák et al., 1995). Such studies will always be

Table 13.1. Estimated relative risk of melanoma in immigrants to Australia by age at arrival in Australia when compared against Australian-born and adjusted for age, period, cohort and State (Khlat et al., 1992)

Region of birth	Age (years) at arrival		
	<15	15–24	25+
New Zealand			
Males	0.87	1.30	0.82
Females	0.19	1.00	0.96
Other Oceania			
Males	0.72	0.60	0.25
Females	1.43	0.58	0.23
England			
Males	0.90	0.41	0.32
Females	0.79	0.43	0.33
Ireland/Scotland/Wales			
Males	0.77	0.46	0.31
Females	0.70	0.52	0.29

limited because of possible selection bias and other confounding factors, but they may serve as useful indicators for more refined studies.

As well as providing us with pointers to the role of environmental factors in causing AD, migrant studies may also give us important insights into critical periods of exposure to various harmful environmental factors. In a study of mortality from melanoma in migrants to Australia, children of British descent, born in Australia, who were subsequently followed-up, demonstrated much higher rates of malignant melanoma when compared with older children and young adults who migrated to Australia from Britain (Khlat et al., 1992). As shown in Table 13.1, the risk of melanoma was also shown to depend on the duration of stay and the age at migration. This study suggests that the critical period of exposure for carcinogenesis in melanoma could be in the first 20 years of life, a finding which has been very helpful in targeting primary prevention policies. By analogy, the study of AD rates in populations who migrate to countries at different ages may provide us with important clues as to the

critical periods for sensitization to allergens which could inform public health intervention strategies.

The study of migrant populations therefore provides a basis for examining several aspects of the role of environmental factors in the aetiology and expression of AD.

Defining migrant groups

The task of defining migrant groups is a difficult one as there is no clear-cut definition of what constitutes a 'migrant' person and what is 'long enough' in terms of duration of residency in another country. A person who has lived in a country long enough to become a legal immigrant is an easy definition to choose, but perhaps not such a useful one for examining biological phenomena, since legal processes such as residency and naturalization can take anything from two months to 20 years. Definitions based on such status might miss some of the most relevant migrant groups who have only temporary legal status, or no legal status at all. In one sense, any person who decides to set up an abode in another country may be considered to be a 'migrant'. However, persons who have only just arrived in their new country would hardly have resided there for sufficient time to be exposed to some important environmental risk factors. Studying these individuals would be unlikely to yield valuable information concerning the effects of the new environment on disease processes. On the other hand, people who have resided in a country for a few generations may have experienced some physiological tolerance to certain harmful environmental exposures, or some degree of behavioural or genetic adaptation may have occurred. The situation might be further compounded in offspring by genetic mixing through intercultural marriage.

The term 'migrant' in epidemiological studies of AD therefore needs to: (*a*) encompass an element of moving from one place with a distinct set of cultural and geophysical exposures to another with a different constellation of exposures; and (*b*) include an exposure period to the newly purported risk factors of sufficient duration to substantially increase the risk of disease. The corollary is that the definition of migrant groups is best thought of in terms of the specific exposures of interest. For studies of strong risk factors which require only a short exposure time, such as sulphur dioxide emissions and upper respiratory tract symptoms, then a study of people who have lived in an area of high SO_2 fallout for a period of a few months, compared with similar people from their town or country of origin, will probably be sufficient for a 'migrant' study. On the other hand, more insidious exposures such as cumulative ultraviolet light radiation (UVR) and basal cell carcinoma requires the study of groups who reside in a country with low UVR compared with those who migrate from such a country to another with high UVR exposure for *decades* before it becomes a 'useful' migrant study.

We believe it is reasonable to consider that the term 'migrant' can be applied to children born in the new country to which their parents have migrated, e.g. Black Caribbean children born in London to parents who have migrated from the Caribbean. These children would be exposed to environmental factors in the new environment and their only link to their parents' country of origin would be genetic plus cultural factors which they take with them. We make such a recommendation reservedly because we know so little about the risk factors for AD and the duration and timing of exposure in order for the disease to manifest itself. For example, it is possible that a child migrating from a hot and humid country such as Malaysia, who has never suffered from AD, but who is predisposed to atopy genetically, might begin to express AD for the first time within a few months of moving to a cold country with low humidity such as northern Scandinavia (e.g. because of dry skin leading to disruption of barrier function). As a minimum, it is clearly important to state how long 'migrants' have lived in their adopted country when referring to migrant studies.

Migrant studies have traditionally referred to populations who migrate from one country to another. However, the study of any well defined group of people who move from one geographical area to another (e.g. rural to urban), where they experience

Table 13.2. Relative risk of death from cancers of specific sites among Japanese men aged 45–64 years compared with white Californians (Buell & Dunn, 1965)

Site	Californian whites	Sons of Japanese immigrants	Japanese immigrants	Japanese in Japan
Stomach	1.0	2.8	3.8	8.4
Colon	1.0	0.9	0.4	0.2
All sites	1.0	0.7	0.9	1.1

a different range of exposures and different disease rates, may be considered as a migrant study. We should not, therefore, be constrained into defining migrant studies as those which study groups who migrate between countries. In some cases, differences in exposures may be larger *within* one country (e.g. UVR in southern and northern USA) than *between* countries (e.g. climatic conditions in southern Spain and Portugal). What matters is the change and constancy of a new set of exposures which can be measured in a well defined group of people who move from one area to another.

Migrant studies of other diseases

Before investing time and energy into exploring migrant groups with respect to AD it is worthwhile examining whether migrant studies have been successful in contributing to our understanding of other diseases.

In Japan, mortality rates from stomach cancer are amongst the highest in the world. In a study of stomach cancer mortality among Japanese living in California, first generation Japanese men were found to have rates that were intermediate between those of males in Japan and those of white Californian males (Buell & Dunn, 1965). Their male offspring, brought up in Californian, were found to have rates closer to those for white California males (Table 13.2). These results strongly suggest the possibility of environmental carcinogens being

Table 13.3. Average annual mortality rates per 1000 Japanese men in the Japan, Honolulu and San Francisco areas by age and underlying cause of death (Worth et al., 1975)

Age at death (years)	Cause of death	Japan rate	Honolulu rate	San Francisco rate
50–54	All strokes	1.4	0.5	–
	All CHD	0.4	1.1	1.3
	All causes	9.4	4.5	3.3
55–59	All strokes	1.5	0.9	0.5
	All CHD	1.4	1.7	4.8
	All causes	13.9	7.6	13.9
60–64	All strokes	5.4	1.1	2.5
	All CHD	2.1	3.9	4.9
	All causes	24.5	13.7	14.8

responsible for the higher rates of cancer of the stomach in Japan (Kolonel et al., 1981).

In the late nineteenth and early twentieth century large numbers of Japanese migrated to Hawaii and California. They provided an easily accessible group of immigrants in whom the effect of environmental factors could be studied. The mortality from coronary heart disease (CHD) in Japan is relatively low while in the USA it is high. Epidemiological studies of CHD in Japanese men living in Japan, Hawaii and California (Table 13.3) showed a gradient in CHD mortality increasing from Japan to Hawaii to California (Syme et al., 1975; Worth et al., 1975). When the Japanese in Hawaii were divided according to place of birth, recent Japanese migrants had higher rates than Japanese born in Hawaii. The converse was true of Caucasian migrants to Hawaii who had lower rates than Caucasians born in Hawaii.

Migrant studies can also suggest whether age of exposure is important. Studies of multiple sclerosis in South Africa have shown that recent white immigrants have a much higher rate of disease when compared with similar whites born in South Africa. One possible explanation for this is that an initiating factor occurs some years before the onset of symptoms and that people who migrate from the UK to

South Africa take some of their higher risk with them (Barker & Rose, 1984).

Thus, migrant studies have provided us with important clues as to the role of the environment in several common noncommunicable diseases to date. We see no reason why migrant studies should not be similarly helpful for the study of AD and related diseases.

What have migrant studies informed us about atopic dermatitis?

Earlier studies of AD in migrant groups have referred to those attending clinics as opposed to entire populations in the community. Interpreting such studies has been almost impossible since differences detected between populations living in different locations may have resulted in differences in the use of diagnostic criteria (which were often not defined at all), cultural differences in the use of disease labels, and differences in the use of and accessibility to medical care. True comparisons between individuals of the same genetic background living in different parts of the world with respect to AD were inadequate until quite recently.

Studies of ethnic groups in one location

Strictly speaking, studies of rates of disease in different ethnic groups living in one location are not true migrant studies because they do not compare disease rates in the corresponding countries of origin of the migrant populations. Studies of variation of disease according to ethnicity (Figure 13.1) tell us something about the disease burden experienced by certain ethnic groups when compared with the indigenous population, and they may also hint that migrant studies may be worthwhile if it is suspected that disease rates are much lower in the country of origin of these people. Alternatively, if different ethnic groups of similar genetic origin experience very different disease rates following migration to another country, then it is worth investigating lifestyle factors as a possible explanation for such differences in disease rates.

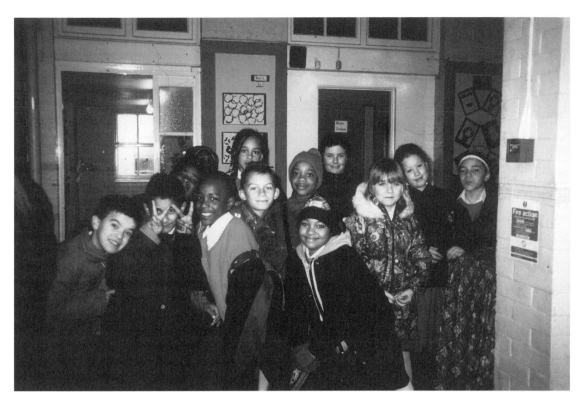

Fig. 13.1. Studies of variation of atopic dermatitis prevalence according to ethnic group are not true migrant studies, but they may hint that further migrant studies may be worthwhile

A study of the prevalence of AD referrals to the Dermatology Department of the Leicester Royal Infirmary in the UK found that Asian children were three times more likely to be referred when compared with nonAsian children (Sladden et al., 1991). However, when a subsequent population-based study was carried out, no difference in the prevalence of AD was detected amongst the different ethnic groups (Neame et al., 1995). In this later study, three samples were utilized: examination of children attending obligatory routine surveillance clinics at the ages of 18 and 42 months; interviews of parents of children attending Social Services day nurseries, and examination of medical records of children aged 1–4 at one primary care health centre. In the three samples, the prevalence rates of AD among all groups were 14%, 27% and 32%, respectively. This study has therefore also demonstrated that the method used to define AD may affect the prevalence estimates and emphasizes the importance of using standardized methods for comparative studies. It also underscores the importance of conducting a population study as opposed to a clinic-based study because differences in ethnic groups described in clinic-based studies may be due to differences in referral rates. Such differences in referral rates could be due to factors such as unfamiliarity of British general practitioners with the appearance of AD in a dark skin, or it may reflect parental unfamiliarity with the condition (George et al., 1997). Although such studies cannot be classified as true migrant studies as the prevalence of AD in the country of origin was not measured, Kanwar & Dhar (1995) hinted that the true prevalence of AD in India may be a lot lower than that of Indian children in the UK, a finding echoed by preliminary results from the International Study of Asthma and Allergies in Childhood (ISAAC) (Williams et al., 1999).

Some comparative studies between Black Caribbean children and European children have been conducted in South London. An early study by Davis, Martin & Sarkany (1961) documented a much higher 'incidence' of eczema among the children of Black Caribbean origin attending a paediatric casualty department when compared with white children. Although there were no identical studies of demand incidence performed in the countries of origin of these children, workers in Jamaica suggested that the incidence was significantly less there (Lawrence & Segree, 1981). Golding & Peters (1987), in a British cohort study of five-year-olds born in 1970, sought to identify major associations between the medical, social, environmental and behavioural background of children with eczema and to identify independent early predictors of eczema. They found that children born to mothers of West Indian origin had a higher prevalence of reported eczema at the age of five, occurring in 17.4% of such children compared with 9.3% of children whose mothers were born in the UK ($p<0.001$) (Peters & Golding, 1987).

These earlier studies, which hinted that being a child of Afro-Caribbean origin in the UK is associated with a higher risk of disease when compared with indigenous white children, have been supported by a recent population survey in Lambeth (an area of London with a large Afro-Caribbean population). In this community-based study (Williams et al., 1995), the prevalence of AD according to examination by a dermatologist was 16.3% in Black Caribbean children and 8.7% in white children (Table 13.4). The odds ratio of having AD if the child was of Afro-Caribbean background was 2.1 (95% confidence intervals 1.1 to 3.9, $p=0.03$). This difference persisted regardless of how AD was defined. In that same study, children of mixed race (predominantly Black Caribbean and white intermarriage) also had prevalence values similar to the Black Caribbean group, whilst children from the Indian subcontinent had prevalence values similar to White children. It is unclear what counts for these differences in prevalence but one explanation could be a higher rate of allergic skin reactivity in Blacks (Gergen, Turkeltaub & Kovar, 1987).

Table 13.4. Ethnic group and prevalence of atopic dermatitis on the basis of a dermatologist's examination of 693 schoolchildren aged 4–11 years in West Lambeth, London (Williams et al., 1995)

Ethnic group*	Prevalence of atopic dermatitis % (n/N)	95% CI
White	8.7 (26/300)	5.7 to 12.4
Black Caribbean	16.3 (23/141)	10.6 to 23.5
Mixed[†]	14.9 (15/101)	8.6 to 23.3
Black other	22.0 (9/41)	10.6 to 37.6
Black African	4.7 (2/43)	0.6 to 15.8
Indian	7.4 (2/27)	0.9 to 24.3
Bangladeshi	9.1 (1/11)	0.2 to 41.3
Pakistani	7.1 (1/14)	0.2 to 33.9
Chinese and other	13.3 (2/15)	1.7 to 40.5
Overall prevalence of atopic dermatitis	11.7 (81/693)	9.3 to 14.0

* As nominated by parents.

[†] More than 90% of these children had one white and one Black parent.

Worth (1962), in his study of AD among Chinese infants in Honolulu and San Francisco, was also able to detect major ethnic group differences in the prevalence of AD. He was consistently able to show that Chinese infants had a higher prevalence of AD when compared with their white counterparts, and that within the Chinese infants there was a tendency for AD to be more common in males and in families of higher socioeconomic classes. In the Chinese infants born to Chinese parents in San Francisco, there was a clear relationship between atopic eczema incidence in the first year of life and the Americanization of the parents, viz: 14% if both parents were born in China, 23% if one parent born in China and 34% if both parents born in the US. These differences could not be explained easily on the basis of genetic, intra-uterine or psychiatric factors and tended to point to some extrinsic physical agent preferentially offered to Chinese infants, possibly dietary.

Another recent study has followed-up 61 ethnic

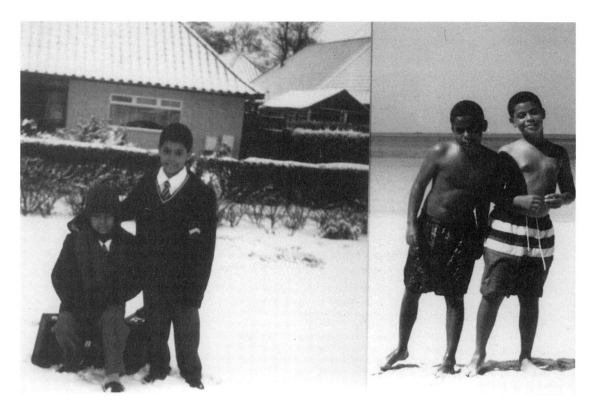

Fig. 13.2. There may be vast differences in the range of environmental exposures experienced by those who migrate from one country to another

Chinese, 59 Vietnamese and 62 Caucasian children born in Melbourne, Australia, and found that 44%, 17% and 21% developed atopic eczema in the first year, respectively (Mar & Marks, 1998). The authors found that the lifestyles of Chinese and Caucasians were very similar in terms of proportion of families with detached homes and plush pile carpets, and suggested that the higher incidence of AD in Chinese children may reflect genetic factors. On the other hand, they argued that the difference in AD incidence between Chinese and Vietnamese children (who have a common genetic pool in the distant past) could be due to differences in environmental exposures, on the basis that Vietnamese families were more likely to live in nondetached homes, were less likely to have carpets in the home and they were less likely to continue prolonged breast feeding. This

important study assumes that Chinese and Vietnamese children are sufficiently similar in genetic terms to tease out the relative contribution of environmental factors. Perhaps a more direct approach which could be used in future studies of such infants would be to measure allergens such as house dust mite levels in the homes of such children, and to see whether the relative or attributable risk of AD incidence differs according to ethnic status, i.e. to see whether there is an interaction between ethnicity and an important environmental risk factor.

Studies of migrants in two locations

Studies of migrants in two locations (i.e. the country of origin and the adopted country) are true migrant studies which are designed to tell us something about the *aetiology* of disease and to what extent genetics and environmental factors may be significant (Figure 13.2). Studies of migrant populations have shown increases in the prevalence of AD when compared with similar populations living in their country of origin. A study of Tokelaun children who migrated to New Zealand (Waite et al., 1980) found that only one (0.1%) of 706 children examined in Tokelau was classified as having eczema on the basis of a 'physical examination' (no further details are given), compared with 99 (8.5%) of 1160 Tokelauan children who had migrated to the Wellington area of New Zealand. Similar large differences were found for asthma (11.0% compared with 25.3%, respectively). This study supports the idea that environmental factors associated with the transition from a traditional island lifestyle to a modern urban society may be important in the aetiology of atopic eczema and asthma. Leung & Ho (1994) further confirmed the effect of 'westernization' on the prevalence of expression of asthma and allergic diseases by showing considerable prevalence differences between three south-east Asian populations (Chinese living in Malaysia, mainland China and Australia) despite similar rates of atopy.

The authors have recently conducted a population-based study of the prevalence of AD in Black Caribbean children who live in Lambeth and similar children living in a comparable urban setting of Kingston, Jamaica (Burrell-Morris et al., 1997). Using the UK refinement of Hanifin and Rajka's diagnostic criteria, the study showed a prevalence of 5.6% in Black Caribbean children in Jamaica and 14.9% in London, representing a relative risk of AD of more than 2½ times greater for children living in London. Similar differences were observed for other methods of defining AD (Table 13.5). A major strength of this study was that cases were defined in both locations using well defined criteria by the same observer in both locations. This study represents a true migrant study.

So far, migrant studies relating to AD have limited themselves to making simple observations of increased risk in adopted countries when compared with the country of origin. They have also all been conducted on socioeconomically disadvantaged populations moving to developed Western-style cultures as opposed to the other way around, where a decrease in AD might be possible. Collectively, these studies have been helpful by suggesting that the environment plays a key role in AD. Theoretically, migrant studies could be taken one step further by simply stating that disease risk is higher in one country when compared with another and seeing whether specific risk factors such as house dust mites might account for the *excess* risk of disease. The analysis of such data is problematic as there are so many differences between countries which could serve as potential confounders between candidate exposures and disease. One possible solution to this problem is to quantify the risk of AD attributable to common specific risk factors by analysing cases and controls in each country separately, rather than conducting a simple analysis of predictors of risk difference between countries. Environmental factors such as house dust mite allergen levels, staphylococcal colonization, skin hydration, exposure to ultraviolet light, and water hardness may be just a few of the possible important factors responsible for producing significant differences in the prevalence of AD between two countries such as Jamaica and England, and these are being studied by the authors at present.

Why do migrants have more atopic dermatitis than those in their country of origin?

It is generally accepted that the aetiology of AD is multifactorial with an interplay of environmental factors and genetic factors. There are several factors such as the increase in prevalence, geographic variation, positive social class gradient and migrant studies which point to the critical role played by the environment in the expression of AD (Williams, 1995). Inhaled or ingested allergens (Tan et al., 1995; Platts-Mills et al., 1983; Norris, Schofield & Camp, 1988; Coloff, 1992; Casimir et al., 1993; David, 1993), irritants (Riedel, 1991), bacteria (Hauser, 1986), skin hydration and environmental temperature and humidity, may all be important factors in determining visible or symptomatic disease in an individual who is genetically susceptible or atopic.

Inhalated or ingested allergens: As Platts-Mills points out in Chapter 14, the most important aller-

Table 13.5. Prevalence of atopic dermatitis in Black Caribbean children in London and Jamaica (Burrell-Morris et al., 1997)

Method of defining AD	London (n = 323)	Jamaica (n = 2087)
UK criteria	48 (14.9%)	117 (5.6%)
Visual flexural dermatitis (point prevalence)	28 (8.6%)	17 (0.8%)
Doctor diagnosed eczema	43 (13.0%)	81 (3.9%)
Severe cases (sleep disturbance >1 night per week)	17 (5.6%)	39 (1.8%)

gen in AD seems to be the house dust mite. Could it be that there are species differences between the countries of origin and the migrant countries? So little is known about the ecology of house dust mite in some countries such as Jamaica. Such knowledge is important to gather before studies are carried out, otherwise there is a danger of not measuring the clinically relevant allergens (e.g. *Euroglyphus mayneii* as opposed to *Dermatophagoides pteronyssinus*) in the new country (Arruda & Chapman, 1992; Hansen et al., 1991). The exposure to relatively new allergens which are uncommon in the countries of origin may be responsible for unmasking the disease in a genetically susceptible individual (Turner et al., 1988). This idea of migrant populations previously naïve to a particular allergen experiencing higher rates of manifest disease than those previously exposed gains some support from studies of IgE reactivity in Turks who have migrated to Sweden (Kalyoncu & Stålenhein, 1992). Such enhanced IgE reactivity may decrease with time, suggesting a degree of adaptation.

Alternatively, it could be that the antigen levels in the migrant countries may simply be much higher or above a certain critical level required for disease expression. This could be related to factors such as building design (e.g. better insulation leading to less air circulation and higher humidity), factors such as differences in house cleaning measures, or a change

in bedding from traditional open wooden structures to sprung fabric-covered mattresses which provide an ideal culture medium for house dust mites (Feather et al., 1993).

Exclusive and prolonged breast feeding is thought to be protective (Saarinen & Kajosaari, 1995) but early introduction of solids and maternal diet are more important (Fergusson, Horwood & Shannon, 1982). It may be that breast feeding may be a less common practice or that maternal diets are richer in chemicals and additives which exacerbate AD in the migrant countries.

Other correlates of 'western' lifestyle such as traffic pollutants, stress, changes in dietary habits, e.g. a reduction in the consumption of free radical scavengers, or changes in family structure are all factors which might contribute to the increased prevalence of AD documented in the industrialized countries.

Changes in skin hydration may also be a contributing factor to the increased prevalence of AD in the migrant population. It may be that skin hydration in the migrant population may be decreased due to an interplay of climatic conditions. Anecdotal experience suggests that people from tropical climates frequently complain that their skin becomes much drier in the cool and less humid climate in the UK. Subclinical inflammation from skin dryness may be only one step away from manifest skin eczematous changes in susceptible individuals.

Bacterial colonization by Staphylococcus aureus may be different in the migrant population, predisposing them to manifesting AD more frequently or more severely than their counterparts in their country of origin. Such a mechanism could be mediated through increased skin dryness in cooler climates due to the increased adherence of the organism on a dry skin.

Loss of helminthic parasites: an inverse relationship between parasitic infestations and the manifestation of allergic diseases has been suggested, atopic subjects having a decreased parasite load. Helminthic infections have been shown to improve established atopic disease (Grove & Forbes, 1975; Turton, 1976). Loss of this helminthic load (or even ectoparasites) following migration to a more developed country may result in a highly activated but displaced IgE–mast cell system which reacts to common but harmless environmental allergens whose epitopes bear some resemblance to previous parasites.

Positive health-related behaviour: it is possible that immunization against common infectious diseases, whilst having unquestionable benefits in reducing mortality, might predispose to precipitation or perpetuation of allergic diseases such as AD. Similarly, fewer infections in early childhood could increase the risk of AD (Strachan, 1989). Following on from this 'hygiene' hypothesis, which has some credence as a possible explanation for the increasing risk of AD in smaller families and birth order, it is possible that excessive washing and showering using a wide array of soaps in developed countries results in a cumulative insult to the skin's barrier function which could directly result in AD through irritation or indirectly by rendering it more susceptible to allergic triggers. It is also possible that many of the pharmacological treatments used for AD in modern countries, such as emollients and topical corticosteroids, actually increase the chronicity of the disease despite helping in the short term.

Potential drawbacks of migrant studies

It should be remembered that most studies of migrant groups are a kind of 'natural experiment' and are thus observational in design. Since the division into people who choose to migrate and those who remain behind is certainly not a random process, and because some knowledge of harmful exposures may lead to avoidance behaviour, such observational studies are subject to all of the limitations of bias and confounding inherent in other observational studies. Some particular problems are worthy of further discussion in relation to migrant studies.

Ethnicity or race?

Race more closely relates to the genetic make-up of an individual, but race cannot be defined in any meaningful way in epidemiological studies (Silver, 1992). The phenotypic characteristics cannot be used to determine the race to which an individual belongs as there is significant variation within any one race. For example: what is Black? (Azuonye, 1996). Within the Black race there is variation of skin colour from light brown to black and significant variation of hair morphology from slightly wavy to tightly curled. The Afro-Caribbean people display significant genetic heterogeneity and represent a mixture of hamiticized Negroes, Chinese, Indian, Northern European and Hispanics. It is far more logical to define people in terms of ethnic group, i.e. a common set of beliefs and customs. Ethnicity is a fluid concept and people change their self assessment over time. Thus, it is possible for a person who is phenotypically 'Indian' to nominate themselves as 'Black Caribbean' if they feel that such an ethnic group best represents their cultural identity.

Intermarriage

Most migrant studies demonstrate a similar pattern of disease rates in the indigenous and migratory populations, e.g. high rates of stomach cancer in Japan, medium rates in recent immigrants and rates similar to indigenous US population in the offspring of the immigrants. It is important to consider to what extent this can be simply explained by intermarriages with the indigenous population. In the Lambeth AD study, for instance (Table 13.4), it was shown that the increased risk of AD was present in children born to exclusive Black Caribbean parents as well as those born to parents of mixed ethnic groups, suggesting that the findings could not simply be explained on the grounds of intermarriage with the local population. It is therefore essential to record the ethnic groups of both parents and to decide beforehand how to deal with those who class themselves as 'mixed'.

Retention of customs

Ethnic groups tend to keep customs after travelling to a new country, e.g. the Muslim and Jewish culture with their unique food, leisure and bathing customs. Therefore, migrant populations are not entirely exposed to a new environment but still maintain some of their original customs such as dietary habits. It is important to take into account, therefore, the degree to which the culture which migrant people take with them may result in behaviour which may modify their exposure to potentially harmful or even protective factors for AD. To some extent, these problems in observing *groups* of people can be overcome by the study of exposures affecting *individuals*.

Migrants are an unusual group

Migrants may not be a representative population as they form a select group of people who choose, or are forced, to leave their homeland for a variety of reasons. It has been shown that the incidence of psychoses is higher in Norwegian immigrants to the USA than in Norway. It is unclear whether this is due to an environmental factor in the USA, or the result of selective migration of people more liable to mental illness, or due to the stresses imposed upon immigrants as they adjust to a foreign culture (Barker & Rose, 1984). Bentham (1988) has pointed out that because young migrants moving large distances are relatively healthy, areas of net out-migration may become less healthy in population terms, whereas areas of net in-migration may appear healthier. Older people tend to migrate shorter distances in order to avoid environmental health hazards or to be closer to medical care. This has the paradoxical effect of increasing morbidity and mortality rates in areas with favourable environmental conditions and good health services.

In the case of AD we feel that it is unlikely that migration is linked with atopic status. Historically, Caribbean migrants to the UK tended to be of the lower socioeconomic group and AD is linked with higher socioeconomic groups. The net effect of selective migration with respect to socioeconomic group should reduce the likelihood of increased disease rates in the UK, rather than the opposite, as found in our study.

Conclusions and future recommendations

So far, migrant studies have been useful in suggesting that the environment has a major role in determining the expression of AD. Further studies of large migrant groups, such as those moving from India and East Africa to the UK and USA, and also studies of people moving away from the US, UK and Australia, are needed to build up a picture of possible harmful and beneficial risk factors. These may be different for different ethnic groups and different migratory routes. Preliminary evidence suggests that examining differences in allergen exposure, dietary differences, differences in parasitic load, infections, immunization rates, family size, water supply, pesticide residues and climatic differences, such as ultraviolet exposure and humidity, may all be worthwhile. Other simple studies which follow the short-term effects of children with AD who return to their country of origin (e.g. Afro-Caribbean children living in the UK returning to Jamaica for holidays) may tell us something about the effects that short-term exposures such as climate might have on AD. Conversely, studies of people with latent atopic disease who travel from a hot, humid country and who spend a long period in a cooler climate (e.g. Malaysian people who come to England to study) may be another interesting group to study.

As Godfrey points out in Chapter 9, we must not be constrained into thinking only about environment or genetics in a binary fashion. Factors operating in the intra-uterine or perinatal environment may also be critical. It is also possible that some 'dormant' genes may be aroused by environmental factors on migration to a new environment, i.e. the changes in disease risk experienced by people who migrate to a new country might be activated through genetic mechanisms which mediate a range of phenomena such as allergic hyper-responsiveness. Such genetic–environmental interaction may demonstrate 'fatigue' with increasing duration of residence in a new country and in subsequent generations. Better genetic markers of atopy, atopic dermatitis and disease severity are obstacles which need to be overcome before much progress can be made in this

Table 13.6. Recommendations for future migrant studies of atopic dermatitis

Migrant studies of atopic dermatitis should:
(1) Be population based
(2) Use valid and repeatable diagnostic criteria
(3) Include more than one measure of disease
(4) Use identical methods of sampling and disease definitions at both sites
(5) Measure ethnic group and not race
(6) Include objective tests of atopy
(7) Include measures of asthma and hay fever
(8) Define age at, and duration of, migration
(9) Record parental ethnic group and atopic status
(10) Consider the time for an exposure to exert its effect.

field. Recommendations for future studies of migrant groups are suggested in Table 13.6.

Acknowledgments

We wish to thank the Wellcome Trust and the British Skin Foundation for supporting the work on which much of this chapter is based.

Summary of points

- Migrant studies offer a powerful means for pointing to the relative contribution of environmental versus genetic factors in the aetiology of atopic dermatitis (AD).
- Genetic and environmental factors are likely to work in concert rather than in competition.
- Migrant studies may also indicate whether timing of migration is important in determining disease expression.
- Studies of variation in AD prevalence according to ethnic group in one country are not true migrant studies, but they may hint that further migrant studies may be worthwhile.
- Most migrant studies of AD to date have suffered from flaws in study design such as unclear sampling frames and disease definitions.
- Three studies have shown that populations who migrate from countries where there is a low preva-

lence of AD, assume disease rates which are similar or higher than those already living in the adopted country.
- Collectively, migrant studies suggest that environmental factors may be critical in AD expression.
- Possible 'risk factors' worthy of further exploration in migrant studies include differences in exposure to aeroallergens, differences in diet, climate, microbial colonization and health-related behaviour.
- Future migrant studies for AD should be population-based, use validated diagnostic criteria for diagnosing cases, record the timing and duration of migration and ethnic group of both parents.
- The identification of migrant groups who develop high rates of AD and related diseases provides us with a unique opportunity to evaluate interventions which could reduce such high disease rates.

References

Arruda, L. & Chapman, M.D. (1992). A review of recent immunochemical studies of *Blomia tropicalis* and *Europglyphus maynei* allergens. *Exp Appl Acarology*, **16**, 129–40.

Azuonye, I.O. (1996). Who is 'black' in medical research? *Br Med J*, **313**, 760.

Barker, D.J.P. & Rose, G. (1984). *Epidemiology in Medical Practice*. London: Churchill Livingstone.

Behrendt, H., Krämer, U., Dolgner, P. et al. (1993). Elevated levels of total serum IgE in East German children: atopy, parasites, or pollutants? *Allergol J*, **2**, 31–40.

Bentham, G. (1988). Migration and morbidity: implications for geographical studies of disease. *Soc Sci Med*, **26**, 49–54.

Bobák, M., Koupilová, I., Williams, H.C. et al. (1995). Prevalence of asthma, atopic eczema and hay fever in five Czech towns with different levels of air pollution. *Epidemiology*, **6**, S35.

Buell, P. & Dunn, J. (1965). Cancer mortality among Japanese Issei and Nisei of California. *Cancer*, **18**, 656–64.

Burrell-Morris, C.E., LaGrenade, L., Williams, H.C. & Hay, R. (1997). The prevalence of atopic dermatitis in black Caribbean children in London and Kingston, Jamaica. *Br J Dermatol*, **137** (Suppl. 50), 22.

Casimir, G.J.A., Duchateau, J., Gossart, B., Cuvelier, Ph., Vandaele, F. & Vis, H.L. (1993). Atopic dermatitis: role of food and house dust mite allergens. *Pediatrics*, **92**, 252–6.

Coloff, M.J. (1992). Exposure to house dust mites in homes of people with atopic dermatitis. *Br J Dermatol*, **127**, 322–7.

David, T.J. (ed.) (1993). Triggers of atopic eczema. In *Food and Food Additive Intolerance in Childhood*, pp. 319–36. Oxford: Blackwell Scientific.

Davis, L.R., Martin, R.H. & Sarkany, I. (1961). Atopic eczema in European and negro West Indian infants in London. *Br J Dermatol*, **73**, 410–14.

Feather, I.H., Warner, J.A., Holgate, S.T., Thompson, P.J. & Stewart, G.A. (1993). Cohabiting with domestic mites. *Thorax*, **48**, 5–9.

Fergusson, D.M., Horwood, L.J. & Shannon, F.T. (1982). Risk factors in childhood eczema. *J Epidemiol Comm Hlth*, **36**, 118–22.

George, S., Berth-Jones, J. & Graham-Brown, R.A.C. (1997). A possible explanation for the increased referral of atopic dermatitis from the Asian community in Leicester. *Br J Dermatol*, **136**, 494–7.

Gergen, P.J., Turkeltaub, P. C. & Kovar, M.G. (1987). The prevalence of allergic skin test reactivity to eight common aeroallergens in the US population: results from the second National Health and Nutrition Examination Survey. *J Allergy Clin Immunol*, **80**, 669–79.

Golding, J. & Peters, T. (1987). The epidemiology of childhood eczema. I: A population based study of associations. *Paediat Perinatal Epidemiol*, **1**, 67–79.

Grove, D.I. & Forbes, I.J. (1975). Increased resistance to helminth infestation in an atopic population. *Med J Aust*, **1**, 336–8.

Hansen, R.L., Marx, J.J., Twiggs, J.T. & Gray, R.L. (1991). House dust mites in the West Indies. *Ann Allergy*, **66**, 320–3.

Hauser, C. (1986). The role of *Staphylococcus aureus* in atopic eczema. *Int J Dermatol*, **25**, 573–4.

Kalyoncu, A.F. & Stålenhein, G. (1992). Serum IgE levels and allergic spectra in immigrants to Sweden. *Allergy*, **47**, 277–80.

Kanwar, A.J. & Dhar, S. (1995). Frequency and significance of major and minor clinical features of atopic dermatitis. *Dermatology*, **190**, 317.

Khlat, M., Vail, A., Parkin, M. & Green, A. (1992). Mortality from melanoma in migrants to Australia: variation by age at arrival and duration of stay. *Am J Epidemiol*, **135**, 1103–13.

Kolonel, L.N., Abraham, M.Y. et al. (1981). Association of diet and place of birth with stomach cancer incidence in Hawaii Japanese and Caucasians. *Am J Clin Nutr*, **34**, 2478–85.

Lawrence, A.W.W. & Segree, W. (1981). The prevalence of allergic disease in Jamaican adolescents. *West Indian Med J*, **30**, 86–9.

Leung, R. & Ho, P. (1994). Asthma, allergy, and atopy in three south-east Asian populations. *Thorax*, **49**, 1205–10.

Mar, A. & Marks, R. (1998). The frequency of atopic dermatitis amongst ethnic Chinese, Vietnamese and Caucasian infants in Australia. *J Invest Dermatol*, **110**, 195.

Neame, R.L., Berth-Jones, J., Kurinczuk, J.J. & Graham-Brown, R.A.C. (1995). Prevalence of atopic dermatitis in Leicester: a study of methodology and examination of possible ethnic variation. *Br J Dermatol*, **132**, 772–7.

Norris, P.G., Schofield, O. & Camp, R.D.R. (1988). A study of the role of house dust mite in atopic eczema. *Br J Dermatol*, **118**, 434–40.

Peters, T. & Golding, J. (1987). The epidemiology of childhood eczema: II: Statistical analyses to identify independent early predictors. *Paediat Perinatal Epidemiol*, **1**, 80–94.

Platts-Mills, T.A.E., Mitchell, E.B., Rowntree, S. et al. (1983). The role of house dust mite allergens in atopic dermatitis. *Clin Exp Dermatol*, **8**, 233.

Riedel, F. (1991). Environmental pollution and atopy. In: Ruzicka, T., Ring, J. & Pryzbilla, B. (eds.) *Handbook of Atopic Eczema*, pp. 319–22. Berlin: Springer-Verlag.

Saarinen, U.M. & Kajosaari, M. (1995). Breastfeeding as prophylaxis against atopic disease: prospective follow-up study until 17 years old. *Lancet*, **346**, 1065–9.

Schultz Larsen, F. (1986). Atopic dermatitis – a genetic epidemiologic study in a population-based twin sample. *J Am Acad Dermatol*, **15**, 487–94.

Schultz Larsen, F., Holm, N.V. & Henningsen, K. (1986). Atopic dermatitis. A genetic–epidemiological study in a population-based twin sample. *J Am Acad Dermatol*, **15**, 487–94.

Silver, S.E. (1992). Melanocytic nevus density in Asian, Indo-Pakistani, and white children. *J Am Acad Dermatol*, **27**, 277–8.

Sladden, M.J., Dure-Smith, B., Berth-Jones, J. & Graham-Brown, R.A.C. (1991). Ethnic differences in the pattern of skin disease seen in a dermatology department – atopic dermatitis is more common among Asian referrals in Leicestershire. *Clin Exp Dermatol*, **16**, 348–9.

Strachan, D.P. (1989). Hay fever, hygiene, and household size. *Br Med J*, **299**, 1259–60.

Syme, S.L., Marmot, M.G. et al. (1975). Epidemiologic studies of coronary heart disease and stroke in Japanese men living in Japan, Hawaii and California: introduction. *Am J Epidemiol*, **102**, 477–90.

Tan, B.B., Strickland, I., Weald, D. et al. (1995). House dust mite allergen avoidance in atopic dermatitis: a double blind controlled study. *Br J Dermatol*, **133** (Suppl. 45), 18.

Turner, K.J., Stewart, G.A., Woolcock, A.J., Green, W. & Alpers, M.P. (1988). Relationship between mite densities and the prevalence of asthma: comparative studies in two populations in the Eastern Highlands of Papua New Guinea. *Clin Allergy*, **18**, 331–40.

Turton, J.A. (1976). IgE, parasites and allergy. *Lancet*, **2**, 686.

Waite, D.A., Eyles, E.F., Tonkin, S.L. & O'Donnell, T.V. (1980).

Asthma prevalence in Tokelauan children in two environments. *Clin Allergy*, **10**, 71–5.

Williams, H.C. (1995). Atopic eczema: we should look to the environment, *Br Med J*, **311**, 1241–2.

Williams, H.C., Pembroke, A.C., Forsdyke, H., Boodoo, G. et al. (1995). London-born black Caribbean children are at increased risk of atopic dermatitis. *J Am Acad Dermatol*, **32**, 212–17.

Williams, H.C., Robertson, C.F., Stewart, A.W. et al. (1999). Worldwide variations in the prevalence of symptoms of atopic eczema in the international study of asthma and allergies in childhood. *J Allergy Clin Immunol*, **103**, 125–38.

Worth, R.M. (1962). Atopic dermatitis among Chinese infants in Honolulu and San Francisco. *Hawaiian Med J*, **22**, 31–6.

Worth, R.M., Kato, H. et al. (1975). Epidemiologic studies of coronary heart disease and stroke in Japanese men living in Japan, Hawaii and California: mortality. *Am J Epidemiol*, **102**, 481–2.

14

The role of inhalant allergens in atopic dermatitis

Harriett Kolmer and Thomas A.E. Platts-Mills

Introduction

It was only after considerable resistance that the name for this form of eczema was changed from 'Besnier's prurigo' – a title reflective of merely the predominant symptom – to 'atopic dermatitis' (AD) which more aptly describes the underlying nature of the disease. Acceptance of this new name in the 1930s reflected not only the growing awareness of an association between the disease and other manifestations of atopy but also the view that exposure to allergens played a significant role in the disease (Atherton, 1981; Sulzberger & Vaughan, 1934; Rost, 1932). In the last century, Vidal reported the association between asthma and a type of dermatitis (Vidal, 1886), and in 1923 Coca suggested a familial role for the development of asthma, eczema and allergic rhinitis (Coca & Cooke, 1923). In 1949, Tuft reported that most adult patients with AD had positive skin tests to autologous house dust (Tuft, 1949). He went on to demonstrate both exacerbation of eczema with inhaled dust, as well as improvement of skin symptoms when houses were 'cleaned'.

Despite the mounting evidence that allergens played a role in the disease, considerable scepticism remained, largely based on (but not limited to) the observation that immunotherapy with suspected allergens failed to elicit improvement in patients' symptoms. This finding could have been attributed to lack of specificity of the allergens used (for example, house dust was simply a 'black liquid' since dust mites were yet to be discovered). These arguments blocked further understanding and investiga-

tion of the allergic aetiology of eczema for many years. Today, with the development of techniques to better define specific allergens, and a clearer understanding of the pathogenesis of eczema, the role of allergens can be studied in detail. It is important to remember, of course, that AD is multifactorial and needs to be approached in this way if successful management is to be achieved.

To further understand the relevance of allergens in AD, we will review the relationship between immunoglobulin E (IgE) levels and AD, results of patch tests in atopic individuals, and the more recent findings related to serum eosinophil cationic protein (ECP) levels in these patients. We will then discuss in more detail the specific inhalant allergens implicated in the disease, namely: dust mites, moulds, pollens, animal dander and, finally, cockroach allergen.

Relationship to immunopathology

Serum IgE concentrations

With the discovery of IgE by Ishizaka in 1967 and the development of the radioallergosorbent test (RAST) in 1971 by Wide and Johannson, it became clear that at least 80% of patients with AD had elevated levels of these antibodies (Juhlin, 1969). Ogawa et al. reported an association between IgE levels and severity of disease which has been supported in subsequent studies (Ogawa et al., 1971; Jones et al., 1974). Furthermore, early studies established that the patients had specific IgE antibodies to a range of

Table 14.1. Cellular infiltrate in the eczematous response to repeated application of aqueous allergen to a patch test over ten days.

Patch applied	Time of biopsy	Basophils	Mast	Eosinophils	Monophils	Neutrophils	Total
Saline	2 days	2	46	0	303	16	367
Der p I	2 days	26	56	337	795	37	1251
Der p I	6 days	22	77	1249	833	13	2194
Der p I	10 days	21	113	96	932	9	1171

Note:

* 5 μg Der p I was applied on a patch of gauze to three separate sites and was reapplied every two days. Biopsies carried out with a 4 mm patch biopsy were fixed with Karnovsky, embedded in plastic and stained with Giemsa. Values for a representative patient.

allergens that are present in the air both outdoors and indoors. With the purification of cat and mite allergens, it was found that AD patients have both specific IgE and IgG antibodies to these allergens, supporting the view that the raised total IgE is part of a specific immune response (Chapman et al., 1983). Nevertheless, there are some confounding issues in the association of high IgE levels and AD. Many of the patients with AD also have respiratory allergy, and some reports have suggested that the 20% of AD patients without elevated levels of IgE represent those with AD alone, without co-existent allergic rhinitis and/or asthma (Jones et al., 1974). Other groups, however, liken the normal or low IgE level seen in some AD patients to the finding of low IgE levels in patients with intrinsic asthma (Leung & Geha, 1986). In our own studies we have identified patients having no respiratory tract symptoms who have very high IgE (Chapman et al., 1983). Confusing the issue, however, is the finding of elevated IgE levels in other dermatoses, such as cutaneous T-cell lymphoma, scabies and psoriasis, as well as helminthic infestations in many developing countries (Guerevitch, Heiner & Reiner, 1973). The elevated IgE in scabies reflects immediate hypersensitivity to *Sarcoptes scabeii*, which is a close relative of Dermatophagoides and has considerable antigenic cross-reactivity (Arlian et al., 1984). The specific IgE antibodies found in AD patients also tend to correlate well with IgG_4 levels, in keeping with the evidence for a specific response of the Th2 type (Chapman et al., 1983). It remains possible that ele-

vated IgE levels in AD patients are simply an incidental finding or are a consequence of altered B-cell regulation. However, it is more likely that they are directly relevant to the pathogenesis of the disease.

Results of patch tests

Exacerbation of skin rash in AD patients has been reported following allergen challenge by nasal provocation, bronchial provocation and skin testing. None of these approaches, however, provided a consistent model in which the response of the skin to allergen exposure could be studied. Indeed, it was often argued that allergens produced an 'urticarial' response in the skin. Perhaps the best technique reported so far for studying the role of inhalant allergens in AD has been the patch test. Mitchell et al., using a technique of 'stripping' the skin (to remove the lipid barrier that would normally prevent penetration of proteins of molecular weight 10 000–35 000) and then applying a patch containing 5 μg of purified mite allergen, found a consistently eczematous response in AD patients at 48 hours (Mitchell et al., 1982). This finding was limited to AD patients who gave a positive immediate skin reaction to the same allergen. Subsequent studies have confirmed the finding of positive patch test results in AD patients. One study, performed in paediatric patients with AD using patch tests of house dust mite, cockroach, mould mix and grass mix, induced an eczematous response in 90% of the children tested with AD. The control group, atopic children without AD, developed an eczematous response in only 10% of the cases, yielding an impressive p value of $<10^{-6}$ (Wananukul, Huiprasert & Pongprasit, 1993).

Biopsy of patch test responses has shown cellular infiltrates of eosinophils and mononuclear cells (Mitchell et al., 1982; Bruijnzeel-Koomen et al., 1988; Henoque & Vargaftig, 1988). Mitchell et al. also reported the finding of basophils in biopsies from patch reactions, although this finding has not been reproduced in all other studies (Mitchell et al., 1982; Bruijnzeel-Koomen et al., 1988; Henoque & Vargaftig, 1988; Reitamo et al., 1986; Gondo, Saeki & Tokuda, 1986). The finding of eosinophils in patch tests was surprising since eosinophils are not present in biopsies of naturally occurring eczematous skin lesions. When the patch test was extended by reapplying allergen every two days, the biopsies showed a progressive increase in eosinophils up to the sixth day but a dramatic decrease at ten days (Mitchell et al., 1986) (Table 14.1). This finding suggested that continued presence of antigen leads to degranulation of eosinophils with release of their toxic contents, substances that go on to perpetuate the eczematous lesions. This view is strongly supported by studies investigating eosinophil major basic protein (MBP) in lesions of patients with AD. Gleich and his colleagues found strong staining in skin biopsies using anti-MBP even though the skin did not have identifiable eosinophils (Leiferman et al., 1985).

Because eosinophils do not generally cause a significant change in the epidermis, one has to postulate that there is some other mechanism contributing to the lesions seen in AD. The finding of basophils in patch test biopsies was interesting, since basophils are typically found in a form of delayed hypersensitivity, and in animal models this recruitment is T-cell dependent. Using serum from patients with AD it was possible to demonstrate that the eosinophil response could be passively transferred with IgE antibody but that the local basophil response could only be transferred with whole serum (Mitchell et al., 1984) (Table 14.2). At present, this experiment is difficult to interpret since there is no general agreement about the existence of T-cell

Table 14.2. Local passive transfer patch test responses to mite allergen *Der p I*: cell count in the dermis after 48 hours*

Transfer	n	Basophils	Eosinophils	Neutrophils
Saline	8	0	1	6
		(0–4)	(0–2)	(0–31)
Serum	7	69	320[†]	59[NS]
		(12–161)	(20–560)	(3–200)
Heated serum	3	6	0	2
		(0–6)	(0–10)	(0–56)
Purified antibody	5	0	99	19
		(0–7)	(45–188)	(13–50)

Notes:

* Serum, saline or antibody was injected into the skin of nonatopic individuals: 24 hours later a patch of gauze containing 5 μg *Der p I* was applied to the site. Biopsies taken at 48 hours were fixed in Karnovsky, medium embedded in methocrylate and stained with Giemsa.

[†] $p < 0.02$ compared to biopsy of patch test following saline injection.

[NS] Not significant.

derived factors that could sensitize the skin to produce a local basophil infiltrate (Borish & Rosenwasser, 1997; Mitchell & Askenase, 1982). Furthermore, the interpretation of a passive transfer is changed by the recent demonstration that IgE antibody can bind to a high affinity receptor on Langerhans cells as well as mast cells (van der Heijden et al., 1993; Bruijnzeel-Koomen et al., 1991).

Clearly, the results of the patch test model support a role for inhalant allergens in the exacerbation and pathophysiology of AD. While it has been shown that eosinophils play a role in this response, the role of mast cells, basophils and T cells is less clear. The issue of whether inhalant allergen-induced inflammation of the skin involves a direct role for T cells remains undecided.

Eosinophilic cationic protein (ECP)

As mentioned above, eosinophil-derived proteins have been found in lesions of patients with AD, even when eosinophils are not visible (Leiferman et al., 1985). More recently, serum ECP levels have been found to be significantly elevated in patients with AD, with levels correlating well with disease activity (Kapp, 1993; Kapp et al., 1991; Czech et al., 1992). Kapp, furthermore, showed that improvement in disease is associated with a decrease of the ECP level (Kapp, 1993). Interestingly, ECP concentrations did not correlate well with the eosinophil count, leading those authors to speculate that the ECP level reflects the activation state of the eosinophil pool rather than a quantitative assessment of eosinophils (Kapp, 1993). Comparing serum ECP levels in AD patients to levels in normal controls and psoriasis patients, they also found a slight increase in some psoriasis patients, although the finding was not statistically significant compared with normal controls. Those authors proposed that ECP is not a nonspecific indicator of skin inflammation but rather is a marker for allergic pathogenesis in skin disease.

Inhalant allergens

Dust mites

As early as 1932, Rost reported that patients with eczema improved when living in dust-free environments (Rost, 1932). Later, Tuft confirmed that most patients improved when taken out of their homes (Tuft, 1949). Despite an impressive amount of anecdotal support for the role of dust allergy in AD, only a few controlled trials have been published. Harving, in 1990, reported some success with a controlled trial of mite avoidance (Harving et al., 1990). True placebo-controlled trials have been difficult. First, it is difficult to standardize avoidance measures, and the degree to which avoidance is carried out by one individual is hard to quantitate. Secondly, there is a marked tendency for patients in both groups to change their cleaning habits, a bias which tends to conceal real responses to the treatment. Finally, one has to expect a large placebo response, which probably includes, but is not limited to, increased compliance with medications. Still, in our experience,

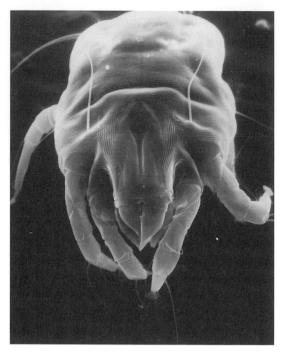

Fig. 14.1. Despite an impressive amount of anecdotal support for the role of dust allergy in AD, only a few controlled trials have been published

there is a subset of patients with severe AD who, despite evidence for immediate hypersensitivity to dust mite allergen, fail to improve even when moved to dust-free environments. The degree to which other factors such as bacterial skin infection, and possibly even fungal colonization of the skin are present probably explain this finding. Despite these problems, Tan et al. reported a controlled trial of dust mite avoidance measures in the treatment of AD, with significant decrease in symptoms and extent of rash (Tan et al., 1996). As with avoidance studies for asthma, there was a large placebo effect, but part of this reflects reduced exposure secondary to increased cleaning by 'placebo' families.

Specific avoidance measures recommended for AD patients with dust mite hypersensitivity include covering the pillow, mattress and box springs with allergen-impermeable covers; removing carpeting (especially from the bedroom and main living area); keeping humidity as low as possible in the house;

and reducing the temperature to less than 70°F. Additionally, bedding should be washed in hot (≥130°F) water every 7–10 days. One could argue that focusing on avoidance measures in the bed is more important for dust mite allergic AD patients than those with respiratory allergy since the major organ involved, the skin, is in direct contact with the bedding. However, it is not clear whether inhalant allergens have their primary role as direct allergens applied to the skin, or whether inhalation and absorption through the respiratory tract is equally important. This second possible explanation is easy to propose, given our understanding of food allergens exacerbating eczema by absorption through the gastrointestinal mucosa. Indeed, some experience suggests that inhaled allergen is an important route by which the severe itching is induced (Tupker et al., 1996). Comparatively, the patch test produces only moderate itching.

In addition to patch test results involving dust mites, mentioned earlier in this chapter, further support for the role of these inhalant allergens has come from studies involving T-cell responses. Although no significant quantitative difference was found between proliferative responses in AD patients compared with those with respiratory allergy, there is no dispute that patients with AD have circulating T cells that proliferate in response to mite allergens (Rawle, Mitchell & Platts-Mills, 1984). These circulating T cells have the characteristics of Th2 cells which secrete IL-4 (important in IgE regulation) and IL-5 (important in eosinophil recruitment). It seems reasonable, therefore, to propose that allergen-specific T cells are a driving force behind the pathogenesis of AD.

Moulds

One of the earliest reports of a possible role for moulds in AD was by Hopkins in 1930. He reported worsening of skin rash in an AD patient following the inhalation of Alternaria (Hopkins, Kesten & Benham, 1930). Rajka confirmed this finding in several AD patients, demonstrating the induction of eczematous lesions following inhalation of a mould

mix extract (Rajka, 1963). Additionally, exacerbations of eczema have been noted in some reports to occur during seasons of elevated mould spore levels (Jillson & Adami, 1955). Patch test results have also supported a role for mould allergen in AD, although not to the degree that dust mite has been shown to be important. Wananukul reported that 50% of paediatric patients with AD had positive patch test results to a mould mix compared with only 7% of nonatopic children (Wananukul et al., 1993). In addition, there have been anecdotal reports of improvement in AD with mould immunotherapy although, again, controlled trials are necessary.

Pollens

Seasonal allergens such as ragweed and grass pollens have been implicated in AD in several case studies, the earliest of which was in 1918 by Walker. He reported two patients who demonstrated significant clearing of their skin following pollen avoidance. Both of these patients had been noted previously to suffer seasonal exacerbations (Walker, 1918). Tuft reported immediate itching of the skin in two ragweed allergic AD patients inhaling ragweed allergen, following by an exacerbation of skin rash that persisted for several days (Tuft & Heck, 1952). Despite these reports, we believe that the majority of patients with AD are not influenced by pollen seasons. This is supported by the observation that many AD patients actually improve during the spring and summer months (i.e. at the time when most pollen levels are elevated). This finding would seem to suggest that pollens are important in only a minority of cases, although in those cases results of challenges and avoidance interventions can be rather dramatic.

Animal dander

As with moulds and pollens, a clear role for animal dander in AD has been supported mainly by isolated reports rather than in large controlled trials. Walker, in addition to reporting a role for pollens in AD, also noted worsening of rash following inhalation of horse dander in a horse-allergic AD patient (Walker, 1918). More recent studies have reported elevated specific IgE to animal danders, namely cat or dog (Haatela & Jaakonmaki, 1981). Many patients will report an increase in pruritus when exposed to cat or dog danders in their environment, although the degree to which there is a psychological component here is not known. While it is possible that animal dander can act as a topical irritant, there is no doubt that many patients have very high titre IgE antibody to purified animal allergen. In our own experience, these patients improve when removed from exposure, but it remains to be shown that avoidance measures for animal dander in the home can produce improvement in AD (Warner, 1992).

Cockroach allergen

Although cockroach allergen has gained recent attention in its role in asthma (particularly asthma in inner-city children), its contribution to AD has only recently begun to be investigated (Call et al., 1992; Arruda et al., 1995; Wananukul et al., 1993). In the paediatric study mentioned earlier in this chapter, positive intradermal reactions to cockroach were found in 86% of paediatric AD patients. Additionally, 70% of these children had positive patch test results to cockroach (Wananukul et al., 1993). Because purification of the allergens has been fairly recent, further studies dealing solely with cockroach allergy and AD have yet to be done. Given its fairly impressive role in asthma, however, one might predict that cockroach allergen may come to be seen as playing an important role in AD, particularly among inner-city patients.

Serum IgE antibodies as epidemiological risk factors for atopic dermatitis

In general, it has been very difficult to carry out epidemiological studies of AD, because it is difficult to define eczema objectively in a study based on questionnaires. Two studies have suggested that exposure to allergens contributes to the early development of eczema. Arshad & Hide (1992)

Table 14.3. Prevalence and quantities of total IgE and specific IgE antibodies in patients with atopic dermatitis, asthma and controls (data from Scalabrin et al., 1999)

	AD ($n = 65$)	Asthma ($n = 70$)	Controls ($n = 70$)
Mean serum total IgE (IU/ml)	2640	135.5	40.5
IgE ab to D. pteronyssinis (IU/ml)	143*[†] (88%)	1.05 (17%)	0.62 (16%)
IgE ab to Alternaria	3.74 (49%)	1.14 (26%)	0.77 (16%)
IgE ab to P. ovale	2.19 (41%)*[†]	<0.03 (0%)	<0.03 (0%)

Notes:

* IgE ab to D. pteronyssinis expressed as a percentage of total IgE was significantly higher in patients with AD compared with asthma or controls.

[†] The prevalence of IgE antibodies significantly higher than controls.

reported the effect of dust mite exposure while Bener et al. (1995) reported evidence on the effects of pet ownership. Although dermatitis is common in early childhood (i.e. ~10%), the disease in its more severe form is not common enough to obtain data through population-based studies on schoolchildren. In addition, random presentation to an emergency room is not a common event. Thus, populations of patients are most often obtained from referrals to a dermatology or allergy clinic. Studies based on referral to subspecialty clinics should be interpreted with care because the severe patients may not reflect the population in general. However, with a large enough patient base (i.e. ≥50) it is possible to compare patients with eczema to random populations of normal controls or individuals presenting to an ER with asthma. Results were recently reported for mite, Alternaria, *Pitirosporium ovale* and Trichophyton (Bavbek et al., 1997) (Table 14.3). The results provide three models that illustrate the difficulty of evaluating positive serology.

IgE antibodies to dust mite allergens were present in ~85% of the patients with AD. Both the prevalence of raised IgE and the mean concentration were higher than in asthmatics and controls. The concentration of IgE antibody to mite in sera from patients with AD was ~100 fold greater than in the other patients. Furthermore, IgE antibody to mite as a percentage of total IgE was significantly higher than in the other groups. For Alternaria, IgE antibodies were present in a large proportion of sera from patients with AD, and the levels were higher than in the other two groups. However, neither the prevalence nor the absolute levels were as high as for IgE antibody to dust mites. When IgE antibody to Alternaria was expressed relative to total IgE, the levels in patients with AD were not higher than in patients with asthma or controls. As has been reported elsewhere, IgE antibodies to *P. ovale* are common in patients with AD. However, by contrast with Alternaria, in our study these antibodies were not found in sera from asthmatics or controls. Finally, IgE and IgG antibodies to Trichophyton were not significantly associated with AD. Thus, the interpretation of positive IgE antibodies should consider how common these antibodies are in other patients, the absolute levels and the quantity of IgE antibody relative to total IgE. Judged by these standards sensitization to dust mite and *P. ovale* were very strongly associated with AD.

The time course of atopic dermatitis

Exposure to allergens starts before birth since it is quite clear that food allergens can be absorbed and can be transferred across the placenta. After birth, food antigen exposure occurs through eating or through breast milk. Given the quantities inhaled per day, i.e. ~5–50 ng of mite allergen *Der p I*, it seems very unlikely that the fetus is exposed to sufficient mite allergen to produce an immune response before birth. The T-cell proliferative responses that have been reported in cord blood have not convincingly been shown to relate to exposure or to a subsequent allergic response. Exposure to dust mite and other indoor allergens is generally low in the first few months. Obviously, the great majority of children do not go on to develop allergic disease and only a small minority, i.e. ~1%, have persistent trouble with AD. This makes prospective studies difficult and also implies that most children reach a state of 'tolerance'. For food antigens it is clear that the infant, and subsequently the child, is exposed to sufficient allergen to produce an immune response. Thus, the nonallergic state must indeed be tolerance. By contrast, for inhalant allergens including dust mites, exposure is low or very low and the nonallergic state may be either some form of tolerance or a failure to make an immune response. In general, antibodies to mite allergens become measurable only in allergic children during the third year of life (Sporik et al., 1990). Specific T cells are present in allergic children but different groups have provided different answers about their presence in the blood of nonallergic individuals (Rawle et al., 1984). In children with AD T-cell responses are exaggerated and antibody levels are very high. The problem is to understand how the normal processes of tolerance become deregulated. At present, it is not clear whether severe AD develops because of excessive environmental exposure, infection of the skin, or some other event that leads to an exaggerated immune response and the associated excessive inflammatory response in the skin.

Conclusions

Louis Tuft concluded that sensitization to foods was the major factor in AD in young children but that by the age of seven years most patients were sensitive to inhalants (Tuft, 1949). Since the discovery of IgE most of his observations have been confirmed – in particular, the prevalence of IgE antibodies to inhalants and the effect of reducing exposure to house dust (Chapman et al., 1983; Platts-Mills et al., 1983; Adinoff & Clark, 1989). Taken together, the case that inhalants contribute to AD is extremely strong:

(1) Patients with AD have very high titre IgE antibodies to dust mites and other inhalants. In keeping with this they have specific T cells of the Th2 type and specific IgG_4 antibodies.

(2) Application of dust mite allergens to the skin can produce a patch of eczema with a marked infiltrate including eosinophils, basophils and T cells. In uncontrolled experiments, inhaling allergens can exacerbate the skin rash.

(3) Reducing exposure to dust mite allergens produces improvement in the rash. This has been demonstrated both with hospital admission and in controlled trials of avoidance measures in the patients' houses.

Atopic dermatitis, like all allergic diseases, ranges from mild (or very mild) to severe and sometimes debilitating. In mild cases a change in the environment or modest doses of topical steroids may provide adequate treatment. Among cases with moderate disease careful avoidance of dust mite allergens has been proven to be effective treatment (Tan et al., 1996), and it is safe to assume that avoidance measures can help with other inhalants. However, as cases become more severe they also become more complex with multiple factors contributing to severity. It is well recognized that skin infection with *Staphylococcus aureus* can exacerbate the disease. However, it is less well recognized that colonization of the skin with so-called 'nonpathogenic bacteria' or a wide range of fungi, may contribute to the disease. Thus, managing the most severe cases may require attention to dietary factors, control of environmental exposure, antibiotics and even anti-fungal treatment (Kolmer et al., 1996). Establishing specific sensitization of patients with AD to inhalants and foods using skin testing or in vitro assays should be a routine part of treatment. The results should be used to help in defining which allergens should be avoided.

Summary of key points

- Chronic pruritic eczema in children and adults is called atopic dermatitis (AD) because it is very strongly associated with other atopic diseases such as allergic rhinitis and extrinsic asthma.
- A large proportion of patients with AD who are over the age of five years have evidence of immediate hypersensitivity to dust mites and/or other common allergens found in house dust.

- The immune response to mite proteins such as *Der p 1* and *Der p 2* includes T cells which characteristically produce IL-4 and IL-5, as well as IgG$_4$ and IgE antibodies.

- The evidence that exposure to common indoor allergens contributes to the disease comes from:

(1) The association between high levels of IgE antibodies to mites and this skin disease.

(2) Patch test showing that application of allergens to the skin can produce an eczematous response over 24–48 hours.

(3) Seasonal exacerbations of dermatitis.

(4) Evidence that reducing exposure to dust mites by simple techniques in the home can improve symptoms and skin lesions.

Acknowledgment

The research for this work was supported by NIH Grants AI 30840 and AI 34607.

References

Adinoff, A.D. & Clark, R.A.E. (1989). The allergic nature of atopic dermatitis. *Immunol Allergy Pract*, **ii**, 17–28.

Arlian, L.G., Geis, D.P., Vyszenski-Moher, D.L., Bernstein, I.L. & Gallagher, J.S. (1984). Crossed antigenic and allergenic properties of the house dust mite *Dermatophagoides farinae* and the storage mite *Tyrophagus putrescentiae*. *J Allergy Clin Immunol*, **74**, 172–9.

Arruda, L.K., Vailes, L.D., Mann, B.J., Shannon, J., Fox, J.W., Vedvick, T.S., Hayden, M.L. & Chapman, M.D. (1995). Molecular cloning of a major cockroach (Blattelle germanica) allergen, Bla g 2: sequence homology to the aspartic proteases. *J Biol Chem*, **270**, 19563–8.

Arshad, S.H. & Hide, D.W. (1992). Effect of environment factors on the development of allergic disorders in infancy. *J Allergy Clin Immunol*, **90**, 235–41.

Atherton, D.J. (1981). Allergy and atopic eczema, I and II. *Clin Exp Dermatol*, **6**, 191, 317–26.

Bavbek, S., Woodfolk, J., Scalabrin, D. & Platts-Mills, T.A.E. (1997). Fungal allergen specific IgE Ab in patients with atopic dermatitis. *J Allergy Clin Immunol*, **99**, No. 1, Part 2.

Bener, A., Galadari, I. & Naser, K.A. (1995). Pets allergy and respiratory symptoms in children living in a desert country. *Allergie et Immunologie*, **27**, 190–95.

Borish, L. & Rosenwasser, L. (1997). T_{H1}/T_{H2} lymphocytes: doubt some more. *J Allergy Clin Immunol*, **99**, 161–4.

Bruijnzeel-Koomen, C.A.F.M., van Wichesn, D.F., Spry, C.J.F., Venge, P. & Bruijnzeel, P.L.B. (1988). Active participation of eosinophils in patch test reactions to inhalant allergens in patients with atopic dermatitis. *Br J Dermatol*, **1118**, 229–38.

Bruijnzeel-Koomen, C.A.F.M., Mudde, G., Bruijnzeel, P. & Beiber, T. (1991). IgE receptors on Langerhans cells: their significance in the pathophysiology of atopic eczema. In: Rozicka, T., Ring, J. & Przybilla, B. (eds.) *Handbook of Atopic Eczema*, pp. 154–65. London: Springer-Verlag.

Call, R.S., Smith, T.F., Morris, E., Chapman, M.D. & Platts-Mills, T.A.E. (1992). Risk factors for asthma in inner city children. *J Pediat*, **121**, 862–6.

Chapman, M.D., Rowntree, S., Mitchell, E.B., Di Priso de Fuenmajor, M.C. & Platts-Mills, T.A.E. (1983). Quantitative assessments of IgG and IgE antibodies to inhalant allergens in patients with atopic dermatitis. *J Allergy Clin Immunol*, **72**, 27–33.

Coca, A. & Cooke, R. (1923). On the classification of the phenomena of hypersensitiveness. *J Immunol*, **8**, 163–82.

Czech, W., Krutmann, J., Schopf, E. & Kapp, A. (1992). Serum eosinophilic cationic protein (ECP) is a sensitive measure for disease activity in atopic dermatitis. *Br J Dermatol*, **126**, 351–5.

Gondo, A., Saeki, N. & Tokuda, Y. (1986). Challenge reactions in atopic dermatitis after percutaneous entry of mite allergen. *J Dermatol*, **115**, 485–93.

Guerevitch, A., Heiner, D. & Reiner, R. (1973). IgE in atopic dermatitis and other common dermatoses. *Arch Dermatol Forsch*, **2**, 712–15.

Haatela, T. & Jaakonmaki, I. (1981). Relationship of allergen-specific IgE antibodies, skin prick tests and allergic disorders in unselected adolescents. *Allergy*, **36**, 251–6.

Harving, H., Korsgaard, J., Dahl, R., Beck, H.I. & Bjerring, P. (1990). House dust mites and atopic dermatitis. A case-control study on the significance of house dust mites as etiologic allergens in atopic dermatitis. *Ann Allergy*, **65**, 25–31.

Henoque, E. & Vargaftig, B.B. (1988). Skin eosinophilia in atopic dermatitis. *J Allergy Clin Immunol*, **81**, 691–5.

Hopkins, J., Kesten, B. & Benham, R. (1930). Sensitization to saprophytic fungi in a case of eczema. *Proc Soc Exp Biol Med*, **27**, 342–4.

Jillson, O. & Adami, M. (1955). Allergic dermatitis produced by inhalant molds. *Arch Dermatol*, **72**, 411–19.

Jones, H.E., Inouye, J.C., McGerity, J.L. & Lewis, C.W. (1974). Atopic disease and serum immunoglobulin E. *Br J Dermatol*, **92**, 17–25.

Juhlin, L., Johansson, G.O., Bennich, H., Hogman, C. & Thyresson, N. (1969). Immunoglobulin E in dermatoses. *Arch Dermatol*, **100**, 12–16.

Kapp, A., Czech, W., Krutmann, J. & Schopf, E. (1991). Eosinophil cationic protein in sera of patients with atopic dermatitis. *J Am Acad Dermatol*, **24**, 555–8.

Kapp, A. (1993). The role of eosinophils in the pathogenesis of atopic dermatitis – eosinophil granule proteins as markers of disease activity. *Allergy*, **48**, 1–5.

Kolmer, H.L., Taketomi, E.A., Hazen, K.C., Hughs, E., Wilson, B.B. & Platts-Mills, T.A.E. (1996). Effect of combined antibacterial and antifugal treatment in severe atopic dermatitis. *J Allergy Clin Immunol*, **98**, 702–7.

Leiferman, K.M., Ackerman, S.J., Sampson, H.A., Haugen, H.S., Venencie, P.Y. & Gleich, G.J. (1985). Dermal deposition of eosinophil granule major basic protein in atopic dermatitis. *N Engl J Med*, **313**, 282–5.

Leung, D. & Geha, R. (1986). Immunoregulatory abnormalities in atopic dermatitis. *Clin Rev Allergy*, **4**, 47–86.

Mitchell, E.B., & Askenase, P.W. (1982). Suppression of T cell mediated cutaneous basophil hypersensitivity by serum from guinea pigs immunized with meobacterial adjuvant. *J Exp Med*, **156**, 159–72.

Mitchell, E.B., Crow, J., Chapman, M.D., Jouhal, S.S., Pope, F.M. & Platts-Mills, T.A.E. (1982). Basophils in allergen-induced patch tests sites in atopic dermatitis. *Lancet* i, 127–301.

Mitchell, E.B., Crow, J., Rowntree, S., Webster, A.D. & Platts-Mills, T.A.E. (1984). Cutaneous basophil hypersensitivity to inhalant allergens: local transfer of basophil accumulation with immune serum but not IgE antibody. *J Invest Dermatol*, **83**, 290–5.

Mitchell, E.B., Crow, J., Williams, G. & Platts-Mills, T.A.E. (1986). Increase in skin mast cells following chronic house dust mite exposure. *Br J Dermatol*, **114**, 65–73.

Ogawa, M., Berger, P.A., McIntyre, O.R., Clendenning, W.F. & Ishizaka, K. (1971). IgE in atopic dermatitis. *Arch Dermatol*, **103**, 578–80.

Platts-Mills, T.A.E., Mitchell, E.B., Rowntree, S., Chapman, M.D. & Wilkins, S.R. (1983). The role of dust mite allergens in atopic dermatitis. *Clin Exp Dermatol*, **8**, 233–47.

Rajka, G. (1963). Studies in hypersensitivity to molds and staphylococci in prurigo Besnier (atopic dermatitis). *Acta Derm Venereol*, **43**, Suppl. 54, 21–39, 86–102.

Rawle, F.C., Mitchell, F.B. & Platts-Mills, T.A.E. (1984). T cell responses to the major allergen from the house dust mite

Dermatophagoides pteronyssimus antigen P1: comparison of patients with asthma, atopic dermatitis, and perennial rhinitis. *J Immunol*, **133**, 195–201.

Reitamo, S., Visak, K., Kahonen, K., Kaynko, K., Stubbs, S. & Salo, O.P. (1986). Eczematous reactions in atopic patients caused by epicutaneous testing with inhalant allergens. *Br J Dermatol*, **114**, 303–9.

Rost, G.A. (1932). UberErfahrungen mit der alhergenfreien Kammer Nach Storm von Leeuwen: insbesondere in der Spatperiode der exsudatmen Diatnese. *Arch Dermatol Syphilol*, **155**, 297–308.

Scalabrin, D.M.F., Bavbek, S., Perzanowski, M.S., Wilson, B.B., Platts-Mills, T.A.E. & Wheatley, L.M. (1999). Use of specific IgE in assessing the relevance of fungal and dust mite allergens to atopic dermatitis: a comparison with asthmatic and non-asthmatic control. *J Allergy Clin Immunol*, In Press.

Sporik, R.B., Holgate, S.T., Platts-Mills, T.A.E. & Cogswell, J. (1990). Exposure to house dust mite allergen (Der p 1) and the development of asthma in childhood: a prospective study. *N Eng J Med*, **323**, 502–7.

Sulzberger, M.B. & Vaughan, W.T. (1934). Experiments in silk hypersensitivity and inhalation of allergen in atopic dermatitis (neurodermatitis disseminatus). *J Allergy*, **5**, 544–60.

Tan, B.B., Weald, D., Strickland, I. & Friedman, P.S. (1996). Double blind controlled trial of effect of housedust mite allergen avoidance on atopic dermatitis. *Lancet*, **347**, 15–18.

Tuft, L.A. (1949). Importance of inhalant allergen in atopic dermatitis. *J Invest Dermatol*, **12**, 211–19.

Tuft, L. & Heck, V. (1952). Studies in atopic dermatitis. IV. Importance of seasonal inhalant allergens, especially ragweed. *J Allergy*, **23**, 528–40.

Tupker, R.A., De Monchy, J.G.R., Coenraads, P.J., Homan, A. & Van De Meer, J. (1996). Induction of atopic dermatitis by inhalation of house dust mite. *J Allergy Clin Immunol*, **97**, 1064–70.

van der Heijden, F.L., Joost van Neerven, R.J., van Katwijk, M., Bos, J.D. & Kapsenberg, M.L. (1993). Serum IgE facilitated allergen presentation in atopic dermatitis. *J Immunol*, **150**, 3642–50.

Vidal, E. (1886). Du lichen (lichen, prurigo, strophulus). *Ann Dermat Syph*, **17**, 131–54.

Walker, C. (1918). Causation of eczema, urticaria and angioneurotic edema. *J Am Med Ass*, **70**, 897–900.

Wananukul, S., Huiprasert, P. & Pongprasit, P. (1993). Eczematous skin reaction from patch testing with aeroallergens in atopic children with and without atopic dermatitis. *Pediat Dermatol*, **10**, 209–13.

Warner, J.A. (1992). Environmental allergen exposure in homes and schools. *Clin Exp Allergy*, **22**, 1044–5.

15

Dietary factors in established atopic dermatitis

Tim J. David, Leena Patel, Carol I. Ewing and R.H.J. Stanton

Basic concepts

The first concept, the *terra firma*, is that in certain individuals, eating specific food triggers can cause preexisting atopic dermatitis (AD) to worsen. The second concept, which by no means follows from the first, is that avoidance of selected foods can cause AD to improve. This chapter tests the strength of the data that underpin these two assertions.

Food triggers can worsen preexisting atopic dermatitis

This concept is the result of two merged themes. The first is that some children with AD react adversely to certain foods. The second is that such reactions can cause worsening of preexisting dermatitis.

Some children with atopic dermatitis react adversely to foods

The key data come from Hugh Sampson and colleagues at Johns Hopkins Hospital in Baltimore, who used the double-blind placebo-controlled food challenge (DBPCFC) as a strategy to make the diagnosis of food allergy in children with AD. Despite great strengths, it is important to be aware of some inherent weaknesses in this study design.

In 1988, Sampson reported on 514 DBPCFCs in 160 selected patients with severe AD that was refractory to conventional therapy (Broadbent & Sampson, 1988; Sampson, 1988). The ages of the patients ranged from three months to 24 years, with

a median age of 5.3 years; 96% of patients had a family history of atopic disease. At the time of study, 21% of patients had AD as their sole atopic disease, while the remainder also had asthma, rhinitis or both. The serum IgE concentration was 'elevated' (the term was undefined) in 85%.

The way the patients were selected, or how they would compare with patients with AD seen in hospital in the UK, was unclear. 'Most' patients had a history of dermatitis dating back to infancy, and their condition was uncontrolled with regimens of lubricating creams, topical steroids and antihistamines (Sampson, 1987). 'About 75%' had been given systemic steroids on at least one occasion for control of skin symptoms (Sampson, 1987). 'Almost all' had been placed on 'various elimination diets' but 'without notable success' (Sampson, 1987).

Between 7 and 10 days before admission to hospital for study, suspected food triggers were avoided and antihistamines discontinued. Beta-agonists were stopped 12 hours before admission. No patient had received oral steroids for at least one month prior to admission.

On the day of admission, a battery of skin prick tests was performed, using commercial glycerinated extracts. A weal reaction 3 mm in diameter greater than the control was regarded as positive. There were 575 positive skin prick test results in 160 children evaluated. Egg, peanut, milk, wheat, soya and fish accounted for 56% of the positive skin tests. Foods such as strawberry, tomato, corn (maize) and chocolate 'rarely' elicited a positive result. Of the 575 positive skin test results, 334 (65%) were 'clinically insignificant or false positive' in diagnosing food allergy. Conversely a negative skin prick test 'was found to be an excellent means of excluding immediate food hypersensitivity in the pathogenesis of a patient's AD'.

Patients were often treated for several days with an intensive topical regimen to 'clear cutaneous erythema and pruritus' (Sampson, 1988). In this respect, these patients are different from the type of patient referred to hospital in the UK with refractory AD, in whom clearing of the lesions cannot easily be achieved with simple topical therapy.

For DBPCFCs, 400 to 500 mg dehydrated food per capsule was used (Sampson, 1983), and the food or placebo was administered to the patient on an empty stomach (Sampson, 1987). Up to 8 g of powdered food (up to 18 capsules per challenge) or up to 10 g in broth or juice (up to 150 ml per challenge) was given over a one-hour period. Two challenges were performed each day, one at 8 a.m. and one at 1 p.m. One of the daily challenges was with a placebo (sucrose or corn starch), and one was with a suspect food. Dietitians randomized the challenges, and the investigators were blinded. If there were no symptoms then the code was broken the following day, and the food given in an open fashion. Equivocal reactions, or those that occurred in individuals with negative skin prick test results, were repeated at least once. A standard sheet was used to score all studies.

All those who experienced a negative DBPCFC were fed the food openly before discharge to confirm the results of the DBPCFC. Three children, aged four years, four years and two years, had cutaneous reactions only after drinking milk openly. One child aged five developed symptoms after openly eating peas (Sampson, 1988).

DBPCFCs were not performed in 25 instances, on the basis of a previous history of an anaphylactic reaction to a food. In all cases the patient had a 'strongly positive' skin test to the food in question. The symptoms induced by food challenge all occurred within 10 to 90 minutes of the oral challenge. Cutaneous reactions occurred in 143 of 180 (79%) of positive challenges and consisted of pruritus and an erythematous, macular, maculopapular

or morbilliform rash involving 5% or more of the body area (Sampson, 1983; 1988). Skin symptoms occurred most commonly in areas where the patients' eczema lesions typically flared. Urticarial lesions were very uncommon (Sampson, 1983) and generally consisted of only two or three lesions (Sampson, 1988). Only 29% of challenges elicited exclusively cutaneous symptoms. Gastrointestinal symptoms occurred in 43% of challenges, and respiratory symptoms occurred in 28% of challenges. Most (78%) of the children with documented food hypersensitivity by DBPCFC were symptomatic to only one or two foods. Only 19% reacted to three foods, and only 3% reacted to four or more different foods. The numerator, the number of challenges that were done in each case, and the number of foods selected for DBPCFC, were not stated.

All reactions occurred within three hours of initiating the food challenge (Sampson, 1988). However, many patients who experienced immediate skin symptoms developed pruritus and, less frequently, a macular, pruritic rash in reaction sites six to eight hours after the initial response. Although pruritus associated with the immediate reaction was severe and generally short-lived (less than two hours), pruritus associated with the later response was less intense but longer lasting (often four to six hours) (Sampson, 1988).

Broadbent and Sampson concluded that 'the type of food the parents and child thought caused allergic symptoms was not predictive of which foods actually elicited a positive food challenge' (Broadbent & Sampson, 1988). Elsewhere it was concluded that routine laboratory studies, such as skin prick tests and RAST tests, were of 'marginal value in identifying children who will exhibit symptoms of food hypersensitivity' (Sampson, 1987). Referring to the skin prick test, Sampson wrote 'Positive results are useful only for limiting the number of food antigens that must be confirmed or excluded in a more definitive study, such as the blinded oral food challenge. In our experience, children generally have positive skin prick test reactions to 3 to 6 food antigens of a standard battery of 20 food antigens, although 10 to 12 positive skin reactions are not unheard of. When challenged, however, most of these children will experience a positive clinical reaction to only one or two foods. A positive skin prick test reaction merely confirms the presence of antigen-specific IgE bound to cutaneous mast cells and does not necessarily correlate with clinical hypersensitivity.' (Sampson, 1987.)

One question that arises is why patients should exhibit marked reactions to single foods when exposed under the controlled conditions of a DBPCFC, but appear not to react to the same food in normal everyday life. Sampson (1987) concluded: 'In daily life, these children receive several exposures each day to allergens such as egg, milk, soy, and wheat; symptoms, which appear dramatically when foods are eaten in isolation or on an empty stomach during a challenge, are less pronounced and blend into each other. Repeated consumption of the offending food establishes and maintains a chronic hypersensitive state, which results in reactions to very small doses of antigen and nonantigenic irritant stimuli. Moreover, children scratch vigorously for one to two hours after a brief allergen exposure, often excoriating the affected area.'

Comment

Although the patients were highly selected, Sampson's data clearly show that some children with AD experience adverse reactions to individual foods when tested under controlled conditions. The reactions can be cutaneous, or noncutaneous, or both. The cutaneous reactions were neither urticarial nor eczematous. Given that acute urticaria is one of the most common features of acute reactions to food in those who are allergic (David, 1993), its absence in these studies is extraordinary.

There are difficulties with the study design, particularly the very short period (four hours) allowed for observation following a challenge, with each patient receiving two challenges per day, one in the morning and one in the afternoon. This design, on the one hand, precluded the detection or documentation of delayed reactions and, on the other, allowed any such reactions to interfere with the observations that were made. One of the observations made in Sampson's studies was of a pruritic rash occurring six to eight hours after the initial response, sometimes accompanied by longer lasting pruritus. If such reaction occurred to a morning challenge it is hard to see how it could have failed to interfere with the outcome of the afternoon challenge. It is odd, therefore, that there were no reactions to the placebo. Furthermore, there were in effect a number of simultaneous challenges in progress, for if a test challenge was negative for a food, then that food was openly introduced into the diet, with the ever-present possibility that a reaction to an open challenge could be confused with a reaction to a simultaneous blind challenge.

The strategy used in Sampson's studies was to get through a maximum number of DBPCFCs while the child was in hospital, and the short observation period and the need for two challenges per day were essential for this approach. The difficulty is that this design virtually precluded the detection of delayed reactions, which may be of equal or greater relevance to patients with AD. Delayed reactions are far harder to demonstrate under blind and controlled conditions, and may require much larger quantities of food than can be given in a capsule, but the evidence of their existence is strong. For example, Hill, Ball & Hosking (1988) found that, whereas 8–10 g of milk powder (corresponding to 60–70 ml of cow's milk) was adequate to provoke a response in some patients with cow's milk protein allergy, other patients (with late onset symptoms) required up to ten times this volume of milk daily for more than 48 hours before symptoms developed. Similarly, Goldman in his classic study reported a subset of children with cow's milk allergy who reacted adversely only when given more than 100 ml of cow's milk, and whose reactions tended to be delayed (Goldman et al., 1963). More recently, Seidman and his colleagues described a subset of children with cow's milk allergy who required as much as 2700 ml before a reaction occurred, the onset of the reaction being delayed for as much as 48 to 72 hours after ingestion (Baehler et al., 1996). A further example is the eczematous lesions which occur one to eight days after eating incorrectly processed cashew nuts which had become contaminated with oil from the shell of the nut (Marks et al., 1984). The delayed nature of these reactions is important, not least because it makes it far more difficult to identify food triggers from the history.

One is left accepting that many children with AD experience adverse reactions to selected foods, but being uncertain (on the basis of the Sampson studies alone) as to the relationship between these reported reactions and the subsequent development of eczematous skin lesions. Other studies employing various types of challenges, however, have documented the development of eczematous skin lesions when large amounts of a trigger food have been given (Goldman et al., 1963; Hill, Ball & Hosking, 1988; Hill et al., 1984; Baehler et al., 1996). In 1936, Engman and his colleagues reported a two-year-old child with AD and allergy to wheat (Engman, Weiss & Engman, 1936). Ingestion of a wheat cracker would produce intense itching. In an experiment, the child was admitted to hospital, wheat eliminated from the diet, and when the skin had cleared his left arm and leg were dressed in a thick and stiff crinoline bandage. The child was given two wheat crackers, and within two hours he had intense pruritus. The following morning, the boy had typical eczematous lesions, except under the bandages, where the skin remained clear. The conclusion from that is that the cutaneous reaction to food produced intense pruritus, scatching and rubbing, leading to eczematous skin lesions.

Subsequently, Hammar reported the induction of eczematous skin lesions in 15 out of 81 hospitalized children less than five years of age after two to three days of ingesting 100 ml of cow's milk daily (Hammar, 1977).

Reactions to foods cause worsening of preexisting atopic dermatitis

There is clear evidence from studies which have used double-blind placebo-controlled food challenges that selected food triggers can in certain individuals cause eczematous rashes or cause worsening of preexisting AD. The clear link between food triggers and AD comes best from challenge studies done in children with cow's milk allergy (Goldman et al., 1963; Hill, Ball & Hosking, 1988; Hill et al., 1984; Baehler et al., 1996), which include patients with AD, rather than studies of children with AD. It is not known exactly what proportion of children with AD experience worsening of skin lesions after ingestion of specific food triggers. Nor is it known whether the severity or extent of the skin lesions has any relationship with the chances of having one or more food triggers. Although it is not proven, age is likely to be an important determinant of the importance of food triggers, for it is well documented that most children with food allergy (other than nut allergy) grow out of their food allergy, sometimes by the age of one year, often by the age of three years, and usually by the age of five years (David, 1993).

Avoidance of selected foods can cause atopic dermatitis to improve

The literature is replete with claims that dietary elimination causes improvement of AD in some cases, but in most cases the evidence fails to withstand close scrutiny. In Sampson's studies, having identified food triggers by DBPCFC, the patients were then put on a diet which completely excluded these triggers. The authors reported that after the food-allergic children were placed on the appropriate diet, there was a marked and rapid improvement in the patient's AD in most cases. Some children's skin lesions 'cleared entirely and required little if any additional treatment.' Unfortunately no data were provided to support these conclusions, and there was no control group for comparison. It is impossible to tell, therefore, how much of the improvement was due to a placebo effect.

Patients who did not have proven food allergy, and who are therefore presumably in a different category altogether, were not treated with a diet, but this cannot be regarded as a control group. A controlled design would have required that some patients with proven food allergy were randomized to receive, for a trial period, no diet or some alternative diet. Understandably enough, having proven that certain patients had food allergy, there was a reluctance to allow continued exposure to trigger foods. The authors concluded 'patients appropriately diagnosed and maintained on an antigen-free diet have been shown to improve compared to those children who are not found to be allergic to any food, or to those food-allergic children who are noncompliant with the avoidance diet.' The course of 34 children with AD followed for three or four years (it is unclear how this subgroup was selected) was reviewed. Group 1 contained 17 children with AD and food allergy who were maintained on appropriate elimination diets. Group 2 comprised 12 children with AD who did not have food allergy and 5 children with AD and food allergy who were noncompliant with their diet. The initial symptom scores (these were not defined) of the two groups were not significantly different. The symptom scores were significantly better at mid-study and post-study in group 1 when compared with the scores of group 2. However, a puzzling and notable feature, which makes it impossible to generalize from these limited data, is that the symptom scores hardly fell at all in group 2. This is most odd, because one most striking feature of childhood AD is its very strong tendency to improve with time in the majority of cases.

The UK approach is to make no attempt to prove a diagnosis of food allergy, but simply to try elimination of one or more foods for a defined period of time and observe the effect on the skin condition. The drawback is the lack of proof of food allergy, but the advantage is that a placebo-controlled design is permitted. There are three main types of dietary strategy, the simple elimination of cow's milk protein and egg, the few food diet, and the so-called elemental diet. These will be briefly described.

Cow's milk protein- and egg-free diet

This approach has been tested by controlled trial. Atherton and colleagues studied 36 children with AD, using a control diet which contained cow's milk and dried egg (Atherton et al., 1978). Twenty chil-

dren, median age six years, completed the study; 14 patients responded more favourably to the milk- and egg-free diet, whereas only 1 patient responded more favourably to the control diet than the milk- and egg-free diet. Three patients experienced a severe exacerbation of eczema within a few days of starting the control diet period, probably because the control diet included added egg, and these cases were excluded. Furthermore, there appeared to be relatively little benefit associated with the control diet, an unusual feature for diets usually have a marked placebo effect (David, 1993). It has been suggested that this study showed a placebo effect from a milk- and egg-free diet, this effect being masked in the control diet by the inclusion of added egg which exacerbated the eczema. A further controlled study of dietary avoidance of cow's milk protein and egg in 53 patients of varying ages with AD failed to show significant benefit (Neild et al., 1986).

The few food diet

This is a diet in which all but a handful of foods is excluded (David, 1993). An example used in Manchester permits the child to eat lamb, potato, rice (and Rice Crispies), one of the brassica family (cauliflower, cabbage, Brussels sprouts or broccoli), pears (in restricted quantities, to avoid loose stools caused by the high fructose content) and tap water. This diet is used for an initial period (in our unit six weeks, but four to six weeks in some other units), before the child is reassessed. Dietetic supervision and family motivation are both essential. Early uncontrolled studies suggested benefit from this regimen. Thus, Pike et al. studied 66 selected children with AD, mean age 4.2 years, and found an unquantified benefit associated with a few food diet in 24 (36%), this benefit being sustained in 12 (18%) (Pike et al., 1989). Forty one (62%) patients were unresponsive to this treatment. There was no control group.

In a prospective but uncontrolled follow-up study in Manchester, 63 children (median age 2.9 years) with AD were selected for treatment with a few food

Table 15.1. *Results of few foods diet in atopic dermatitis (Devlin, David & Stanton 1991a)*

		Prediet	Six weeks	Six months	One year
Number attending follow-up					
Diet	success	33	33	32	24
Diet	failure	21	21	20	15
	N.C.	9	7	6	4
Median disease severity score					
Diet	success	70	20	10	15
Diet	failure	60	60	16	16
	N.C.	50	36	10	17
Percentage of patients receiving any topical steroid					
Diet	success	82	79	78	75
Diet	failure	95	76	90	80
	N.C.	100	86	100	100

Note:

N.C. = Patients who were unable to comply with diet.

diet (Devlin, David & Stanton, 1991a). Nine patients (14%) abandoned the diet before the initial six-week treatment period had been completed. Of the 54 patients who completed six weeks of treatment, 33 (52%) showed a greater than 20% improvement in the disease severity score and were categorized as having improved. Twenty one (39%) failed to show a greater than 20% improvement, and were classed as treatment failures. Compliance data were not available. All groups were followed up, and the key finding (see Table 15.1) was that at 12 months *all three groups* had markedly improved, regardless of whether they had responded to the diet or not. The conclusion was that, although the diet was associated with short-term benefit in some patients, there was no evidence of long-term benefit, all patients showing a marked tendency to improvement over time.

In the only randomized controlled trial of a few food diet, 85 children (median age 2.3 years) with refractory AD affecting more than 12% of the body surface area, were randomly allocated to receive a few foods diet supplemented with either a whey hydrolysate ($n = 27$), or a casein hydrolysate formula ($n = 32$), or to remain on their usual diet and act as controls ($n = 26$), for a six-week period (Mabin, Sykes & David, 1995). Thirty five patients who received the diet and four controls had to be withdrawn because of nonadherence with the diet or intercurrent illness. The change in dermatitis severity was evaluated by a blinded observer who estimated the extent of the dermatitis and severity, using a skin severity score. After six weeks, there was a significant reduction in all three groups in the percentage of surface area involved. Sixteen (73%) of the 22 controls and 15 (63%) of the 24 who received the diet showed a greater than 20% improvement in the skin severity score. This study failed to show benefit from a few foods diet. The main difficulty with the study design was one of numbers. To give an extreme example, if one started out with the assumption (say) that only 1% of patients had food allergy and would therefore stand to benefit from a diet, then clearly the sample size was insufficient.

Elemental diet

In the so-called elemental diet, more accurately described as a nonmacromolecular diet, ordinary foodstuffs are all avoided, and the patient receives a liquid diet which contains amino acids, carbohydrate, fat, minerals and vitamins. The chances of an allergic reaction are minimal, but the palatability of so-called elemental formulae such as Vivonex (now renamed Tolerex, and not available in the UK) or Elemental 028 is very poor. Because of this, some units administer these formulae by nasogastric tube.

Munkvad et al. (1984) reported on a controlled study of an elemental formula Vivasorb. Thirty three adults with AD entered the study, and 23 patients completed the study. The patients were hospitalized and randomized to receive the elemental diet or a control diet which comprised normal food that had been liquidized. The conclusion was that there was no significant difference between the two groups. Studies of eosinophil count, IgE concentration, orosomucoid and skin biopsies showed no significant difference between the two groups. The conclusion was that food intolerance plays little role in adults with AD.

The only substantial study of elemental diets in children with AD was uncontrolled. Thirty seven children, median age three years, with refractory and widespread AD, were admitted to hospital and received an elemental formula (Vivonex) for a mean duration of 29 days (Devlin, David & Stanton, 1991b). Complications included greater than 10% body weight loss in ten patients, loose stools in seven, and a mean fall in the serum albumin of 9.6 g/l. Food challenges were performed at intervals of seven days, and the patients followed-up for at least 12 months; 40 of 185 food challenges in hospital were positive, and 28 of 40 were delayed reactions only detectable one to seven days after a food was introduced. After discharge, 19 of 37 patients experienced allergic reactions to pets, house dust or grass; 10 of 37 (27%) either failed to respond to the regimen or relapsed within 12 months. Sustained improvement in the dermatitis was seen in 27 of 37 (73%) patients, and by discharge from hospital their disease severity score had fallen to a mean of 29% of the pretreatment figure and only 1 of 27 required topical corticosteroids. There were no clinical or laboratory findings which could be used to predict the outcome. The lack of a control group means that it is impossible to tell how much of the benefit was a placebo effect associated with diet, hospitalization and pet avoidance.

Maternal dietary exclusion in breast-fed infants with atopic dermatitis

Cant et al. (1986) studied 37 breast-fed infants with AD; 19 mothers and babies took part in a double-blind cross-over trial of exclusion of egg and cow's milk, and 18 took part in open exclusion of 11 foods followed by double-blind challenge to those mothers whose infants seemed to respond. Nearly half (46%) of the babies showed an improvement in their dermatitis during the exclusion periods, but the authors admitted that, had the mothers not returned to a normal diet, they would have thought that dietary exclusion was beneficial when 'in fact

the improvement was probably spontaneous'. In 6 of the 37 babies, however, the eczema did seem to respond by both improving when the mothers avoided egg and cow's milk and relapsing when these foods were reintroduced. No specific factors predicted which babies would respond to maternal dietary exclusion, and skin prick tests were unhelpful. The authors concluded that AD in breast-fed infants has a high rate of spontaneous improvement, which is often wrongly attributed to maternal dietary exclusion, but that nevertheless a subgroup of such babies do seem to be genuinely affected by foods in their mothers' diets.

Reasons for improvement of dermatitis on an elimination diet

Although in a proportion of children with AD, the elimination of certain foods from the diet may be associated with improvement of the dermatitis (Devlin, David & Stanton, 1991a, 1991b) without randomized controlled studies it is impossible to tell how much of this improvement is due to a placebo effect. Some studies of dietary therapy have incorporated challenges of selected single foods, but the finding of positive challenges is no proof that the benefit of the diet was solely due to specific food avoidance (Juto, Engberg & Winberg, 1978; Veien et al., 1987; Pike et al., 1989; Van Bever, Docx & Stevens, 1989; Devlin, David & Stanton, 1991a, 1991b).

These and other uncontrolled observational studies have been conducted on highly selected groups of patients. The problem is that such studies fail to provide information about what sort of success can be expected from the general clinical application of elimination diets in the treatment of AD in childhood.

It is important to remember that diets are associated with a marked placebo effect. A good example of this is a controlled study of the exclusion of dietary vasoactive amines in children with migraine (Salfield et al., 1987). Patients were randomly allocated to either a high fibre diet low in dietary amines (the treatment group) or a high fibre diet alone (the placebo group). Both groups showed a highly significant decrease in the number of headaches, emphasizing the need for a control diet in studies designed to show that dietary manipulation improves disease.

A common fallacy is to assume that a positive food challenge proves that improvement on a diet was caused by the diet. Most studies of treatment with exclusion diets (including many studies of AD) have opted for an open study of the diet, followed by some blind challenges. Unfortunately, positive food challenges do not prove that the improvement was caused by the diet. One has to remember that food allergy and AD commonly co-exist in the same patient, so that if a child with AD improves on a diet as a placebo effect or as a coincidence, there is still quite a high chance that the child will react adversely to selected foods when challenged.

Even if an elimination diet is associated with improvement, an important area of uncertainty is whether such treatment has any long-term effect on the outcome. One study suggests that any benefit from diets may be in the short term (i.e. first few weeks of diet) rather than the long term (Devlin, David & Stanton, 1991a).

The lack of reliable tests to diagnose food allergy is an important handicap. The subject is discussed in detail elsewhere (David, 1993), but skin prick tests for food allergy are notoriously unreliable, because of the large number of false positive and false negative reactions (Bock et al., 1977; Aas, 1978; Lessof et al., 1980; Bousquet, 1988; Hill et al., 1988; Meglio et al., 1988). The clinical interpretation of in vitro IgE antibody tests (e.g. RAST tests) is subject to the same caveats and pitfalls as the interpretation of skin prick testing, so that as with skin testing, tests to detect circulating IgE antibody are of little practical use. Unfortunately, there is no test that can be done to predict the outcome of dietary elimination (David, 1993).

Conclusion

It is well established that many children with AD have food allergy, and it is clear that in these subjects ingestion of trigger foods in sufficient quantities may cause worsening of the eczematous skin lesions. Whilst some of these cases are quite dramatic, and stand out by obviously being made ill by trigger foods, the place of elimination diets in the management of established AD has yet to be established by controlled trial.

Summary of key points

- There is clear evidence from studies that have used double-blind placebo-controlled food challenges that some (but not all) children with atopic dermatitis (AD) have food allergy.
- There is clear evidence from studies that have used double-blind placebo-controlled food challenges that selected food triggers can, in certain individuals, cause eczematous rashes or cause worsening of preexisting AD.
- Reasons for improvement of AD in association with an elimination diet include removal of food triggers, coincidental improvement of the skin disease, or a placebo effect.
- Whilst one continues to see a few individual subjects with AD in whom there is dramatic improvement of severe intractable disease in association with an elimination diet, the place for dietary elimination in the management of AD has yet to be established by controlled trials.
- There are no reliable simple tests for the identification of individual food triggers or for the prediction of outcome after dietary elimination.
- There is no evidence of long-term benefit from dietary elimination.

References

Aas, K. (1978). The diagnosis of hypersensitivity to ingested foods. Reliability of skin-prick testing and the radioallergosorbent test with different materials. *Clin Allergy*, **8**, 39–50.

Atherton, D.J., Sewell, M., Soothill, J.F. & Wells, R.S. (1978). A double-blind controlled crossover trial of an antigen-avoidance diet in atopic eczema. *Lancet*, **1**, 401–3.

Baehler, P., Chad, Z., Gurbindo, C., Bonin, A.P., Bouthillier, L. & Seidman, E.G. (1996). Distinct patterns of cow's milk allergy in infancy defined prolonged, two-stage double-blind, placebo-controlled food challenges. *Clin Exp Allergy*, **26**, 254–61.

Bock, S.A., Buckley, J., Holst, A. & May, C.D. (1977). Proper use of skin tests with food extracts in diagnosis of hypersensitivity to food in children. *Clin Allergy*, **7**, 375–83.

Bousquet, J. (1988). In vivo methods for study of allergy: skin tests, techniques, and interpretation. In: Middleton, E., Reed, C.E., Ellis, E.F., Adkinson, N.F. & Yunginger, J.W. (eds.) *Allergy. Principles and Practice*, pp. 419–36. St Louis: Mosby.

Broadbent, J.B. & Sampson, H.A. (1988). Food hypersensitivity and atopic dermatitis. *Pediat Clin N Am*, **35**, 1115–30.

Cant, A.J., Bailes, J.A., Marsden, R.A. & Hewitt, D. (1986). Effect of maternal dietary exclusion on breast fed infants with eczema: two controlled studies. *Br Med J*, **293**, 231–3.

David, T.J. (1993). *Food and Food Additive Intolerance in Childhood*. Oxford: Blackwell Scientific.

Devlin, J., David, T.J. & Stanton, R.H.J. (1991a). Six food diet for childhood atopic dermatitis. *Acta Dematol Venereol (Scand.)*, **71**, 20–24.

Devlin, J., David, T.J. & Stanton, R.H.J. (1991b). Elemental diet for refractory atopic eczema. *Arch Dis Childh*, **66**, 93–9.

Engman, M.F., Weiss, R.S. & Engman, M.F.J. (1936). Eczema and environment. *Med Clin N Am*, **20**, 651–63.

Goldman, A.S., Anderson, D.W., Sellers, W.A., Saperstein, S., Kniker, W.T. & Halpern, S.R. (1963). 1. Oral challenge with milk and isolated milk proteins in allergic children. *Pediatrics*, **32**, 425–43.

Hammar, H. (1977). Provocation with cow's milk and cereals in atopic dermatitis. *Acta Dermatol Venereol (Scand.)*, **57**, 159–63.

Hill, D.J., Ball, G. & Hosking, C.S. (1988). Clinical manifestations of cows' milk allergy in childhood. I. Associations with in-vitro cellular immune responses. *Clin Allergy*, **18**, 469–79.

Hill, D.J., Ford, R.P.K., Shelton, M.J. & Hosking, C.S. (1984). A study of 100 infants and young children with cow's milk allergy. *Clin Rev Allergy*, **2**, 125–42.

Hill, D.J., Duke, A.M., Hosking, C.S. & Hudson, I.L. (1988). Clinical manifestations of cows' milk allergy in childhood. II. The diagnostic value of skin tests and RAST. *Clin Allergy*, **18**, 481–90.

Juto, P., Engberg, S. & Winberg, J. (1978). Treatment of infantile atopic dermatitis with a strict elimination diet. *Clin Allergy*, **8**, 493–500.

Lessof, M.H., Buisseret, P.D., Merrett, J., Merrett, T.G. & Wraith, D.G. (1980). Assessing the value of skin tests. *Clin Allergy*, **10**, 115–20.

Mabin, D.C., Sykes, A.E. & David, T.J. (1995). Controlled trial of a few foods diet in severe atopic dermatitis. *Arch Dis Childh*, **73**, 202–7.

Marks, J.G., DeMelfi, T., McCarthy, M.A., Witte, E.J., Castagnoli, N., Epstein, W.L. & Aber, R.C. (1984). Dermatitis from cashew nuts. *J Am Acad Dermatol*, **10**, 627–31.

Meglio, P., Farinella, F., Trogolo, E. & Giampietro, P.G. (1988). Immediate reactions following challenge-tests in children with atopic dermatitis. *Allergie Immunologie*, **20**, 57–62.

Munkvad, M., Danielsen, L., Hoj, L., Povlsen, C.O., Secher, L., Svejgaard, E., Bundgaard, A. & Larsen, P. (1984). Antigen-free diet in adult patients with atopic dermatitis. A double-blind controlled study. *Acta Dermatol Venereol (Scand.)*, **64**, 524–8.

Neild, V.A., Marsden, R.A., Bailes, J.A. & Bland, J.M. (1986). Egg and milk exclusion diets in atopic eczema. *Br J Dermatol*, **114**, 117–23.

Pike, M.G., Carter, C.M., Boulton, P., Turner, M.W., Soothill, J.F. & Atherton, D.J. (1989). Few food diets in the treatment of atopic eczema. *Arch Dis Childh*, **64**, 1691–8.

Salfield, S.A.W., Wardley, B.L., Houlsby, W.T., Turner, S.L., Spalton, A.P., Beckles-Wilson, N.R. & Herber, S.M. (1987). Controlled study of exclusion of dietary vasoactive amines in migraine. *Arch Dis Childh*, **62**, 458–60.

Sampson, H.A. (1983). Role of immediate food hypersensitivity in the pathogenesis of atopic dermatitis. *J Allergy Clin Immunol*, **71**, 473–80.

Sampson, H.A. (1987). Late-phase response to food in atopic dermatitis. *Hosp Pract*, **22**, 111–28.

Sampson, H.A. (1988). The role of food allergy and mediator release in atopic dermatitis. *J Allergy Clin Immunol*, **81**, 635–45.

Van Bever, H.P., Docx, M. & Stevens, W.J. (1989). Food and food additives in severe atopic dermatitis. *Allergy*, **44**, 588–94.

Veien, N.K., Hattel, T., Justesen, O. & Norholm, A. (1987). Dermatitis induced or aggravated by selected foodstuffs. *Acta Dermatol Venereol (Scand.)*, **67**, 133–8.

PART IV

Intervention studies

16

Prevention of atopic dermatitis

Adrian Mar and Robin Marks

Introduction

Previous chapters have outlined the evidence suggesting that both genetic and environmental factors are important in the causation of atopic dermatitis (AD). In light of the commonly held belief, particularly amongst layfolk, that AD may be initiated by exposure to certain foods and environmental conditions during childhood, it is not surprising that attempts are often made by parents or medical practitioners to prevent the disease. However, it is clear that AD is a condition of complex aetiology, ensuring that such efforts are unlikely to be straightforward.

Before considering preventive measures it is necessary to obtain an understanding of disease causation, or at least to devise a conceptual model on which prevention strategies can be based. The first part of this chapter suggests a model for AD causation and then, using this model, outlines some theoretical strategies for prevention. The second part provides a summary of recent studies which have attempted to evaluate the prophylactic benefit of early intervention measures (mostly dietary manipulation), and discusses current recommendations for AD prevention and the implications for future research and public health planning.

Model of atopic dermatitis causation

A conceptual model of AD causation is shown in Figure 16.1. It assumes that the development of AD

is a stepwise progression from a state of susceptibility through preclinical to clinical disease. Genetic and environmental factors contribute to the alterations in systemic immune function and local cutaneous physiology that are characteristic of this condition. As an extension of this model, AD may be considered as a systemic condition (the immunologically related 'atopic state') which, due to cutaneous localizing factors, is manifest as a disease of the skin. The relative importance of genetic, environmental, immunological and local cutaneous factors in AD causation probably differs between individual cases, accounting for the variation seen in clinical presentation and prognosis. AD may represent a spectrum of disease processes: the pathogenesis in some cases may be largely related to environmental exposures, whereas in others endogenous factors may be more important.

Genetic factors

Genotype is an important risk factor for the development of AD (see Chapter 8). Although the exact genetic basis of AD is still to be identified, it seems that complex interactions between multiple gene products, rather than a single gene defect, are responsible for the disease expression. It is likely that the degree of susceptibility is at least partly the result of variance of genotype, with some individuals inheriting a 'high-risk' gene or genetic pattern (perhaps for some of these individuals prevention by environmental manipulation is futile), while others

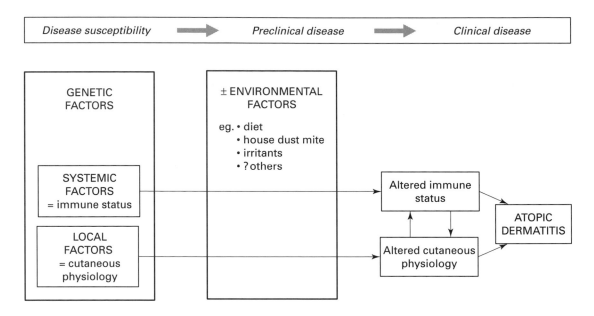

Fig. 16.1. Model of atopic dermatitis causation

have a 'low-risk' genotype in which AD might be manifest only under adverse environmental conditions.

Environmental factors

Strong evidence for the causative role of environmental factors is provided by epidemiological studies as outlined in previous chapters. Population-based studies have demonstrated a dramatic increase in disease prevalence over the past several decades (Williams, 1992) (see Chapter 7). Such changes over a short period of time cannot be explained on the basis of genetic selection and must be assumed to be secondary to changes in the environment. AD is more frequent in cities compared with rural areas (Pöysä et al., 1991; Kjellman, Pettersson & Hyensjö, 1982) (see Chapter 5) and amongst migrants to industrialized countries compared with those still living in the country of origin (Waite et al., 1980) (see Chapter 13). Furthermore, a social gradient in prevalence rates exists: AD is a disease of the higher social classes (Golding & Peters,

1987) (see Chapter 10), an observation which is also reflected in differences in housing conditions (Williams, Strachan & Hay, 1994).

Immunological factors

Atopic dermatitis is generally accepted as being a disease occurring within the context of an altered immune response. Its clinical course, which is often relapsing but tending towards spontaneous improvement, is suggestive of immunologically-mediated hypersensitivity and tolerance responses, respectively. However, AD cannot be characterized according to classical hypersensitivity reactions. Efforts to find the fundamental immunological defect have been frustrated by the lack of an animal model and the observation that laboratory evidence of altered immune function is inconsistent and usually found in some but not all cases. Various indicators of immune dysfunction have been described in patients with AD. Depression of cell-mediated responses has been repeatedly demonstrated in both in vitro and in vivo experiments (McGready & Buckley, 1975; Young, Bruijnzeel-Koomen & Berrens, 1985). However, a study by Uehara & Sawai (1989) found that the diminished contact sensitivity to dinitrochlorobenzene in patients with severe AD could no longer be demonstrated once the dermatitis had been actively treated, suggesting that altered contact sensitivity responses may be secondary to the disease. Recent studies have focused on abnormalities of cytokine production, in particular the enhancement of interleukin-4 production (Renz et al., 1992) and the apparent reduction in interferon-γ secretion (Reinhold et al., 1990; Jujo et al., 1992).

'Atopy' includes in its definition the development of IgE antibodies in response to antigen exposure. Although IgE has a clear causative role in allergic rhinitis (and less so in asthma), its significance in AD is still unclear. A correlation between elevation of serum IgE levels and severity of AD is well documented (Ogawa, Berger & McIntyre, 1971; Johnson, Irons & Patterson, 1974); however, in one study levels were raised in only 37% of patients with severe 'pure' AD (i.e. those with no personal or family history of respiratory atopy) and this elevation was only mild to moderate (Uehara, 1989). Furthermore, cases have been reported of classic AD in the virtual absence of circulating IgE (Peterson, Page & Good, 1962). Clinical studies also fail to support a mechanism of specific allergen sensitization as an important component of AD in the majority of cases: flare-ups of the rash cannot usually be induced by allergen challenge tests in patients with established disease (Sampson, 1992).

Nonetheless, the notion has prevailed amongst some investigators that priming of the immune system by specific allergens via an IgE response (i.e. 'sensitization') is an essential step in AD causation, and this has been the basis for attempts at AD prevention by allergen avoidance. Recently, evidence has appeared which may enable a possible link to be made between IgE production and immunologically cell-mediated inflammation in the skin. It has been shown that Langerhans cells in the skin of AD patients express receptors for IgE (Bruijnzeel-Koomen et al., 1986). There is evidence to suggest that IgE may play a part in the presentation of antigens by Langerhans cells and that IgE-positive Langerhans cells preferentially activate the subset of T cells (Th2 cells in the mouse) thought to be involved in AD skin lesions (Mudde et al., 1990; Hauser et al., 1989). IgE-bearing Langerhans cells, however, may not be specific to AD and the precise role of these cells in AD awaits further clarification (Bieber & Braun-Falco, 1991).

In a discussion of AD prevention, therefore, it is necessary to retain the concept of 'sensitization' although the immunological mechanisms involved in AD are not understood and likely to be of a complex nature.

Local cutaneous factors

Atopic dermatitis is associated with physiological changes in the skin. Patients with AD typically have dry skin and demonstrate clinical signs such as facial pallor and white dermographism. These features are indicative of an associated abnormality of skin barrier function and vascular reactivity, respectively. Changes in transepidermal water loss (Werner & Lindberg, 1985; Watanabe et al., 1991), lipid fractions (Yamamoto et al., 1991) and delivery of lamellar bodies (Fartasch, Bassukas & Diepgen, 1992) have been observed in the uninvolved skin of AD patients. Others have noted abnormal cutaneous responses to acetylcholine (Lobitz & Campbell, 1953) and histamine (Uehara, 1982). Szentivanyi (1968) proposed that β-adrenergic blockade could be an underlying process in those predisposed to atopic diseases.

There is still insufficient evidence to establish whether the abnormalities of immune function and cutaneous physiology described in patients with AD are primary genetic defects or secondary changes resulting from environmental influences. For instance, a cutaneous barrier defect may facilitate penetration of allergens or irritants but, on the other hand, inflammation resulting from an altered immune response causes alterations in the barrier function. It is conceivable that environmental factors which alter the physiological properties of the skin may act as 'enhancers' of the immunological abnormalities, but evidence that such a process is necessary for the development of AD is lacking. Recent studies have demonstrated a reduction in interferon-γ secretion (Tang et al., 1994) and membrane-associated arachidonic acid in cord blood mononuclear cells of newborns (Ioppi et al., 1994) who subsequently develop atopic disease. It has been suggested that such abnormalities are intrinsic and therefore may have a causative role. However, the possibility of these findings being due to environmental influences in utero cannot as yet be excluded.

Potential targets for atopic dermatitis prevention

In this chapter the term 'prevention' will be considered as any interventional measure which results in a healthy individual remaining unaffected by the disease. This encompasses the notions of so-called primary and secondary prevention, which in the case of AD are difficult to define. Primary prevention can refer to preventing occurrence of the disease in healthy individuals by eliminating disease susceptibility. Secondary prevention can mean intervention at a 'preclinical stage' of the disease process to halt further progression to clinical disease. The term tertiary prevention is sometimes used to refer to optimizing management of established clinical disease of a chronic nature to reduce the severity or likelihood of relapse. Some authors have considered primary prevention of AD as inhibition of IgE sensitization and secondary prevention as deterrence of disease expression in previously sensitized individuals. However, since the pathogenesis of AD cannot currently be described purely in terms of specific IgE sensitization, the use of this definition seems inappropriate. Until a better understanding of causative mechanisms is gained, the distinction between the states of susceptibility and preclinical disease, and hence primary and secondary prevention, is somewhat arbitrary in the case of AD and serves little practical purpose.

Genetic engineering

Some might suggest that the ultimate form of prevention is by means of intervention at the genetic level. In theory, once the disease can be defined in terms of specific gene defects, it should be amenable to prevention by way of manipulation using genetic engineering techniques. Although currently speculative, development in this area is advancing rapidly and offers exciting potential application in the management of skin disease.

Genetic intervention could take place at the earliest stage of development (i.e. the gamete or early fetus) or, alternatively, specific cell lines could be targeted in the mature subject. The technology required for the latter approach is already being developed as a means of cancer treatment in cases such as malignant melanoma (so-called 'gene therapy'). In this method host immune cells are modified in vitro (by exogenous gene transfer techniques) and then reintroduced into the body of the patient (in cancer therapy the cells are modified to target the neoplastic cells and then to secrete large amounts of cytokines) (Rosenberg, 1990). The potential for a similar approach of immune system modification in AD is suggested by reports of clearing of dermatitis in patients with Wiskott–Aldrich syndrome who had received bone marrow transplantation from nonatopic donors (Saurat, 1985). In addition to these methods of altering the systemic immunological response, it is conceivable that genetic manipulation techniques could also be directed at correcting local cutaneous abnormalities such as barrier structure and function. Such an approach awaits future development.

An important use of DNA technology in disease prevention is the development of diagnostic tests which can accurately predict disease. Such tests are already available for the detection of inherited conditions such as cystic fibrosis, and in the future mass screening or target population screening for a wide range of diseases may be possible. For AD we may one day be able to offer specific preventive lifestyle advice on the basis of genotypic pattern.

Environmental engineering

Until technology allows easy access to manipulation at the genetic or cellular level, our attempts at disease prevention are limited to modifying the environmental component of the causative process. Candidate risk factors for AD which are potential targets for preventive strategies are outlined in the following section.

Due to the lack of a proven model for AD causation, the rationale behind any attempt at AD prevention must be based on notion rather than scientific fact. Most efforts to prevent AD by manipulation of the environment have been conducted on the assumption that avoiding IgE-mediated allergen sensitization may eliminate a key step in the causative process. Using this theory it follows that allergen exposure must occur in early development in order to explain the occurrence of disease in the first several months of life. Possible routes of antigen exposure are transplacental (i.e. in utero), through infant diet (either breast milk, formula feeds or solid foods) or by inhalation of aeroallergens.

It is possible, of course, that environmental factors may influence AD causation in other ways. There is evidence that early allergen exposure may induce immunological tolerance under certain conditions and therefore be of importance in *reducing* the risk of sensitization. The condition of the infant's skin, particularly the extent of dryness, may also be a critical factor in determining whether or not AD develops. Further research is required to address these issues.

Skin barrier function

Xerosis, the clinical condition of dryness of the skin, is associated with altered skin barrier function and may have a causative role in AD either as an initiating event or by enhancing the inflammatory response induced by immunological or irritant factors (Tupka et al., 1990). There is probably a genetic tendency towards developing xerosis in many cases but environmental irritants such as exposure to soaps and detergents, central heating and climate may also play an important role. It has been suggested that an increase in the use and diversity of household cleaning materials over the past 30 years may have contributed to the increase in AD prevalence (Williams, 1992).

Prevention of dryness may therefore have a prophylactic effect in some individuals. A small case-control study in Kenya suggested that the use of Vaseline in infancy might have protected against the development of AD (Macharia, Anabwani & Owili, 1991). However, further prospective randomized controlled studies are required to evaluate the true protective benefit of emollient use or avoidance of dryness caused by the use of soaps and central heating in infants with normal appearing skin.

In utero sensitization

An elevation of IgE in the newborn has been shown to be a risk factor for the development of atopy (Croner & Kjellman, 1990), although recent studies have demonstrated that cord blood IgE measurements lack sufficient sensitivity for their routine use as a predictor of atopic disease (Ruiz et al., 1991) (see Chapter 9). As IgE is unable to cross the placental barrier, cord blood IgE is thought to be of fetal origin, and it has been postulated that sensitization to transplacental allergens may occur in utero. Maternal avoidance of allergenic foods during pregnancy has therefore been considered as a possible means of reducing in utero sensitization of the fetus. On the other hand, it has been suggested that antigen exposure in utero may actually benefit the newborn based on evidence from animal experiments that demonstrate the importance of this process in the induction of immunological tolerance (Pathirana et al., 1981). More work is necessary to explore these apparent contradictions.

Breast feeding

Breast feeding may reduce allergen sensitization in two ways. First, by feeding exclusively with breast milk direct exposure to food allergens is reduced. It must be noted, however, that small amounts of dietary allergens can be detected in breast milk (Cant, Narsden & Kilshaw, 1985; Cavagni et al., 1988) and the potential for these to cause sensitization is suggested by the observation of immediate food hypersensitivity reactions occurring on initial food exposure in exclusively breast-fed infants (Van Asperen, Kemp & Mellis, 1983), and the demonstration of specific IgE to egg and cow's milk in a similar group of infants fed solely on breast milk (Hattevig et al., 1984; Kaplan & Solli, 1979). Maternal diet during lactation may therefore be of importance.

The second benefit from breast feeding may be the protective effect of secretory IgA (sIgA) and other breast milk constituents. It has been proposed that sIgA binding to food allergens may inhibit the absorption of these antigenic substances across the immature gut mucosa (Walker & Hanson, 1985). Others have suggested that growth factors found in the milk may facilitate early maturation of the infant gut (Kleinman & Walker, 1984).

Hypoallergenic formula feeding

Cow's milk is well recognized as a source of potential 'food allergy' in infants. β-lactoglobulin is the major antigen found in cow's milk although all proteins, including casein, are potentially allergenic (Freir, 1973). Animal studies show that the capacity of different infant formula preparations to cause IgE-mediated sensitization relates to the presence of high-molecular-weight peptides. In an attempt to reduce the immunogenicity of the protein constituents, hydrolysates of cow's milk, soy or beef collagen have been developed. Recent interest has focused on casein hydrolysate formulas which appear to be the least allergenic whilst maintaining adequate nutritional value (Sampson et al., 1991).

Delayed introduction of solid foods

The idea has arisen that exposure to antigenic food substances early in life may increase the risk of developing food-related allergies. Studies in mice have demonstrated sensitization of both humoral and cell-mediated immune responses to the egg protein ovalbumin following ingestion by the newborn or introduction into the amniotic sac of the fetus. This is in contrast to a tolerance response in adult animals exposed to ovalbumin for the first time (Strobel & Ferguson, 1984). It has been pro-

posed that a defect in the normal mucosal barrier of the gut is present in susceptible infants, allowing excessive absorption of macromolecules which in turn leads to stimulation of an IgE response. Mucosal barrier dysfunction has been suggested to be a manifestation of a generalized abnormality of the skin and mucosa of AD patients (Ogawa & Yoshiike, 1993). Increased permeability of the gut in patients with AD has been demonstrated (Ukabam, Mann & Cooper, 1984; Pike et al., 1986) but is still controversial (Barba et al., 1989).

The putative beneficial role of sIgA from breast milk has been mentioned. The possibility that atopic individuals may have an inherent deficiency of sIgA has also been raised. Decreased levels of serum and secretory IgA have been found in atopy-prone infants during the first few months of life (Taylor et al., 1973) and there have been reports of an increased incidence of atopy in IgA-deficient individuals (Schwartz & Buchley, 1971).

The foods most commonly implicated in eliciting IgE responses in infants are egg, cow's milk, fish and peanuts. Based on the premise that an immature gut and immune system can be the cause of excessive sensitization during infancy, it has been considered that atopic disease may be preventable by strict dietary avoidance of these foods during this period. The age at which potentially allergenic food substances can be 'safely' introduced is not known but 12 months of age is typically recommended. However, a report by Saarinen & Kajosaari (1980) raises doubts about the effectiveness of such an approach in preventing food allergies. In this study of 375 children followed-up at three years, a similar frequency of fish and citrus allergy, defined by positive challenge tests, was found in children with and without first-year elimination of the foods.

House dust mite

A sensitivity to house dust mite antigen can be demonstrated in many patients with AD and this may have significance in the clinical setting (see Chapter 14). In the case of asthma, exposure to mite antigen (*Der p I*) during infancy has been related to the subsequent development of clinical disease in a cohort study over 11 years (Sporik et al., 1990). Whether early sensitization is a risk factor for the development of AD remains to be established.

Intervention studies

Over the past several decades many clinical studies have been performed with the purpose of evaluating the effect of dietary and other environmental interventions on the subsequent development of atopic disease including AD. Most have had important flaws in their methodology and the resulting inconsistency in published data has only fuelled ongoing debate. This has been most notably the case in breast feeding studies. A major difficulty in studying the benefits of breast feeding is the inability to randomize subjects. It has been demonstrated in some reports that prolonged breast feeding is associated with a strong history of atopic disease (bilateral versus unilateral parentage), higher educational level and greater awareness of health issues. In the absence of a definitive study which includes controls for such confounding variables the issue of breast feeding remains unresolved (Kramer, 1988). Similarly randomized controlled studies are needed to confirm reports of a benefit from delayed solid feeding. A birth cohort study by Fergusson & Horwood (1994) which found a linear relationship between the number of solid foods given at four months of age and lifetime prevalence rates of AD at two and ten years did adjust for confounding factors but has been criticized for using medical records and maternal recall for the diagnosis of positive cases.

Preventive strategies can be adequately tested only by carefully conducted prospective randomized studies which compare the prevalence of disease in an intervention group with that of a control group, taking into consideration the following aspects of study design:
• *randomization* of the two groups is essential in order to avoid selection bias. There are a number of potential confounding factors relating to the background history of the subject which can influence the outcome of AD frequency. The most important of these are family history of atopic disease, social class and racial background. It is critical that both the intervention and control groups are comparable with regard to these variables. Randomization also ensures to some degree that many of the unforeseen confounders are adjusted for.
• a *validated set of diagnostic criteria* should be used by the investigator to record positive cases of AD and this person should ideally be *blinded* to the knowledge of group allocation. AD is diagnosed on clinical grounds as there are no specific laboratory markers for the disease. Therefore, it is important to have in place measures which will reduce the likelihood of observation bias.
• *frequent follow-up assessments* are required to record accurately the cumulative incidence of AD. Since AD is a disease which characteristically fluctuates in severity and site during its course, an estimate of cumulative incidence must often rely on a history of the rash given by the parent. Interviews of mothers need to be conducted at intervals which minimize recall bias.
• *sufficient length of follow-up* is required to assess adequately whether a difference in cumulative incidence at a certain age represents a true reduction in lifetime incidence or simply a delay in onset of the disease.

Recently a number of excellent randomized controlled studies have investigated the effect of dietary manipulation and aeroallergen control during infancy on the subsequent development of AD (Table 16.1). These studies have recruited subjects at high risk for AD, both to increase the chances of observing a positive outcome and, importantly, to improve compliance amongst participating mothers. Most investigators used a definition of 'high risk' based on parental history of atopic disease (positive skin prick tests were required in some studies) or elevated cord IgE levels.

Fälth-Magnusson & Kjellman (1992) conducted a study to evaluate the effect of dietary modification during pregnancy on the risk of developing atopic disease in the newborn child. In this study, the intervention group totally abstained from cow's milk and

Table 16.1. Prospective randomized controlled studies of early intervention measures on the development of AD in high risk infants

Study (reference)	Subjects (n)	Intervention measures	Follow-up	Atopic dermatitis (cumulative incidence in intervention group)	Comments
Pregnancy dietary restriction					
Fälth-Magnusson & Kjellman (1992)	198	No egg or cow's milk during third trimester	5 years	No significant difference between intervention and control groups	AD diagnosed according to criteria of Hanifin & Rajka (1980). Observer blinded
Lilja et al. (1989)	162	No egg or cow's milk during third trimester	1.5 years	No significant difference between intervention and control groups	No objective diagnostic criteria. Observer blinded
Hypoallergenic formula feeding					
Mallet & Henocq (1992)	177	Casein hydrolysate (vs. adapted cow's milk formula) for 4 months	4 years	Reduced at 2 and 4 years ($p<0.001$)	No objective diagnostic criteria. Observer not blinded
Chandra et al. (1989)	124	Casein hydrolysate (vs. cow's milk or soy milk) for 6 months	1.5 years	Reduced at 1.5 years ($p<0.05$)	Diagnostic criteria not validated. Observer blinded. Short length of follow-up
Lactation dietary restriction and delayed solid feeding					
Zeiger & Heller (1995)	288	No egg, cow's milk or peanuts during third trimester and lactation. Breast feeding +/or casein hydrolysate for 12 months. Solids >6 months; cow's milk, soy, citrus, corn (>12 months); egg, fish, peanut (>24 months)	7 years	Reduced at 1 year ($p<0.05$) but no significant reduction at 2, 4 and 7 years	Diagnostic criteria not validated. Observer blinded. Severity of AD not assessed
Hide et al. (1994)	120	No egg, cow's milk, fish or nuts during lactation. Breast feeding +/or soy hydrolysate for 9 months. Cow's milk (9 months); egg (11 months); all others (12 months)	2 years	Reduced at 1 year ($p<0.05$) but no significant reduction at 2 years	Diagnostic criteria not validated. Observer blinded. Severity of AD not assessed
Chandra et al. (1989)	97	No egg, cow's milk, peanuts, soy or fish during lactation. Breast feeding for ~6 months. Solid foods ~6 months	1.5 years	Reduced at 1.5 years ($p<0.05$). Reduced severity	Diagnostic criteria not validated. Observer blinded. Compliance assessed by breast milk antigen measurement. Severity score used

egg during the third trimester of pregnancy. There was no difference in the point prevalence rates for AD, asthma and hay fever at 18 months and 5 years of age. Likewise, skin prick testing and total IgE levels were similar between the two groups. The finding that dietary modification during pregnancy has no effect on subsequent atopic disease in the child has also been supported by a similar study by Lilja et al. (1989). Furthermore, concern has been raised that dietary restriction during pregnancy may lead to nutritional deficiencies in the mother and a lower birth weight of the newborn child.

Mallet & Henocq (1992) studied the benefit of casein hydrolysate formula feeding of 'high risk' infants comparing the frequency of AD in this group with a group of infants fed an adapted cow's milk formula. The assigned formula was fed to the infant for four months either exclusively or as a complement to breast milk. During this time no other food was allowed. The point prevalence of AD was significantly less in the hydrolysate formula group compared with the cow's milk formula at two years (11.5% versus 42.6%) and four years (7.1% versus 25%) and the severity of AD was also less in the former group. A similar protective effect of casein hydrolysate was found by Chandra, Shakuntla & Hamed (1989) in infants followed to 18 months.

Three well-conducted studies have investigated the effect of strict food allergen avoidance during infancy by way of restricting the diet of mothers during lactation, using hypoallergenic formula feeds for those not breast fed, and delaying the introduction of solid foods. Zeiger and co-workers followed a cohort of 165 'high-risk' children over seven years (Zeiger et al., 1989; Zeiger & Heller, 1995). In the intervention group mothers avoided cow's milk, egg and peanut during the last trimester of pregnancy and lactation. Infants not breast fed were given a casein hydrolysate formula (instead of a cow's milk-based whey infant formula) and avoided cow's milk until the age of one year, egg until two years of age and peanut and fish until three years old. The cumulative incidence of AD was significantly lower in the intervention group at 12 months of age but was no longer significant at two, four and seven years.

A similar study was performed by Hide and colleagues on the Isle of Wight (Arshad et al., 1992; Hide et al., 1994; Hide, 1995). These investigators reported a follow-up of 120 newborns over two years. Breast-feeding mothers in the intervention group were placed on an exclusion diet free of dairy products, eggs, fish and nuts. Breast feeds were supplemented if necessary with a soya-based protein hydrolysate formula and infant solid feeding was delayed (cow's milk and soya until nine months, wheat until ten months and egg until eleven months). In addition, the houses of subjects in the intervention group were treated with anti-dust mite foams and powders for nine months and special mattress covers were used. Dust sampling confirmed a reduction of house dust mite antigen in these cases. The results of this study matched those of the previous study: a significant reduction in AD was observed in the intervention group at the 12-month follow-up but this difference was no longer significant at two years.

The third study by Chandra et al. (1989) reported a significant reduction of AD at the end of an 18-month follow-up in a group of 97 infants whose mothers were on a restricted diet during lactation (no egg, cow's milk, peanuts, soy or fish) and who delayed introduction of solid foods until six months. Compliance was assessed by examining daily diaries for food consumed and testing by enzyme-linked immuno-assay (ELISA) for β-lactoglobulin and ovalbumin in random samples of breast milk and was found to be satisfactory. A reduction in AD severity (based on a system developed at the St John's Hospital for Diseases of the Skin, London) was also noted in the intervention group. Further follow-up would have been of interest in determining whether AD was prevented or delayed in this cohort.

To summarize these findings:
- Dietary restriction during pregnancy appears to have no influence on the risk of AD in newborn children.
- Restricting the diet of breast feeding mothers together with introducing allergenic foods late in infancy may delay the onset of AD rather than prevent AD from developing.

- A role for house dust mite control in the prevention of AD cannot be established from current studies and awaits further investigation.

The use of hypoallergenic formula feeding during infancy to prevent AD requires additional confirmation. The study by Mallet & Henocq (1992) was weakened by the lack of validated diagnostic criteria for AD and the nonblinding of the observer. The similar findings of Chandra et al. (1989) are of interest but follow-up was short in this study.

Although the results of these studies suggest that allergen avoidance during infancy may not be sufficient to prevent AD, the observation that the disease can be delayed by these measures does lend support for the role of food allergen sensitization in the causation of at least some cases of AD. The period during which this 'pathogenic sensitization' process can occur is unknown, but appears to be beyond the first year of life. It could be speculated that delaying antigenic food exposure beyond infancy may result in a reduction in lifetime incidence of AD. However, practical and nutritional considerations may preclude such measures.

Most of the research on AD prevention has been concerned with demonstrating a reduction in disease incidence without assessing severity of disease. It is possible that interventional measures may lessen the severity of AD without necessarily lowering its incidence. Objective criteria for both diagnosis and severity of AD are required to achieve adequate assessment of outcome.

Recommendations for the prevention of atopic dermatitis and implications for future strategies

Based on current evidence, routine intervention measures during infancy cannot be recommended as a means of preventing AD. However, it is possible that the interventional studies which have so far failed to demonstrate a benefit from dietary intervention may have lacked sufficient statistical power to detect a small difference between the intervention and control groups. Further research is needed, including in the areas of house dust mite avoidance

Table 16.2. High risk versus low risk approach in the prevention of AD (adapted from Williams, 1997)

In a population of 1000 children

	High risk (40%) (i.e. children born to atopic parents)	Low risk (60%)
No. of children	400	600
No. of children who will express AD	160 (40% of 400)	102 (17% of 600)
No. of children in whom AD is preventable (assuming 50% prevention rate)	80	51

- Total children with AD = 160 + 102 = 262
- Percentage of AD preventable by targeting high risk group = 80/262 = 31%

and prophylactic skin care, before the notion of AD as a preventable disease is abandoned altogether. In the absence of definitive studies some authors have suggested that it is reasonable to offer parents of high risk infants advice such as prolonged breast feeding, maternal lactation diet without egg, milk or peanut (supplemented with calcium tablets), use of hypoallergenic formula feeds, delayed introduction of solid foods and avoidance of house dust mite (Zeiger, 1994).

It is worth noting the implications that future research on AD prevention may have on health care planning. As AD is a very common condition in the community and the source of substantial morbidity and public health costs, even small gains in preventing the disease may prove to be worthwhile. In order to assess the cost-effectiveness of preventive strategies, it is necessary to estimate the proportion of AD which can be attributed to preventable factors (i.e. the *attributable fraction*) and to evaluate the relative benefits of targeting high risk groups versus the general population.

The attributable fraction could be considered to

be 100% in the case of genetic factors, meaning that in theory all cases of AD might be preventable by genetic engineering techniques. On the other hand, the proportion of AD which is preventable by practical intervention measures may be substantially less and cannot be ascertained from current data. Early findings from the Isle of Wight study (which were not borne out by subsequent follow-up) suggested that up to 50% of AD cases were preventable (Arshad et al., 1992). Using this estimate, Williams calculated the proportion of AD cases which could be potentially prevented by adopting a high risk strategy (directed only towards children with a family history of atopy), and compared this outcome to that of a population-based approach (Williams, 1997). As Table 16.2 shows, it is assumed in this hypothetical example that children born to atopic parents represent 40% of the general population, and these high risk children have about a 40% chance of developing AD compared with 17% in those considered to be of low risk (Luoma, Koivikko & Viander, 1983). In this situation, only 31% of all cases of AD could be potentially prevented by targeting the high risk group (80 of 262 cases in Table 16.2) compared with a rate of 50% when preventive measures are aimed at the whole population. Thus, adopting a high risk strategy based on a family history of atopy will lead to two fifths of preventable AD cases being missed.

Should the actual proportion of AD which is preventable be closer to say 20%, the practical and financial costs involved for both participant and public health provider may outweigh the small potential yield in preventing the disease. The success rate of such allergy prevention programmes is likely to be even lower outside the setting of a clinical trial. Strong motivation is required in undertaking lifestyle intervention measures, especially when strict adherence to a specific diet is required. Compliance is most likely to occur when the perceived risk of developing the disease is high and also a high 'success rate' can be claimed for the recommended regimen. If only a small percentage of AD cases can be prevented by allergen avoidance it becomes even more important, for the sake of cost efficiency and ensuring compliance, to be able to

better identify those who are most likely to benefit from early intervention; that is, an accurate predictor of food or aeroallergen-induced AD is required. Zeiger (1994) has suggested that the presence of allergen-specific IgE in the infant may be a reliable marker of this disease risk. He has proposed that periodic screening of asymptomatic infants with skin prick testing or RAST/ELISA tests could be used as a possible means of identifying suitable candidates for prevention programmes. Such screening might be aimed at infants with atopic family history or elevated cord IgE levels. The value of this approach awaits further investigation.

Finally, if the benefits of early intervention programmes can be demonstrated in terms of a significant reduction in disease severity, despite only a small chance of prevention, they may yet become widely accepted as an important strategy in lessening the burden of AD in the community. Emphasis on this aspect of disease prevention may be more rewarding in the short term than attempts at complete eradication of disease expression.

Summary of key points

- A strategy for atopic dermatitis (AD) prevention is based on a conceptual model which supposes that both genetic and environmental factors contribute to alterations in systemic immune function and local cutaneous physiology.
- Although the immunological mechanism in AD is unknown, the notion of allergen sensitization is a useful one when considering preventive strategies.
- In the absence of genetic engineering techniques, potential targets for environmental manipulation include the avoidance of skin drying agents or irritants, and the reduction of exposure to allergens via transplacental, dietary or inhalational routes.
- Factors contributing to xerosis may alter the skin barrier function, thereby initiating or enhancing the causative process, although the prophylactic use of skin emollients is not yet of proven value.
- Breast feeding has the theoretical benefit of reducing allergen absorption through the immature

infant gut; however, the findings of previous studies have been inconsistent due to differences in methodology, and the effect of breast feeding on the subsequent development of AD remains uncertain.

- Prospective randomized controlled studies in high risk groups are the best means of assessing the benefit of early intervention measures in preventing AD.

- Evidence from these studies suggests that dietary modification during pregnancy has no effect on AD risk, whereas there may be some advantage in the use of hypoallergenic feeds in early infancy.

- Intervention studies in which a combination of allergen avoidance regimes have been employed (by lactating mothers avoiding allergenic foods, using hypoallergenic formula feeds, delaying the introduction of solid feeding and reducing house dust mite numbers) have shown a greater effect in delaying rather than preventing AD.

- Further studies are required to determine the relative contribution of preventable factors in AD and to develop a means of identifying those individuals who are most likely to benefit from intervention programmes.

- A reduction in disease severity rather than prevalence may be a more acceptable aim for those attempting to lessen the burden of AD in the community by public health measures.

References

Arshad, S.H., Matthews, S., Gant, C. & Hide, D.W. (1992). Effect of allergen avoidance on development of allergic disorders in infancy. *Lancet*, **339**, 1493–7.

Barba, A., Schena, D., Andreaus, M.C., Faccini, G., Pasini, F., Brocco, G., Cavallini, G., Scuro, L.A. & Chieregato, G.C. (1989). Intestinal permeability in patients with atopic eczema. *Br J Dermatol*, **120**, 71–5.

Bieber, T. & Braun-Falco, O. (1991). IgE-bearing Langerhans cells are not specific to atopic eczema but are found in inflammatory skin diseases. *J Am Acad Dermatol*, **24**, 658–9.

Bruijnzeel-Koomen, C.A., Van Wichen, D.F., Toonstra, J., Berrens, L. & Bruijnzeel, P.L. (1986). The presence of IgE molecules on epidermal Langerhans cells in patients with atopic dermatitis. *Arch Dermatol Res*, **278**, 199–205.

Cant, A., Narsden, R.A. & Kilshaw, P.J. (1985). Egg and cow's milk hypersensitivity in exclusively breast-fed infants with eczema and detection of egg protein in breast milk. *Br Med J*, **291**, 932–5.

Cavagni, G., Paganelli, R., Caffarelli, C., D'Offizi, G.P., Bertolini, P., Aiuti, F. & Giovannelli, G. (1988). Passage of food antigens into circulation of breast-fed infants with atopic dermatitis. *Ann Allergy*, **61**, 361–5.

Chandra, R.K., Shakuntla, P. & Hamed, A. (1989). Influence of maternal diet during lactation and use of formula feeds on development of atopic eczema in high risk infants. *Br Med J*, **299**, 228–30.

Croner, S. & Kjellman, N.I.H. (1990). Development of atopic disease in relation to family history and cord blood IgE levels. Eleven-year follow-up in 1654 children. *Pediat Allergy Immunol*, **1**, 14.

Fälth-Magnusson, K. & Kjellman, N.I.M. (1992). Allergy prevention by maternal elimination diet during late pregnancy – a 5-year follow-up of a randomized study. *J Allergy Clin Immunol*, **89**, 709–13.

Fartasch, M., Bassukas, I.D. & Diepgen, T.L. (1992). Disturbed extracting mechanism of lamellar bodies in dry non-eczematous skin of atopics. *Br J Dermatol*, **127**, 221–77.

Fergusson, D.M. & Horwood, L.J. (1994). Early solid food diet and eczema in childhood: a 10-year longitudinal study. *Pediat Allergy Immunol*, **5** (Suppl. 1), 44–7.

Freir, S. (1973). Paediatric gastrointestinal allergy. *Clin Allergy*, **3**, 597–618.

Golding, J. & Peters, T.J. (1987). The epidemiology of childhood eczema: I. A population based study of associations. *Paediat Perinatal Epidemiol*, **1**, 67–79.

Hanifin, J.M. & Rajka, G. (1980). Diagnostic features of atopic dermatitis. *Acta Dermatol Venereol (Scand.)*, Suppl. 92, 44–7.

Hattevig, G., Kjellman, B., Johansson, S.G.O. & Bjorksten, B. (1984). Clinical symptoms and IgE responses to common food problems in atopic and healthy children. *Clin Allergy*, **14**, 551–9.

Hauser, C., Snapper, C.M., Ohara, J., Paul, W.E. & Katz, S.I. (1989). T-helper cells grown with hapten-modified cultural Langerhans cells produce interleukin 4 and stimulate IgE production by B cells. *Europ J Immunol*, **19**, 245–51.

Hide, D.W. (1995). Allergy prevention – an attainable objective? *Europ J Clin Nutr*, **49** (Suppl 1), S71–6.

Hide, D.W., Matthew, S., Matthew, L., Stevens, M., Ridout, S., Twiselton, R., Gant, C. & Arshad, S.H. (1994). Effect of allergen avoidance in infancy on allergic manifestations at age two years. *J Allergy Clin Immunol*, **93**, 842–6.

Ioppi, M., Businco, L., Arcese, G., Ziruolo, G. & Nisini, R. (1994). Cord blood mononuclear leukocytes of neonates at risk of atopy have a deficiency of arachidonic acid. *J Invest Allergol Clin Immunol*, **4**, 272–6.

Johnson, E., Irons, J. & Patterson, R. (1974). Serum IgE concentration in atopic dermatitis. *J Allergy Clin Immunol*, **54**, 94–9.

Jujo, K., Renz, H., Abe, J., Gelfand, E.W. & Leung, D.Y. (1992). Decreased interferon gamma and increased interleukin-4 production in atopic dermatitis promotes IgE synthesis. *J Allergy Clin Immunol*, **90**, 323–31.

Kaplan, M.S. & Solli, N.J. (1979). Immunoglobulin E to cow's milk protein in breast fed atopic children. *J Allergy Clin Immunol*, **64**, 122–6.

Kjellman, B., Pettersson, R. & Hyensjö, B. (1982). Allergy among school children in a Swedish county. *Allergy*, **37** (Suppl 1), 5.

Kleinman, R.E. & Walker, W.A. (1984). Antigen processing and uptake from the intestinal tract. *Clin Rev Allergy*, **2**, 25–37.

Kramer, M.S. (1988). Does breast feeding help protect against atopic disease? Biology, methodology and a golden jubilee of controversy. *J Pediat*, **112**, 181–90.

Lilja, G., Dannaeus, A., Foucard, T., Graff-Lonnevig, V., Johansson, S.G. & Öman, H. (1989). Effects of maternal diet during late pregnancy and lactation on the development of atopic diseases in infants up to 18 months of age – in vivo results. *Clin Exp Allergy*, **19**, 473–9.

Lobitz, W.C. & Campbell, C.J. (1953). Physiologic studies in atopic dermatitis (disseminated neurodermatitis), 1. Local cutaneous response to intradermally injected acetylcholine and epinephrine. *Arch Dermatol Syphilol*, **67**, 575–89.

Luoma, R., Koivikko, A. & Viander, M. (1983). Development of asthma, allergic rhinitis and atopic dermatitis by the age of five years. *Allergy*, **38**, 339–46.

Macharia, W.M., Anabwani, G.M. & Owili, D.M. (1991). Effects of skin contactants on evolution of atopic dermatitis in children: a case control study. *Trop Doct*, **21**, 104–6.

Mallet, E. & Henocq, A. (1992). Long-term prevention of allergic disease by using protein hydrolysate formula in at-risk infants. *J Pediat*, **121**, S95–S100.

McGready, S.J. & Buckley, R.H. (1975). Depression of cell-mediated immunity in atopic eczema. *J Allergy Clin Immunol*, **56**, 393–406.

Mudde, G.C., van Reijsen, F.C., Boland, G.J., de Gast, G.C., Bruijnzeel, P.L. & Bruijnzeel-Koomen, C.A. (1990). Allergen presentation by epidermal Langerhans' cells from patients with atopic dermatitis is mediated by IgE. *Immunology*, **69**, 335–41.

Ogawa, H. & Yoshiike, T. (1993). A speculative view of atopic dermatitis: barrier dysfunction in pathogenesis. *J Dermatol Sci*, **5**, 197–204.

Ogawa, M., Berger, P.A. & McIntyre, R. (1971). IgE in atopic dermatitis. *Arch Dermatol*, **103**, 575–80.

Pathirana, C., Goulding, N.J., Gibney, M.J., Pitts, J.M., Gallagher, P.J. & Taylor, T.G. (1981). Immune tolerance produced by pre- and postnatal exposure to dietary antigen. *Int Arch Allergy Appl Immunol*, **66**, 114–8.

Peterson, R.D.A., Page, A.R.P. & Good, R.A. (1962). Wheal and erythema allergy in patients with agammaglobulinaemia. *J Allergy*, **33**, 406–11.

Pike, M.G., Heddle, R.J., Boulton, P., Turner, M.W. & Atherton, D.J. (1986). Increased intestinal permeability in atopic eczema. *J Invest Dermatol*, **86**, 101–4.

Pöysä, L., Korppi, M., Pietikäinen, M., Remes, K. & Juntunen-Backman, K. (1991). Asthma, allergic rhinitis and atopic eczema in Finnish children and adolescents. *Allergy*, **46**, 161–4.

Reinhold, U., Wehrmann, W., Kukel, S. & Kreysel, H.W. (1990). Evidence that defective interferon-gamma production in atopic dermatitis patients is due to intrinsic abnormalities. *Clin Exp Immunol*, **79**, 374–9.

Renz, H., Jujo, K., Bradley, K.L., Domenicl, J., Gelfand, E.W. & Leung, D.Y. (1992). Enhanced IL-4 production and IL-4 receptor expression in atopic dermatitis and their modulation by interferon gamma. *J Invest Dermatol*, **99**, 403–8.

Rosenberg, S.A. (1990). TNF/TIL human gene therapy clinical protocol. *Hum Gene Ther*, **1**, 441–80.

Ruiz, R.G., Richards, D., Kemeny, D.M. & Price, J.F. (1991). Neonatal IgE: a poor screen for atopic disease. *Clin Exp Allergy*, **21**, 467–72.

Saarinen, U.M. & Kajosaari, M. (1980). Does dietary elimination in infancy prevent or only postpone a food allergy? A study of fish and citrus allergy in 375 children. *Lancet*, **i**, 166–7.

Sampson, H.A. (1992). The immunopathogenic role of food hypersensitivity in atopic dermatitis. *Acta Dermatol Venereol (Scand.)*, Suppl., **176**, 34–37.

Sampson, H.A., Bernhisel-Broadbent, J., Yang, E. & Scanlon, S.M. (1991). Safety of casein hydrolysate formula in children with cow milk allergy. *J Pediat*, **118**, 520–5.

Saurat, J-H. (1985). Eczema in primary immune deficiencies. Clues to the pathogenesis of atopic dermatitis with special reference to the Wiskott Aldrich syndrome. *Acta Dermatol Venereol (Scand.)*, Suppl., **114**, 125–8.

Schwartz, D.P. & Buchley, M.D. (1971). Serum IgE concentrations and skin reactivity to anti-IgE antibody in IgA-deficient patients. *New Engl J Med*, **284**, 513–7.

Sporik, R., Holgate, S.T., Platts-Mills, T.A.E. & Cogswell, J.J. (1990). Exposure to house-dust mite allergen (Der p I) and the development of asthma in childhood. *New Engl J Med*, **323**, 502–7.

Strobel, S.M.D. & Ferguson, A. (1984). Immune responses to fed protein antigen in mice. 3. Systemic tolerance or priming is related to age at which antigen is first encountered. *Pediat Res*, **18**, 588.

Szentivanyi, A. (1968). The beta adrenergic theory of the atopic abnormality in bronchial asthma. *J Allergy*, **42**, 203–32.

Tang, M.L.K., Kemp, A.S., Thorburn, J. & Hill, D.J. (1994). Reduced interferon-γ secretion in neonates and subsequent atopy. *Lancet*, **344**, 983–5.

Taylor, B., Norman, A.P., Orgel, H.A., Stokes, C.R., Turner, M.W. & Soothill, J.F. (1973). Transient IgA deficiency and pathogenesis of infantile atopy. *Lancet*, **ii**, 111–3.

Tupka, R.A., Pinnagoda, J., Coenraads, P.J. & Nater, J.P. (1990). Susceptibility to irritants: role of barrier function, skin dryness and history of atopic dermatitis. *Br J Dermatol*, **123**, 199–205.

Uehara, M. (1982). Reduced histamine reaction in atopic dermatitis. *Arch Dermatol*, **118**, 244–5.

Uehara, M. (1989). Family background of respiratory atopy: a factor of serum IgE elevation in atopic dermatitis. *Acta Dermatol Venereol (Scand.)*, Suppl. 144, 78–82.

Uehara, M. & Sawai, T. (1989). A longitudinal study of contact sensitivity in patients with atopic dermatitis. *Arch Dermatol*, **125**, 366–8.

Ukabam, S.O., Mann, R.I. & Cooper, B.T. (1984). Small intestinal permeability to sugars in patients with atopic eczema. *Br J Dermatol*, **110**, 649–52.

Van Asperen, P.P., Kemp, S.S. & Mellis, C.M. (1983). Immediate food hypersensitivity reactions on the first known exposure to the food. *Arch Dis Childh*, **58**, 253–6.

Waite, D., Eyles, E.F., Tonkin, S.L. & O'Donnell, T.V. (1980). Asthma prevalence in Tokelauan children in two environments. *Clin Allergy*, **10**, 71–5.

Walker, W.A. & Hanson, D. (1985). The mechanisms of allergic reactions and local antibody production in infancy. *Clin Dis Pediatr Nutr*, **4**, 75–95.

Watanabe, M., Tagami, H., Horii, I., Takahashi, M. & Kligman, A.M. (1991). Functional analyses of the superficial stratum corneum in atopic xerosis. *Arch Dermatol*, **127**, 1689–92.

Werner, Y. & Lindberg, M. (1985). Transepidermal water loss in dry and clinically normal skin in patients with atopic dermatitis. *Acta Dermatol Venereol (Scand.)*, **65**, 102.

Williams, H.C. (1992). Is the prevalence of atopic dermatitis increasing? *Clin Exp Dermatol*, **17**, 385–91.

Williams, H.C. (1997). Inflammatory skin diseases I: Atopic dermatitis. In: Williams, H.C. & Strachan, D.P. (eds.) *The Challenge of Dermato-epidemiology*. Boca Raton: CRC Press.

Williams, H.C., Strachan, D.P. & Hay, R.J. (1994). Childhood eczema: disease of the advantaged? *Br Med J*, **308**, 1132–5.

Yamamoto, A., Serizawa, S., Ito, M. & Sato, Y. (1991). Stratum corneum lipid abnormalities in atopic dermatitis. *Arch Dermatol Res*, **283**, 219–23.

Young, E., Bruynzeel-Koomen, C. & Berrens, L. (1985). Delayed type hypersensitivity in atopic dermatitis. *Acta Dermatol Venereol (Scand.)*, Suppl. **114**, 77–81.

Zeiger, R.S. (1994). Dietary manipulation in infants and their mothers and the natural course of atopic disease. *Pediat Allergy Immunol*, **5** (Suppl 1), 33–43.

Zeiger, R.S. & Heller, S. (1995). The development and prediction of atopy in high-risk children: follow-up at age seven years in a prospective randomized study of combined maternal and infant food allergen avoidance. *J Allergy Clin Immunol*, **95**, 1179–90.

Zeiger, R.S., Heller, S., Mellon, M.H., Forsythe, A.B., O'Connor, R.D., Hamberger, R.N. & Schatz, M. (1989). Effect of combined maternal and infant food-allergen avoidance on development of atopy in early infancy. *J Allergy Clin Immunol*, **84**, 72–89.

PART V

Lessons from other fields of research

17

Parallels with the epidemiology of other allergic diseases

David P. Strachan

Introduction

For many years, atopic dermatitis (AD) has been the 'poor relation' in epidemiological studies of allergic diseases. In many ways this is puzzling, as the condition is more visible and amenable to objective assessment than asthma, rhinitis or food allergy and, arguably, it causes more misery than any of these. The epidemiology of asthma has received most attention, perhaps because it is occasionally a fatal disease, and accounts for a high proportion of paediatric hospital admissions.

This mass of epidemiological research has not been rewarded by clear advances in our understanding of what causes asthma. Instead, it has raised serious questions about the nature of the disease, the distinction between initiating and provoking factors, and the determinants of incidence and prognosis. These will be discussed and related to similar issues concerning AD.

In contrast, fewer studies have investigated the epidemiology of allergic rhinitis, but these have been more productive in generating novel hypotheses about environmental determinants of allergic sensitization. In general, the epidemiological features of hay fever parallel those of AD more closely than asthma, and may be particularly relevant to investigation of the causes of AD.

Finally, building on the themes introduced in Chapter 7, time trends in asthma, hay fever and AD will be reviewed together, with the aim of proposing a unifying hypothesis to explain the apparent rise in prevalence of all three atopic conditions worldwide in recent years.

One disease or many?

Dermatologists are familiar with the overlapping syndromes of 'endogenous eczema' (including AD), irritant contact dermatitis and allergic contact dermatitis. They have the luxury (compared to respiratory physicians) of being able to inspect the diseased organ easily, thus deriving clues about the likely aetiology and pathophysiology from direct observations of the natural history and distribution of the lesions. Respiratory clinicians and epidemiologists have debated long, hard and generally fruitlessly about whether childhood asthma should be regarded as a unitary disorder or as several overlapping syndromes (Wilson, 1989). There have been similar debates about the nature of chronic respiratory disease in adults (Fletcher & Pride, 1984).

Early population studies of schoolchildren distinguished 'asthma' (presumed to be allergic in nature) from 'wheezy bronchitis' (presumed to be caused by infection) largely on the basis of the disease label reported by parents or assigned by doctors. Others classified as 'asthmatic' children with a history of wheezing in the absence of upper respiratory tract infection, and as 'wheezy bronchitics' those who wheezed only in association with colds. During the 1970s this distinction was challenged on both epidemiological and therapeutic grounds (Williams & McNicol, 1969; Speight, Lee & Hey, 1983).

Pioneering studies of wheezy schoolchildren in Melbourne (Williams & McNicol, 1969) suggested that abnormalities of lung function and allergic markers among children with infrequent attacks of wheezing, triggered only by viral infection ('wheezy bronchitis') were qualitatively similar, although less extreme, than among children who wheezed at times in the absence of infection ('asthma'). The authors suggested that 'wheezy bronchitis' and 'asthma' should be regarded as part of a single spectrum of wheezing illness, with varying severity but similar underlying pathophysiology. Dermatologists might similarly debate whether 'cradle cap' and 'atopic dermatitis' should be included in a wider spectrum of 'infant eczema'.

The unitary view was further supported by therapeutic evidence that inhaled bronchodilators are effective in most children with wheeze (Speight et al., 1983) and some nonwheezy children with nocturnal cough (Spelman, 1984). At a time when asthma was infrequently used as a label for childhood wheezing, the concern was of widespread underdiagnosis and consequent undertreatment of asthma (Speight et al., 1983). In more recent British surveys, the asthma diagnosis appears to have been more widely applied and no longer seems to be a prerequisite for prescription of bronchodilators (Strachan et al., 1994), but there is still some evidence of avoidable morbidity and school absence (Anderson, Butland & Strachan, 1994). However, response to a common therapy may be a poor guide to common cause or mechanisms: topical steroids are effective in both atopic and contact dermatitis, and in several unrelated skin conditions.

The pragmatic convenience of considering all wheezing illnesses as a single disease category tended to obscure the obvious variability in the clinical characteristics and natural history of wheezing in childhood. More recently, the unitary view has been challenged (Wilson, 1989; Silverman, 1993; Martinez et al., 1995), and a number of different phenotypes have been proposed: transient early wheezing (common in young infants, with a benign prognosis); a more persistent tendency to virus-associated wheezing (previously 'wheezy bronchitis', tending to resolve before or during adolescence); and atopic asthma (rare in preschoolchildren, more closely related to atopic manifestations, and with a poorer long-term prognosis). These distinctions appear to have some validity in terms of natural history (Martinez et al., 1995), although it remains to be seen whether the definitions prove useful in aetiological investigations or clinical management. There is clearly scope for investigation of similar subcategorization of infant eczema on the basis of disease pattern, natural history, associated asthma or hay fever, and various cutaneous or circulating markers of allergy.

A distinction between different forms of wheezing illness or infant eczema may become particularly relevant in searching for specific genotypes associated with asthma and AD. Furthermore, if genetic subtypes are identified, the epidemiological investigation of environmental causes should logically proceed among subgroups of children with demonstrable genetic predisposition. Investigation of all types of AD together might obscure associations of major importance with specific subtypes.

Prognosis and natural history

Although short-term prognosis has been proposed as one criterion for distinguishing wheezing phenotypes, the long-term outcome of childhood asthma remains uncertain (Sears, 1994). Many studies of the natural history of childhood asthma have been based on patients (Strachan, 1996a). These are difficult to interpret because they sample an unknown proportion of all wheezy children, probably skewed towards the more severe cases. There are few prognostic studies of population-based samples of wheezing illness in childhood (Strachan, 1996a), and only three of these extend from early childhood into adult life (Oswald et al., 1994; Jenkins et al., 1994; Strachan, Butland & Anderson, 1996).

Each of these three studies recruited their cohort at age seven years. Some children with early episodes of wheezing will have been omitted due to incomplete recall and exclusion of wheezing not labelled as asthma or wheezy bronchitis. These exclusions tend to bias estimates of prognosis in an unfavourable direction (Strachan, 1985). Studies of the natural history of AD from early childhood would be most informative if they were established early in infancy and based on a representative sample of all eczematous children, rather than those attending out-patient clinics or identified later with persistent disease (see Chapter 3)

By definition, measurement of long-term outcomes requires long-term follow-up. The results therefore relate to cohorts among whom the causes of wheezing illness, and access to and use of medical care, are likely to be different from those of later generations. This is an intractable problem which limits the generalizability of prognostic studies. A further difficulty posed by long-term follow-up is possible biases related to sample attrition. The proportion of wheezy children on whom measurements of ventilatory function have been obtained in adult life ranges from 53 to 70%, with somewhat greater numbers providing questionnaire information (Strachan, 1996a). It is likely that similar losses to follow-up would apply in studies of the long-term outcome of childhood eczema. Thus, it is important that sufficient information is obtained at baseline to evaluate possible differences between responders and nonresponders at subsequent follow-ups, for instance with respect to disease severity, family history of eczema, socioeconomic status and ethnic group.

One of the problems in measuring an episodic condition such as asthma or eczema is to determine when the disease may be considered in remission. Many epidemiological studies use the occurrence of one or more attacks of wheezing over the last 12 months to define the presence of childhood asthma (Lenney, Wells & O'Neill, 1994). This raises the question whether children who have been free of wheezing for one year have 'grown out of' their asthma. The findings from the Melbourne study (Oswald et al., 1994) and the British 1958 cohort (Strachan, Butland & Anderson, 1996) suggest that this is not the case. There is a tendency for symptoms to relapse in adult life after a period of remission in adolescence, particularly in subjects who take up cigarette smoking, and this relapse rate is greater than the incidence of first-ever wheezing in adult life (Strachan, Butland & Anderson, 1996). As discussed in Chapter 4, there is some evidence of a similar continuity of susceptibility in children who have apparently outgrown early AD, but remain at increased risk of occupational dermatitis.

The apparent relapse of wheezing in a significant minority of children after prolonged remission raises the issue of how asymptomatic persistence of the asthmatic trait may be assessed. Nonspecific bronchial hyper-responsiveness is detectable prior to the onset of wheeze in childhood (Jones & Bowen, 1994) and has been proposed as such an indicator. However, in the Melbourne cohort, reactivity to methacholine among subjects who had been wheeze-free for at least three years did not differ significantly from the levels among control subjects without a history of wheezing in early childhood (Kelly et al., 1988). Development of objective indicators of latent disease (such as increased transepidermal water loss, or abnormal pharmacological responses) may be easier for eczema than for asthma, because the skin is more accessible than the lung to challenge tests and biopsy.

A comprehensive study of disease prognosis should include a range of outcomes (Strachan, 1996a). For example, studies have described the association of childhood wheezing with later respiratory symptoms; ventilatory function; other respiratory diseases; employment prospects and achieved socioeconomic status. Asthma in adult life has been analysed in relation to subsequent risk of cancer and mortality, but no similar studies have been conducted of childhood wheezing. A similar portfolio of outcomes could be considered for AD. For instance, a reduced risk of viral warts among children with atopic disorders (Williams, Pottier & Strachan, 1993), may indicate enhanced cell-mediated immunity which could influence a number of nondermatological diseases.

Initiating and provoking factors

Discussion of the causes of conditions such as asthma or eczema should distinguish clearly between the process whereby healthy people become prone to episodes (disease induction) and the factors which provoke symptomatic episodes or exacerbate the condition (Dolovich & Hargreave, 1981). For asthma, the more convincing evidence relates to known or suspected triggers of symptoms in children who are already susceptible to chest problems. These provoking factors include upper respiratory infections, aeroallergen exposure, airborne irritants, exercise and emotion. Several studies have shown that viral infections are the principal cause of exacerbations even among atopic children and those who also wheeze in response to other triggers (Johnston et al., 1995). There is a clear parallel with AD, which is commonly exacerbated by local irritants, such as soap, wool or microbial organisms, rather than by 'endogenous' or 'exogenous' allergic reactions. These largely clinical observations leave unanswered the question of induction: why healthy children become susceptible to wheezing or eczematous rashes. A further question might also be raised: why do so many children appear to outgrow these diseases? There are a number of possible reasons why epidemiology has failed so far to explain the induction of asthma. Most of these are pertinent to aetiological investigation of AD, although this is at a much earlier stage.

Studies have measured the right exposures imperfectly

Measurements which are imprecise will tend to dilute associations between exposure and disease. Yet for many factors, including virus infections and domestic aeroallergens, measurement of exposure has been extremely crude, especially in relation to exposure during possible 'critical periods' in early childhood (Sporik et al., 1990). The critical period for induction of AD may be shorter than for childhood asthma, as the onset of symptoms usually occurs in infancy, but similar problems arise in the measure-

ment of prenatal exposures and environmental circumstances in the first few weeks of life. Retrospective assessments of maternal exposure during pregnancy may lack specificity (for example, for particular types of viral infections, or their timing during gestation), whereas prospectively collected information will be expensive, laborious and time-consuming, unless the critical period can be clearly specified in the design of cohort studies.

Studies have not adjusted for selective avoidance of exposures

A further problem is the tendency of atopic families to avoid or remove certain exposures which are thought to be hazardous. The risk of wheezing associated with household pets, for instance, may be underestimated if pet avoidance is not addressed in data analysis (Strachan & Carey, 1995). Similar considerations apply to investigation of soap additives or wool clothing in relation to childhood eczema (Luoma, 1984).

Studies have not concentrated on susceptible subgroups

The effect of risk factors which have been adequately measured may have been diluted by studying whole populations, rather than subgroups who are susceptible to the disease. This offers only a partial explanation for lack of success, since at least one-quarter of children experience an attack of wheezing illness at some time in the first two decades of life (Strachan, Butland & Anderson, 1996; Lewis et al., 1995). Thus, it is unlikely that the predisposition to asthma is rare. Atopic dermatitis is also common, but high-risk groups can be defined, for example by parental history of atopy (Burr et al., 1989a; Arshad et al., 1992). It may be that studies of these susceptible infants may be particularly informative.

Studies have addressed the wrong questions

There has been an understandable supposition that the factors which induce asthma are likely to be airborne and that established trigger factors may also be influential in initiating the disease process, but this need not be the case. For instance, diet (Burney, 1987; Schwartz & Weiss, 1990), and obstetric factors (Strachan, Butland & Anderson, 1996) are receiving increasing attention in asthma epidemiology, as they are for AD. Paradoxically, it has recently been suggested that the inhalational route, as opposed to direct contact, may be relevant in the induction of AD by house dust mites (Tupker et al., 1996).

Studies have been of the wrong design

It may be that cross-sectional, case-control and longitudinal studies within populations have failed to detect the major determinants of asthma incidence because these are fairly evenly distributed within a local population. Thus, almost everyone is 'exposed' and studies in a single location can identify only the factors determining individual susceptibility (family history and atopic tendency). Variation in exposure to many of the recognized triggers of asthma is greater between populations than within centres. Some exposures, such as outdoor air pollution (Department of Health, 1995), can only be studied at an 'ecological' (population) level. Ecological studies of AD in relation to, for instance, water quality or house dust mite infestation, should be considered.

There are two or more diseases with different epidemiology

The weak association of wheezing illness with many exposures studied may disguise opposing relationships of two or more distinct diseases with the measured risk factors. While it is hard to believe that all risk factors so far studied should display such opposing trends, it is possible that more detailed study of the epidemiology of wheezing illness in atopic and nonatopic children will clarify whether there are distinct clinical syndromes with characteristic risk factors. One large analysis of this type has recently been published, and remarkably few

differences were observed, although maternal smoking appeared to increase the risk of wheezing only in nonatopic children (Strachan, Butland & Anderson, 1996). Only with more careful attention to the definition of phenotypes in epidemiological studies of wheezing illness will it be possible to determine whether there are aetiologically distinct disease categories within the spectrum of illness presenting in the community.

Risk factors

So far we have discussed epidemiological parallels between asthma and dermatitis in childhood. Although less is known about the distribution of allergic rhinitis within and between populations, a striking feature to emerge from several studies is the epidemiological similarity between hay fever and dermatitis and the contrast between each of these and the patterns displayed for wheezing illness in childhood. Table 17.1 illustrates these similarities and differences for selected risk factors as measured in a large national British cohort, born in March 1958. Parents were asked to recall episodes of asthma or wheezy bronchitis, hay fever or recurrent sneezing, and eczematous rashes in their child at the age of 7 years (Davie, Butler & Goldstein, 1972). School medical officers examined each child for skin disease at the ages of 7, 11 and 16 (Williams, Strachan & Hay, 1994). A subsample of the cohort were skin prick tested as young adults (Strachan et al., 1997b). The epidemiology of immediate cutaneous hypersensitivity to house dust mite, grass pollen and cat fur, mirrors closely the patterns shown here for hay fever.

These data are consistent with other studies in the UK (Golding & Peters, 1986; Strachan, Golding & Anderson, 1990) and elsewhere (Sibbald & Strachan, 1994), which suggest that the epidemiological features of hay fever and AD are different from those of childhood wheezing, showing variations with longitude, family size, birth order, infant feeding and parental social class which are not seen for asthma and wheezy bronchitis. The trends in lifetime prevalence of dermatitis and asthma/wheezy bronchitis

Table 17.1. Prevalence (%) of asthma/wheezy bronchitis, hay fever/recurrent sneezing and eczematous rashes by selected risk factors in the British 1958 birth cohort

Risk factor	No. of subjects	Asthma/WB by age 7	Hay fever by age 7	Eczema by age 7	Eczema seen at 7, 11 or 16	Number examined
Maternal age		***		***		
<20	746	24.7	5.9	7.4	6.1	380
20–24	3981	19.2	5.3	7.7	5.0	2273
25–29	4600	18.0	5.8	8.1	5.4	2708
30–34	2879	17.5	5.5	6.6	5.6	1638
35+	1823	17.0	5.2	4.7	5.5	1017
Birth order			***	***	*	
1st	5152	18.8	6.6	8.6	5.7	3031
2nd	4460	18.2	5.8	7.4	5.5	2600
3rd	2245	18.2	4.9	6.5	5.1	1261
4th	1123	18.3	3.8	5.4	5.1	603
5th or above	1201	17.3	3.5	2.8	3.7	617
Gestation		**		*		
<37 weeks	453	24.1	4.8	5.0	4.7	232
37–38 weeks	1705	20.4	5.3	6.7	5.3	985
39–40 weeks	6053	17.2	5.5	7.7	5.5	3569
41+ weeks	4021	18.8	6.1	7.5	5.5	2305
Birth weight				*		
<2.5 kg	774	17.4	4.5	5.1	6.9	407
2.5–2.9 kg	2546	17.8	5.4	6.8	4.4	1438
3.0–3.4 kg	5084	18.4	5.6	7.5	5.3	2924
3.5–3.9 kg	3909	18.5	5.4	7.4	6.1	2277
4.0+ kg	1266	19.1	6.3	8.1	5.2	726
Place of birth			***	***	*	
Most westerly	3446	17.0	4.7	5.8	4.4	2056
2nd quartile	3659	19.0	4.8	6.2	4.9	2110
3rd quartile	3364	19.1	5.2	8.2	6.7	1888
Most easterly	3568	18.6	7.3	8.8	5.7	1969
Place of birth		***	***	***		
Most southerly	3722	18.9	7.5	8.9	5.9	2113
2nd quartile	3181	20.5	5.8	7.9	6.1	1817
3rd quartile	3793	19.0	4.4	6.3	4.8	2036
Most northerly	3341	15.4	4.4	5.7	4.9	2057
Place of birth						
Conurbation	4292	19.2	6.3	7.5	5.4	2147
Major town	2880	17.6	4.6	6.7	5.5	1705
Urban county	3601	17.6	5.4	6.8	5.2	2138
Rural county	3471	18.8	5.5	7.7	5.4	2151

Table 17.1 (*cont.*)

Risk factor	No. of subjects	Asthma/WEB by age 7	Hay fever by age7	Eczema by age 7	Eczema seen at 7, 11 or 16	Number examined
Sex		***	**			
Male	7463	20.5	6.1	7.3	5.0	4223
Female	7062	16.1	4.9	7.0	5.7	4056
Infant feeding			***	***	***	
Bottle	4560	18.8	4.6	5.6	4.3	2446
Breast <1 month	3579	18.3	5.1	6.8	5.5	2010
Breast ≥1 months	6255	18.1	6.5	8.6	5.9	3746
Mother smoked in pregnancy		***	**	*		
No	9299	17.4	6.0	7.6	5.4	5435
Yes	4578	20.7	4.6	6.4	5.2	2507
Father's social class at age 11			***	***	**	
I (professional)	653	16.7	9.1	9.7	6.5	474
II	2181	17.1	6.8	9.9	6.9	1534
III non-manual	1134	17.6	6.7	8.4	4.5	806
III manual	5163	18.5	5.6	7.3	5.3	3413
IV	2086	18.8	4.6	5.1	4.2	1373
V (unskilled)	723	17.8	2.8	4.4	4.8	435
Siblings at 11			***	***	*	
1	1182	18.9	8.7	7.4	5.8	762
2	4082	18.8	6.6	8.6	6.3	2856
3	3099	17.8	5.3	7.5	4.9	2096
4	1927	18.7	4.4	6.3	4.5	1298
5+	1990	17.2	3.8	5.6	4.2	1226

Note:

Asterisks denote the statistical significance of the linear trend in prevalence across the categories of each risk factor ordered as shown: * $p<0.05$, ** $p<0.01$, *** $p<0.001$.

with latitude, birth weight and maternal age are in a similar direction, but the corresponding relationships with gestational age and maternal smoking during pregnancy run in opposite directions. Gender differences in prevalence of asthma/wheezy bronchitis and hay fever by age 7 are much greater than for eczematous rashes. It is perhaps of interest, as noted above, that maternal smoking is one of the few variables which display a statistically significant difference in effects between atopic and nonatopic wheezers (Strachan, Butland & Anderson, 1996).

Common risk factors do not necessarily imply a common aetiology, but it is reasonable to argue that seasonal allergic rhinitis may be a useful indicator of the distribution of the atopic phenotype (Strachan, 1995a), and where this assumption has been validated by objective measures such as skin prick testing, it appears to be sound (Strachan et al., 1997b; Strachan, Taylor & Carpenter, 1996; von Mutius et al., 1994). The close correspondence between the epidemiology of AD, whether reported by parents, or examined by doctors, and the risk factors for hay fever, suggest that a major influence on the occurrence of AD within Britain, at least, is the distribution of the atopic phenotype. This may be because (as with hay fever) the provoking factors are widespread and therefore the disease pattern is determined by susceptibility. Such an argument raises the question whether recent trends in prevalence of AD and other allergic diseases could reflect changes in this underlying susceptibility (Bousquet et al., 1993; Strachan, 1995b).

Time trends

Over the past 30 years, an upward trend in health care utilization for asthma has been noted in several English-speaking countries (Mitchell, 1985). The rise has been particularly marked in young children. There is some evidence that changes in health service utilization for childhood asthma may have contributed to the upward trend in hospital admissions in the UK (Strachan & Anderson, 1992). On the other hand, there is also substantial evidence from population surveys of a modest increase (by about 50% in relative terms) in the prevalence of all wheezing illnesses among children in Britain (Lenney et al., 1994, Lewis et al., 1996) and Australia (Bauman, 1993) over the past 30 years. Thus, there is evidence of an increase in morbidity, although this may have been exaggerated in routine statistics by changes in diagnosis and medical care.

Studies of British and Swedish children and army recruits suggest that the prevalence of reported hay fever or allergic rhinitis has increased substantially since the 1960s, approximately doubling each decade (Ninan & Russell, 1992; Burr et al., 1989a; Åberg et al., 1995; Taylor et al., 1984). One Swedish study (Åberg et al., 1995) and four British studies (Ninan & Russell, 1992; Burr et al., 1989a; Taylor et al., 1984; Schultz Larsen et al, 1986) have also described a rise in the prevalence of AD among children or adolescents, the magnitude of the increase varying somewhat from 50% to 300% per decade. These studies suggest a more rapid increase in the prevalence of hay fever and AD than for asthma and wheezing taken together. This may be because the former are diagnosic labels which have become more popular over time, or because they are more closely related to allergic mechanisms than the full spectrum of wheezing in childhood.

It would be plausible to relate the simultaneous upward trends in each of the three major allergic diseases to a rise in the underlying prevalence of allergic sensitization. There is some evidence in support of such a trend in Japan (Nakagomi et al., 1994), Britain (Sibbald, Rink & D'Souza, 1990) and the United States (Barbee et al., 1987). In contrast, between the early 1980s and early 1990s there was little change in the proportion of Australian adults (Peat et al., 1992) or children (Peat et al., 1994) who reacted on skin prick testing to local aeroallergens. However, taking a longer term perspective, hay fever appears to have been exceedingly rare before the industrial revolution in Britain (Emanuel, 1988) and Switzerland (Wüthrich, 1989), and emerged earliest among the more privileged urban classes (Emanuel, 1988; Wüthrich, 1989). The recent time trends and persistent socioeconomic variations in prevalence of hay fever and AD may be continuations of these historical changes. In seeking to explain the apparent emergence of allergic diseases as a global epidemic (Strachan, 1989), the current risk factors for hay fever, dermatitis and allergic sensitization may be particularly informative (Strachan, 1995a).

An inverse association between manifestations of allergy and sibship size has been consistently found from an early age (Golding & Peters, 1986; Strachan, 1989) through childhood (von Mutius et al., 1994) and adolescence (Strachan, Taylor & Carpenter, 1996) to adult life (Strachan et al., 1997a, 1997b; Jarvis et al., 1997). Four studies have reported inverse correlations between sibship size and the prevalence of positive skin prick tests (Strachan et al., 1997b; Strachan, Taylor & Carpenter, 1996; von Mutius et al., 1994) or raised levels of specific immunoglobulin E (Jarvis et al., 1997), arguing strongly against a spurious relationship attributable to differential recognition, reporting or diagnosis of symptoms in smaller and larger families. The structure as well as the size of the family may be influential. After allowance for family size, position within the sibship (Strachan et al., 1997b; Golding & Peters, 1986; Strachan, 1995a; Strachan, Taylor & Carpenter, 1996), birth spacing (Strachan, Taylor & Carpenter, 1996), sibling gender (Strachan et al.,

1997a) and maternal age (Strachan, 1995a; Strachan, Taylor & Carpenter, 1996; Strachan et al., 1997a) have been related to hay fever or allergic sensitization. These associations are less consistent than for total sibship size, and require further confirmation. Nevertheless, they may offer useful clues to the biological factors underlying the family size effect.

The most coherent explanation for these associations is that infections acquired by household contact in early childhood protect against the subsequent development of allergic disease (Strachan, 1989). This could also account for the independent associations of hay fever and AD with richer families and breast feeding (Strachan, 1995a) and the apparent increase in allergic diseases over the past century or more (Emanuel, 1988; Wüthrich, 1989). The emergence of allergic disease as a 'post-industrial revolution epidemic' can thus be attributed to the decline in cross-infection within young families, and the current distribution of atopy within and between populations may be explained parsimoniously (Strachan, 1996b).

When it was first proposed (Strachan, 1989), this 'hygiene' hypothesis challenged the immunological opinion prevailing at the time, which proposed that early infection might promote, rather than protect against, allergic sensitization. However, more recent advances in our understanding of T-lymphocyte differentiation (Holt, 1994) have suggested a possible mechanism for such a protective effect. The 'natural' immune response (Romagnani, 1992) to infections occurring in early life, perhaps specifically at the time of first exposure to the relevant allergen, may inhibit the proliferation of Th2-cell clones, and thereby prevent allergy (Martinez, 1994). An alternative hypothesis is that a stable state of Th1-type or Th2-type predominance is not reached for some 5–7 years after birth (Hattevig, Kjellman & Björkstén, 1993) and may be influenced by the cytokine environment prevailing at each of multiple exposures to a specific allergen (Holt, 1994).

Unfortunately, despite these immunological advances, epidemiological evidence directly relating early infection to the subsequent development of allergy is sparse and far from convincing (Shaheen, 1995; Strachan, Taylor & Carpenter, 1996; Backman et al., 1984; Shaheen et al., 1996). Longitudinal studies are required to elucidate the early postnatal influences on sensitization and allergic disease. Atopic dermatitis may prove particularly useful as an early outcome measure, because it is common, can be objectively defined, and occurs soon after birth, yet appears very similar epidemiologically to hay fever and aeroallergen sensitization in young adults (Strachan, 1989; Strachan et al., 1997b).

Thus, rather than being the 'poor relation' in allergic disease epidemiology, AD may in future have much to offer to explaining the global rise in prevalence of all three allergic disorders. An integrated approach to the study of asthma, dermatitis and hay fever is required to elucidate why the contribution of each to the total burden of atopic disease varies by age within individuals, over time within countries, and between countries at a particular point in time.

Summary of key points

- As with dermatitis, there is division of opinion about whether asthma should be regarded as a single entity or multiple diseases.
- Discussion of causes of conditions such as asthma and AD should distinguish clearly between initiating and provoking factors.
- Although all three atopic diseases tend to cluster in individuals, the epidemiological risk factors for AD are more similar to those for hay fever than the risk factors for asthma.
- Eczema, hay fever and skin prick reactivity to common aeroallergens are less common in children from large families and poorer socioeconomic circumstances.
- These patterns may reflect a protective effect of early infections on the development of allergic sensitization.
- Upward trends in the prevalence of childhood wheezing, diagnosed asthma and hay fever in many countries parallel the increase in prevalence of diagnosed AD.
- These trends are plausibly explained by an

increase in the prevalence of allergic sensitization, possibly related to a decline in incidence of infectious illness in early childhood.

- A coherent approach to the epidemiological study of the three atopic diseases is recommended.

References

Åberg, N., Hesselmar, B., Åberg, B. & Eriksson, B. (1995). Increase of asthma, allergic rhinitis and eczema in Swedish school children between 1979 and 1991. *Clin Exp Allergy*, **25**, 815–9.

Anderson, H.R., Butland, B.K. & Strachan, D.P. (1994). Trends in the prevalence and severity of childhood asthma. *Br Med J*, **308**, 1600–4.

Arshad, S.H., Matthews, S., Gant, C. & Hide, D.W. (1992). Effect of allergen avoidance on development of allergic disorders in infancy. *Lancet*, **339**, 1493–7.

Backman, A., Björkstén, F., Ilmonen, S., Juntunen, K. & Suoniemi, I. (1984). Do infections in infancy affect sensitization to airborne allergens and development of allergic disease? *Allergy*, **39**, 309–15.

Barbee, R.A., Kaltenborn, W., Lebowitz, M.D. & Burrows, B. (1987). Longitudinal changes in allergen skin test reactivity in a community population sample. *J Allergy Clin Immunol*, **79**, 16–24.

Bauman, A. (1993). Has the prevalence of asthma symptoms increased in Australian children? *J Paediat Child Hlth*, **29**, 424–8.

Bousquet, J., Burney, P.G.J. et al. (1993). Evidence for an increase in atopic disease and possible causes. *Clin Exp Allergy*, **23**, 484–92.

Burney, P. (1987). A diet rich in sodium may potentiate asthma. Epidemiologic evidence for a new hypothesis. *Chest*, **6** (Suppl.), 143S–148S.

Burr, M.L., Butland, B.K., King, S. & Vaughan-Williams, E. (1989a). Changes in asthma prevalence: two surveys 15 years apart. *Arch Dis Childh*, **64**, 1118–25.

Burr, M.L., Miskelly, F.G., Butland, B.K., Merrett, T.G. & Vaughan-Williams, E. (1989b). Environmental factors and symptoms in infants at high risk of allergy. *J Epidemiol Commun Hlth*, **43**, 125–32.

Davie, R., Butler, N. & Goldstein, H. (1972). *From Birth to Seven. The Second Report of the National Child Development Study (1958 Cohort)*. London: National Children's Bureau.

Department of Health Committee on the Medical Effects of Air Pollutants (1995). *Asthma and Outdoor Air Pollution*. London: HMSO.

Dolovich, J. & Hargreave, F. (1981). The asthma syndrome: inciters, inducers and host characteristics. *Thorax*, **36**, 641–3.

Emanuel, M.B. (1988). Hayfever, a post industrial revolution epidemic: a history of its growth during the 19th century. *Clin Allergy*, **18**, 295–304.

Fletcher, C.M. & Pride, N.B. (1984). Definitions of emphysema, chronic bronchitis, asthma and airflow obstruction: 25 years on from the CIBA symposium. *Thorax*, **39**, 81–5.

Golding, J. & Peters, T. (1986). Eczema and hay fever. In: Butler, N. & Golding, J. (eds.) *From Birth to Five. A Study of the Health and Behaviour of Britain's Five-year-olds*, pp. 171–86. Oxford: Pergamon Press.

Hattevig, G., Kjellman, B. & Björkstén, B. (1993). Appearance of IgE antibodies to ingested and inhaled allergens during the first 12 years of life in atopic and nonatopic children. *Pediat Allergy Immunol*, **4**, 182–6.

Holt, P.G. (1994). A potential vaccine strategy for asthma and allied atopic diseases during early childhood. *Lancet*, **344**, 456–8.

Jarvis, D., Chinn, S., Luczynska, C. & Burney, P. (1997). The association of family size with atopy and atopic disease. *Clin Exp Allergy*, **27**, 240–5.

Jenkins, M.A., Hopper, J.L., Bowes, G., Carlin, J.B., Flander, L.B. & Giles, G.G. (1994). Factors in childhood as predictors of asthma in adult life. *Br Med J*, **309**, 90–3.

Johnston, S.L., Pattemore, P.K., Sanderson, G. et al. (1995). Community study of the role of virus infections in exacerbations of asthma in 9–11 year old children. *Br Med J*, **310**, 1225–9.

Jones, A. & Bowen, M. (1994). Screening for childhood asthma using an exercise test. *Br J Gen Pract*, **44**, 127–31.

Kelly, W.J.W., Hudson, I., Raven, J., Phelan, P.D., Pain, M.C.F. & Olinsky, A. (1988). Childhood asthma and adult lung function. *Am Rev Resp Dis*, **138**, 26–30.

Lenney, W., Wells, N.E.J. & O'Neill, B.A. (1994). The burden of paediatric asthma. *Europ Resp Rev*, **4**, 49–62.

Lewis, S., Richards, D., Bynner, J., Butler, N. & Britton, J. (1995). Prospective study of risk factors for early and persistent wheezing in childhood. *Europ Resp J*, **8**, 349–56.

Lewis, S., Butland, B., Strachan, D., Bynner, J. & Britton, J. (1996). Study of the aetiology of wheezing illness at age 16 in two national British birth cohorts. *Thorax*, **51**, 670–6.

Luoma, R. (1984). Environmental allergens and morbidity in atopic and non-atopic families. *Acta Paediat (Scand.)*, **73**, 448–53.

Martinez, F.D. (1994). Role of viral infections in the inception of asthma and allergies during childhood: could they be protective? *Thorax*, **49**, 1189–91.

Martinez, F.D., Wright, A.L., Taussig, L.M., Holberg, C., Halonen,

M. & Morgan, W.J., Group Health Medical Associates (1995). Asthma and wheezing in the first six years of life. *New Engl J Med*, **332**, 133–8.

Mitchell, E.A. (1985). International trends in hospital admission rates for asthma. *Arch Dis Childh*, **60**, 376–8.

Nakagomi, T., Itaya, H., Tominaga, T., Yamaki, M., Hisamatsu, S. & Nakagomi, N. (1994). Is atopy increasing? *Lancet*, **343**, 121–2.

Ninan, T.K. & Russell, G. (1992). Respiratory symptoms and atopy in Aberdeen schoolchildren: evidence from two surveys 25 years apart. *Br Med J*, **304**, 873–5.

Oswald, H., Phelan, P.D., Lanigan, A., Hibbert, M., Bowes, G. & Olinsky, A. (1994). Outcome of childhood asthma in mid-adult life. *Br Med J*, **309**, 95–6.

Peat, J.K., Haby, M., Spijker, J. et al. (1992). Prevalence of asthma in adults in Busselton, Western Australia. *Br Med J*, **305**, 1326–9.

Peat, J.K., van den Berg, R.H., Green, W.F., Mellis, C.M., Leeder, S.R. & Woolcock, A.J. (1994). Changing prevalence of asthma in Australian children. *Br Med J*, **308**, 1591–6.

Romagnani, S. (1992). Human TH1 and TH2 subsets: regulation of differentiation and role in protection and immunopathology. *Int Arch Allergy Appl Immunol*, **98**, 279–85.

Schultz Larsen, F., Holm, N.V. & Henningsen, K. (1986). Atopic dermatitis. A genetic–epidemiological study in a population-based twin sample. *J Am Acad Dermatol*, **15**, 487–94.

Schwartz, J. & Weiss, S.T. (1990). Dietary factors and their relation to respiratory symptoms. *Am J Epidemiol*, **46**, 624–9.

Sears, M. (1994). Growing up with asthma. *Br Med J*, **309**, 72–3.

Shaheen, S.O. (1995). Changing patterns of childhood infection and the rise in allergic disease. *Clin Exp Allergy*, **25**, 1034–7.

Shaheen, S.O., Aaby, P., Hall, A.J., Barker, D.J.P., Heyes, C.B., Shiell, A.W. & Goudiaby, A. (1996). Measles and atopy in Guinea-Bissau. *Lancet*, **347**, 1792–6.

Sibbald, B. & Strachan, D. (1994). Epidemiology of rhinitis. In: Busse, W. & Holgate, S.T. (eds.) *Mechanisms in Asthma and Rhinitis: Implications for Diagnosis and Treatment*, pp. 32–43. Oxford: Blackwell Scientific.

Sibbald, B., Rink, E. & D'Souza, M. (1990). Is atopy increasing? *Br J Gen Pract*, **40**, 338–40.

Silverman, M. (1993). Out of the mouths of babes and sucklings. Lessons from early childhood asthma. *Thorax*, **48**, 1200–4.

Speight, A.N.P., Lee, D.A. & Hey, E.N. (1983). Underdiagnosis and undertreatment of asthma in childhood. *Br Med J*, **286**, 1253–6.

Spelman, R. (1984). Chronic or recurrent cough in children – presentation of asthma? *J R Coll Gen Practit*, **34**, 221–2.

Sporik, R., Holgate, S.T., Platts-Mills, T.A.E. & Cogswell, J.J. (1990). Exposure to house-dust mite allergen (*Der p1*) and the

development of asthma in childhood. *New Engl J Med*, **323**, 502–7.

Strachan, D.P. (1985). The prevalence and natural history of wheezing in early childhood. *J R Coll Gen Practit*, **35**, 182–4.

Strachan, D.P. (1989). Hay fever, hygiene and household size. *Br Med J*, **299**, 1259–60.

Strachan, D.P. (1995a). Epidemiology of hay fever: towards a community diagnosis. *Clin Exp Allergy*, **25**, 296–303.

Strachan, D.P. (1995b). Time trends in asthma and allergy: ten questions, fewer answers. *Clin Exp Allergy*, **25**, 791–4.

Strachan, D.P. (1996a). Long-term outcome of early childhood wheezing: population data. *Europ Resp J*, **9** (Suppl. 21), S42–S47.

Strachan, D.P. (1996b). Socioeconomic factors and the development of allergy. *Toxicol Lett*, **86**, 199–203.

Strachan, D.P. & Anderson, H.R. (1992). Trends in hospital admission rates for asthma in children. *Br Med J*, **304**, 819–20.

Strachan, D.P. & Carey, I.M. (1995). The home environment and severe asthma in adolescence: a population based case-control study. *Br Med J*, **311**, 1053–6.

Strachan, D.P., Golding, J. & Anderson, H.R. (1990). Regional variations in wheezing illness in British children: the effect of migration during early childhood. *J Epidemiol Comm Hlth*, **44**, 231–76

Strachan, D.P., Anderson, H.R., Limb, E.S., O'Neill, A. & Wells, N. (1994). A national survey of asthma prevalence, severity and treatment in Great Britain. *Arch Dis Childh*, **70**, 174–8.

Strachan, D.P., Butland, B.K. & Anderson, H.R. (1996). The incidence and prognosis of asthma and wheezing illness from early childhood to age 33 in a national British cohort. *Br Med J*, **312**, 1195–9.

Strachan, D.P., Taylor, E.M. & Carpenter, R.G. (1996). Family structure, neonatal infection and hay fever in adolescence. *Arch Dis Childh*, **74**, 422–6.

Strachan, D.P., Harkins, L.S., Golding, J. and the ALSPAC Study Team (1997a). Sibship size and self-reported inhalant allergy among adult women. *Clin Exp Allergy*, **27**, 151–5.

Strachan, D.P., Harkins, L.S., Johnston, I.D.A. & Anderson, H.R. (1997b). Childhood antecedents of allergic sensitisation in young British adults. *J Allergy Clin Immunol*, **99**, 6–12.

Taylor, B., Wadsworth, M., Wadsworth, J. & Peckham, C. (1984). Changes in the reported prevalence of childhood eczema since the 1939–45 war. *Lancet*, **ii**, 1255–7.

Tupker, R.A., de Monchy, J.G.R., Coenrads, P.J., Homan, A. & van der Meer, J.B. (1996). Induction of atopic dermatitis by inhalation of house dust mite. *J Allergy Clin Immunol*, **97**, 1064–70.

von Mutius, E., Martinez, F.D., Fritzsch, C., Nicolai, T., Reitmar, P. & Thiemann, H.H. (1994). Skin test reactivity and number of siblings. *Br Med J*, **308**, 692–5.

Williams, H. & McNicol, K.N. (1969). Prevalence, natural history and relationship of wheezy bronchitis and asthma in children. An epidemiological study. *Br Med J*, **iv**, 321–5.

Williams, H.C., Pottier, A.C. & Strachan, D.P. (1993). Are viral warts seen more commonly in children with eczema? *Arch Dermatol*, **129**, 717–21.

Williams, H.C., Strachan, D.P. & Hay, R.J. (1994). Childhood eczema: disease of the advantaged? *Br Med J*, **308**, 1132–5.

Wilson, N.M. (1989). Wheezy bronchitis revisited. *Arch Dis Childh*, **64**, 1194–9.

Wüthrich B. (1989). Epidemiology of the allergic diseases: are they really on the increase? *Int Arch Allergy Appl Immunol*, **90**, 3–10.

18

Recent developments in atopic dermatitis of companion animals

Susan E. Shaw and Michael J. Day

Introduction

Although atopic dermatitis (AD) is a recognized disease in several animal species, it is best characterized in the dog. In defining the disease, specific clinical and immunological aspects have been variously emphasized. Halliwell & Gorman (1989a) defined canine atopy as an inherited predisposition to develop IgE antibodies to environmental allergens resulting in allergic disease. However, this definition was extended by Scott, Miller & Griffin (1995) to a genetically programmed disease of dogs in which the patient becomes sensitized to environmental allergens that in nonatopic dogs cause no disease. Classically the 'atopic predisposition' was considered to be mediated through IgE, but IgG antibodies are now considered important in the pathogenesis of canine AD (Willemse et al., 1985a, 1985b; Hites et al., 1989; Day, Corato & Shaw, 1996). Although Halliwell & Gorman (1989a) considered that the allergic skin disease associated with canine atopy was not a good model for human atopic dermatitis, Willemse (1986) considers it mimics AD of man both clinically and immunologically.

Feline atopic skin disease has been described clinically although complete characterization of reaginic antibodies including IgE in this species has not been documented (DeBoer et al., 1992; Foster et al., 1995). Atopic dermatitis has not been conclusively indentified in horses or domesticated farm animals although reaginic antibodies, IgE and type I hypersensitivity are well documented in horses, cattle, sheep, swine and goats.

Clinical picture

Canine atopic dermatitis

The clinical picture which most clearly approaches that described in human AD is seen in the dog. The predominant clinical sign is pruritus which may be expressed by scratching, rubbing, biting and licking. The severity of this behaviour often disturbs the sleep of both owner and animal. Willemse (1986) has described major and minor diagnostic criteria for AD in the dog and emphasized the similarity to those described by Hanifin & Rajka (1980) for human AD. In 75% of dogs with AD, clinical signs occur before three years of age. The dermatitis is chronic or chronically relapsing. Although the clinical presentation varies with the chronicity of the disease, 85% of dogs with AD have lichenification of the flexor and/or extensor aspects of their joints and digits as well as involvement of the axillary and inguinal skin creases (Willemse, 1986). Facial pruritus is common in dogs (50–100%) and is considered a major clinical sign by Willemse (1986); 60–70% of dogs with AD have other visible lesions including erythema, papulo-pustular eruption and crusting in the previously described distribution pattern (Willemse, 1986). An individual or family history of AD and/or the presence of a breed predisposition is also characteristic of AD in the dog. Diagnostic features of canine AD have been listed by Willemse (1986) and are given in Table 18.1.

Validation of these major criteria has not been performed in veterinary dermatology. However, the

Table 18.1. Diagnostic features of canine atopic dermatitis (AD) (after Willemse, 1986)

Major features
(1) Pruritus
(2) Chronically relapsing dermatitis
(3) Facial and/or digital pruritus
(4) Lichenification of flexor/extensor surfaces of carpi and tarsi
(5) Individual or family history of atopy or presence of breed predisposition

Minor features
(1) Onset of symptoms before three years of age
(2) Facial erythema and cheilitis
(3) Bilateral conjunctivitis
(4) Superficial staphylococcal pyoderma
(5) Hyperhidrosis
(6) Immediate skin test reactivity to inhalant allergens
(7) Elevated allergen-specific IgE/IgG

approach used by the UK working party on diagnostic criteria for human AD (Williams et al., 1994a, 1994b, 1994c) in determining a minimum list of discriminators, the repeatability of clinical features and independent validation of diagnostic criteria, could be easily adapted to investigating canine AD.

Atopic dermatitis in other companion animal species

Feline AD is recognized as an important clinical entity (Carlotti, 1992; Foster & O'Dair, 1993; Prost, 1998). However, unlike AD in the dog, there is no characteristic presentation other than chronic or recurrent pruritus. A confusing quadrad of syndromes – papular dermatitis, symmetrical alopecia, ulcerative facial dermatitis and eosinophilic granuloma complex – may be present alone or in combination. All of these syndromes have been reported not only in association with feline AD but also with nonatopic, allergic skin disease. Diagnosis of feline AD is still dependent on the history of recurrent pruritus, immediate skin test reactivity to environmental allergens and response to specific immunotherapy (Chalmers & Medleau, 1994; Prost, 1998; Betteny, 1998). No breed predisposition has been documented.

Atopic dermatitis in the horse is also poorly documented. However, the high prevalence of seasonally recurrent allergic dermatitis (Queensland itch, 'sweet itch', Kasen or 'summer eczema') caused by biting insects, particularly the biting flies of the *Culicoides* spp., make clinical characterization of AD difficult. Despite this, it is recognized that there is both an individual and breed predisposition of horses to develop recurrent seasonal pruritic dermatitis in association with respiratory tract disease (Halldordsottir & Larsen, 1991). Recently, Littlewood, Paterson & Shaw (1998) have described a syndrome of atopy-like dermatitis in the horse characterized by chronic, nonseasonal pruritus and/or urticaria without the distribution usually associated with insect bite hypersensitivity. Affected horses have positive intradermal skin test reactivity to dust mites and fungal spores (Littlewood et al., 1998) and respond clinically to decreased specific allergen exposure.

Association of atopic dermatitis with other allergic diseases

There is a variable association between canine AD and allergic disease of the respiratory tract. The prevalence of sneezing in atopic dogs varies between 0% (Griffin, 1993) and 22% (Willemse & Van den Brom, 1983), although control populations have not been studied. In the latter report, sneezing was positively correlated with the presence of conjunctivitis. However, Willemse (1984b) found that less than 4% of dogs with AD had an increase in nasal airway resistance after allergen-specific nasal provocation. Asthma is not a naturally occurring disease in dogs, but in an experimental model for human asthma established in dogs sensitized to *Ascaris suum* antigen, 'atopic-like' dermatitis was reported in association with flares of respiratory disease (Peters, Hirshman & Malley, 1982). In cats with AD, sneezing has been reported in 50% of cases with or without concurrent conjunctivitis (Carlotti & Prost, 1988). However, the feline asthma syndrome, which is believed to have an allergic basis, is not associated

Table 18.2. The prevalence of positive intradermal reactions to fleas (*Ct felis*) in atopic dogs (%)

United Kingdom		France	United States of America		Australia
SE Scotland	SW England	Aquitaine	Illinois	Florida	Queensland
Sture et al. (1995)	Shaw unpublished data	Carlotti & Costargent (1992)	Schick & Fadok (1986)	Schick & Fadok (1986)	Mason, unpublished data
13.8 (*n*= 87)	23.7 (*n*= 100)	35.9 (*n*= 256)	9 (*n*= 130)	79 (*n*= 120)	90 (*n*= 140)

with dermatitis (Corcoran, Foster & Luis Fuentes, 1995).

In animals with AD, the effects of concurrent ectoparasite hypersensitivity must be considered. The association of AD and flea allergy dermatitis (FAD) has been studied in dogs (Table 18.2). In geographical areas where fleas are endemic (e.g. Florida and Queensland), 80–90% of dogs with AD have positive skin reactivity to flea antigen compared with 40% of normal dogs in the same areas (Schick & Fadok, 1986; Halliwell & Gorman, 1989b; Griffin, 1993). In areas of low flea prevalence, such as Illinois, the association decreases proportionately (Schick & Fadok, 1986; Griffin, 1993). However, Carlotti & Costargent (1992) examined both flea allergic dogs and dogs with AD in an area of medium flea prevalence (France) and found that, although 36% of dogs with AD had positive skin test reactivity to fleas, 80% of dogs with FAD had positive skin test reactivity to environmental allergens. This supports the hypothesis that atopic dogs are predisposed to the development and/or maintenance of FAD (Halliwell & Gorman, 1989a).

The relationship between AD and hypersensitivity dermatitis to insects and arachnids other than fleas or house dust mites has been investigated in both dogs and horses. In geographical areas where fleas are rare, up to 42% of dogs with AD had positive intradermal skin test reactivity to arthropods such as biting flies of the *Simulans* spp. (Griffin, 1993), although skin test reactivity for normal dogs was not reported. The prevalence of allergen-specific IgE to insects or arachnids was higher than corresponding skin test prevalence, irrespective of geographical region, suggesting that their role in AD in dogs may

have been underestimated (Griffin, 1993) or that cross-reactivity with house dust mite allergens occurs.

In horses, hypersensitivity to biting flies of the *Culicoides* spp. has been investigated extensively. The allergic dermatitis produced, unlike that of FAD in the dog, has a breed predisposition and a significant association with chronic respiratory tract disease (Halldordsottir & Larsen, 1991). It has been suggested that affected horses have an atopic predisposition and that hypersensitivity to *Culicoides* is one expression (Halldordsottir & Larsen, 1991).

The prevalence of skin test reactivity to specific allergens in canine atopic dermatitis

A range of indoor and outdoor allergens have been incriminated in AD in animals. The largest studies reporting the prevalence of positive intradermal reactions in canine AD have been conducted in Europe (Table 18.3). The most significant groups are those containing the dust mites, *D. farinae* and *D. pteronyssinus*. These in vivo data are supported by serological studies recording the prevalence of allergen-specific IgE and IgG antibodies in atopic dogs which, again, are largely directed against the dust mite group (Day et al., 1996).

Individual atopic dogs react only to specific allergens in a panel on intradermal testing, or ELISA, rather than to all allergens in some degree, which suggests a causative role for those allergens. Moreover, hyposensitization therapy using extracts of these specific allergens is clinically effective when compared with therapy performed using a placebo or clinically irrelevant allergens (Willemse et al., 1984).

Table 18.3. Immediate skin test reactivity in dogs with AD by allergen group expressed as a percentage of positive reactors

	United Kingdom			France		Scandinavia		Holland	United States of America			Australia
	Sture et al. (1995)	Sture et al. (1995)	Shaw unpublished data	Carlotti & Costargent (1992)	Prelaud (1990)	Ohlen (1992) Vollsett (1985)		Willemse (1984a)	Schick & Fadok (1986)	Schick & Fadok (1986)		Mason unpublished data
			SW		Isle de					Florida		Queensland
	SE Scotland (Edinburgh)	SE England (London)	England (Bristol)	Aquitaine	France	Sweden	Norway	Utrecht	Illinois	South	North	SE
Allergen	n=87	n=31	n=100	n=256	n=75	n=204	n=122	n=208	n=130	n=67	n=53	n=140
Mites/dust	62.1	58.1	67.1	80.5	62	54.9	75.5	39	88	71	88	86
Epithelia	80.4	11	<1	35	3	26	59	25–29	1	18	36	ND
Tree pollen	24.1	22.6	<1	5.1	<1	4.1	6.6	23.6	33	41	47	9
Weed pollen	24.1	25.8	5.3	3.5	6	3.3	6.3	13–10.1	31–45	31	47	17.4
Grass pollen	29.9	25.8	11	6.2	11	10.6	21.2	<1	45–61	<1	<1	13.2
Moulds	8.0	12.9	10	9.4	1	3.3	<1	4.3	27–35	15	23	11.8

Pathomechanism of atopic dermatitis

Despite the clinical significance of AD in companion animals, relatively little is known of the specific immunopathogenesis of the disease. To a large extent this reflects the lack of species-specific immunological reagents which are only now becoming available. In the dog, available evidence suggests that classical type I hypersensitivity is the predominant pathomechanism. However, in parallel to some studies in humans, suppressed lymphocyte responses to mitogens and cutaneous reactions to a contact allergen (dinitrochlorbenzene) indicate that altered cell-mediated immunity may be involved in canine AD (Nimmo Wilkie et al., 1991).

Total serum IgE levels in healthy canine reference populations are 1000 times those in humans (Hill et al., 1995). Hill et al. found no significant differences in total serum IgE between healthy dogs, atopic dogs and dogs with intestinal parasites. However, the presence of allergen-specific IgE has been documented in canine AD (Halliwell, 1990; Day et al., 1996).

Although for many years it was believed that the causative allergens in canine AD were inhaled, it is now generally accepted that the major route of exposure is by percutaneous absorption. It has been postulated that changes in the local cutaneous microclimate and epidermal integrity permit allergen translocation (Rhodes et al., 1987; Mason & Lloyd, 1993), the generation of reaginic IgE and IgG antibodies and subsequent sensitization of dermal mast cells. Various pieces of evidence support this hypothesis. Lesional skin biopsies from dogs with AD reveal epidermal hyperplasia and spongiosis, superficial dermal oedema and superficial perivascular dermatitis involving mixed infiltrates of mast cells, eosinophils, macrophages, plasma cells and lymphocytes (Gross, Ihrke & Walder, 1992). To our knowledge there have been no experimental histopathological studies which serially examine the changes in the skin of allergen-sensitized dogs following challenge, and little is known of the 'late phase' response in canine AD. Increased numbers of epidermal Langerhans cells expressing class II major histocompatibility complex molecules and IgE receptors, have been demonstrated in the lesional skin of dogs with AD (Day, 1996; Olivry et al., 1996). IgG-bearing plasma cells are a part of the dermal infiltrate with a dominance of cells containing cytoplasmic IgG2 and IgG4 (Day & Mazza, 1995). Delayed responses (6–24 hours) to intradermal provocation have been reported in the horse (Fadock & Greiner, 1990; Littlewood et al., 1998); however, aeroallergen patch tests have not been performed in companion animals. A single immunohistochemical study of equine insect mediated hypersensitivity has recorded significant numbers of T lymphocytes and class II positive dendritic cells within the inflammatory infiltrate. It has been suggested that this implicates both immediate and delayed hypersensitivity components in the pathogenesis (Kurotaki et al., 1994).

The role of IgG subclasses in canine AD has been investigated. Early studies (Willemse et al., 1985a, 1985b) demonstrated the presence of allergen-specific antibodies of an IgG subclass termed IgGd in atopic dogs and demonstrated that these antibodies were reaginic. More recently (Mazza et al., 1994), it has been proposed that the nomenclature IgG1–IgG4 be adopted for the four canine IgG subclasses based on homology with the subclasses in humans. The human and canine IgG subclasses have similar electrophoretic mobility and relative serum concentration, but to date functional studies have not been performed on the canine immunoglobulins. Dogs reactive to the dust mites (*D. farinae* and/or *D. pteronyssinus*) have a predominance of allergen-specific IgG antibodies of the IgG4 subclass, whereas dogs sensitized to the pollen of Timothy grass produce both an IgG1 and IgG4 antibody reaction (Day et al., 1996).

The demonstration of the presence of allergen-specific IgE, IgG and IgG subclasses in serum of allergic animals has resulted in the development of a plethora of serological tests for the diagnosis of AD in the dog, cat and horse. A polyclonal antiserum specific for feline IgE has been used to develop an allergen-specific ELISA (Gilbert & Halliwell, 1998). Although monoclonal antisera specific for canine IgE have been produced (DeBoer, Ewing & Schultz, 1993; Peng, Simons & Becker, 1993), many commercially available immunodiagnostic tests employ polyclonal antiserum. There is ongoing debate as to the specificity of such reagents and their validity when compared to the 'gold standard' of intradermal skin testing. Serum from clinically healthy dogs (Codner & Lessard, 1993; Bond, Thorogood & Lloyd, 1994) or dogs with parasitic diseases (Paradis & Lecuyer, 1993) produce positive reactions in IgE ELISAs which cloud their interpretation. Many authors have reported a poor correlation between the results of intradermal skin testing in canine AD and commercially available ELISAs for allergen-specific IgE (Codner & Lessard, 1993; Miller et al., 1993; Bond et al., 1994). This may reflect the difference in the kinetics of the cutaneous and systemic antibody response to allergens in the dog. There is generally a good correlation between the levels of allergen-specific IgE and IgG in dogs with AD. However, there is a group of house dust mite-reactive dogs in which only IgE antibodies are found (Day et al., 1996).

IgG antibodies reactive to insect or mould-derived allergens are found in atopic dogs, often in the absence of IgE antibodies of these specificities. These can also be identified in normal dogs (Day & Penhale, 1988; Hites et al., 1989; Day et al., 1996), which suggests that dogs frequently make IgG responses to environmental antigens. It has recently been reported that canine IgE antibodies may bind cross-reactive antigens of different insects including the flea, black ant, fly and cockroach (Pucheu-Haston et al., 1996).

An in vitro leukocyte histamine release assay has been developed for use in the dog (Peters et al., 1982; Jackson, Miller & Halliwell, 1996).

Prevalence and morbidity of atopic dermatitis

The true prevalence of AD in the canine population is unknown. As in human AD differing measures of disease frequency have been used. Although Chamberlain (1974) and Griffin (1993) reported that 10–15% of the canine population are affected with AD, lower estimates are better accepted. Halliwell & Schwartzman (1971) and Scott (1981) reported prev-

alences of 3.3% and 8%, respectively. There are no incidence figures available.

The prevalence of AD alone in horses is unknown. However, the one-year period prevalence of *Culicoides* hypersensitivity dermatitis in the Icelandic breed was 15–17.6% (Brostrom & Larsson, 1987; Halldordsottir & Larsen, 1991).

Risk factors

Risk factors which increase the chance of developing atopic dermatitis

Age and gender

There is general agreement, irrespective of geographical location, that canine AD is a disease of young dogs. The onset of clinical signs occurs before the age of three years in 70–82.5% of dogs (Willemse & Van den Brom, 1983; Griffin, 1993; Scott et al., 1995; Shaw unpublished data); 34% are symptomatic by nine months of age and 10% show signs before the age of six months (Griffin, 1993).

Although earlier reports have emphasized a female predisposition in canine AD (Halliwell & Schwartzman, 1971; Scott, 1981; Schick & Fadok, 1986), this is not a consistent finding. No statistically significant gender predisposition was found for canine AD by Willemse & Van den Brom (1983), Carlotti & Costargent (1992) or Shaw (unpublished data) although there was a trend towards females being more frequently affected in the last study. However, neutered dogs of both sexes had a significantly greater prevalence of AD than those which were entire (Shaw, unpublished data). Hormonal factors may exacerbate AD in humans, and neutering in dogs may allow 'allergic breakthrough' (Katz, 1978) in those dogs with a genetic predisposition to AD.

No gender predisposition has been reported in Icelandic horses with allergic dermatitis (Brostrom & Larsson, 1987; Halldordsottir & Larsen, 1991).

Genetic predisposition

Both breed and familial predispositions are recognized in canine AD. Schwartzman, Rockey &

Halliwell (1971) reported limited breeding studies which showed that all the offspring from a mating between atopic parents developed skin disease and positive skin reactivity to environmental allergens by the age two years. When one parent was affected 50% of the offspring developed AD. Butler (1983) reported an experimental model of AD in a group of related Basenji–Greyhound cross dogs sensitized to *Ascaris* antigen. However, further attempts to establish breeding colonies of affected dogs have been largely unsuccessful (Schwartzman, Massicot & Sogn, 1983). The association of canine AD, serum IgE level and expression of particular dog leukocyte antigens has been examined but no clear relationship was found (Vriesendorp et al., 1975). The susceptibility of Icelandic horses to *Culicoides* hypersensitivity has been positively associated with the expression of a class I equine leukocyte antigen (Halldordsottir & Larsen, 1991).

Numerous studies have identified predisposed breeds of dog. However, such information is biased by the popularity of certain breeds and by the lack of studies comparing breed predisposition of affected dogs to the relevant control populations. There is agreement that certain breeds are predisposed to developing AD at less than six months of age. These include the Golden retriever, Akita and Shar Pei (Scott et al., 1995). Although individual breeds of pure-bred dogs are overrepresented, cross-bred dogs were also significantly affected in the population studied by Shaw (unpublished data).

Month of birth

Van Stee (1983) reported that dogs born during the onset of the pollen season in the USA are predisposed to develop AD. Conversely, Halliwell (1990) reported that birth outside the pollen season was associated with a decreased risk.

Viral infections and vaccination

The use of multivalent viral vaccines is routine in cats, dogs and horses. In addition, the prevalence of viral respiratory tract disease in these species remains high. No information is available in horses or cats but, in dogs, Frick & Brooks (1983) have reported that modified live viral vaccines augment IgE production to pollens, although this was not associated with an increase in prevalence of disease.

The presence of endoparasites

In human AD, there is evidence for an inverse relationship between infestation with helminth parasites and clinical allergic disease. However, this association has not been investigated in animals.

Infestation with helminth parasites is a common occurrence in companion animals, particularly those that are young. The risk of zoonotic infection from nematodes (e.g. *Toxocara canis*, *Ancylostoma caninum*, *Uncinaria stenocephala*) and cestodes (e.g. *Echinococcus granulosus*) has led to rigorous preventive anthelmintic therapy in dogs and cats which is often administered concurrently with vaccination. In geographical areas where heartworm (*Dirofilaria immitus*) is endemic in dogs, monthly prophylactic therapy with broad spectrum anthelmintics is routine. However, there are no studies which compare the prevalence of AD in dogs with a low to zero helminth burden as a result of regular treatment and a comparable nontreated stray or native dog population. In a UK study (Shaw, unpublished data), there was no significant difference between the percentage of dogs with AD that received prophylactic anthelmintic treatment (89.5%) and the nonatopic hospital reference population.

However, as mentioned previously, ectoparasite infestation appears to be positively correlated with AD in both the dog and the horse.

Risk factors exacerbating atopic dermatitis

Season of the year

There is agreement that, although a seasonal pattern may be seen initially in dogs with AD, with chronicity AD becomes perennial. The point prevalence of dogs with a seasonal variation in a UK study (Shaw, unpublished data) was 34%. However, Scott (1981) and Griffin (1993) reported that 80% of dogs with AD will develop nonseasonal variation in

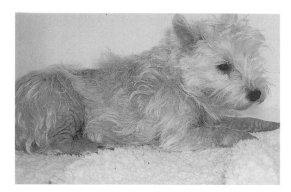

Fig. 18.1. Severe atopic dermatitis in bramble West Highland white terrier. There is lichenification of skin creases and distal limbs. AD is complicated by secondary staphylococcal and malassezial infection.

disease pattern with age. The first onset of clinical signs of AD is less likely in winter than during other seasons of the year (Griffin, 1993; Scott et al., 1995).

Cutaneous bacterial and yeast infections

Atopic dogs are predisposed to secondary infections but this is believed to be a sequel to AD rather than a primary abnormality of immunological function. Atopic dog corneocytes have increased adherence for *Staphylococcus intermedius* (McEwan, 1990) and intradermal histamine promotes percutaneous penetration of Staphylococcal antigen (Mason & Lloyd, 1993). Shearer & Day (1997) reported that 58% of dogs with AD had concurrent Staphylococcal pyoderma. Infection with *Malassezia* spp. complicates AD (Plant et al., 1992), particularly in certain breeds such as the West Highland white terrier (Scott & Miller, 1989) and the German shepherd (Mason, 1993). The prevalence of this infection in 210 dogs with AD was 13% (R. Bond, personal communication).

The relationship of atopic dermatitis with food intolerance

The exacerbation of AD by certain foods is controversial in both veterinary and human dermatology. Although the mechanism is poorly understood, it is accepted that food intolerance contributes to the clinical picture of canine AD and that dietary modification, primarily protein restriction, may reduce the severity of clinical signs (Griffin, 1993). The diagnosis of food intolerance and/or hypersensitivity is complicated by the fact that both intradermal skin testing and serological testing (RAST and ELISA) are unreliable in dogs and cats (Jeffers, Shanley & Meyer, 1991; Kunkle & Horner, 1992; Ferguson & Scheidt, 1993). The most reliable method of diagnosis is dietary restriction followed by provocation, although Griffin (1993) has reported that 10% of dogs with AD have concurrent food intolerance. Carlotti & Costargent (1992), in a large study of dogs with AD, found only 2% in which dietary restriction modified the disease.

Environmental factors

There have been few controlled studies investigating environmental factors in AD in animals.

Local environment

In a UK study of canine AD, Shaw (unpublished data) found no significant association in the prevalence of AD between dogs living in rural or urban areas. All dogs in the study slept inside their owners' house and spent more than 50% of their time in this environment (Shaw, unpublished data); 65% of dogs with AD slept on stuffed bedding (mattress, bean bags, furniture) and 32% slept on carpet. None of these factors was significant when compared with a control nonAD dog population. However, it may be assumed that exposure of the companion dog population to house dust mites mimics that of humans and may be an explanation for the global high prevalence of both skin test and serological reactivity to these allergens (Table 18.3).

Regional and international factors

MIGRANT HORSES   Icelandic horses have become popular in mainland Europe. In Norway and Sweden, the high prevalence of allergic dermatitis ('sweet itch', 'summer eczema') in this breed was unexpected because the disease is unknown in Iceland.

The prevalence of allergic dermatitis in Icelandic

horses exported to Norway and Sweden is significantly higher than in Icelandic horses born in mainland Europe (Brostrom & Larsson, 1987; Halldordsottir & Larsen, 1991). The risk of development of allergic skin disease is six times greater in imported horses than in Icelandic horses born in Sweden. Imported horses have a significantly greater risk of developing prolonged and more severe disease (Brostrom & Larsson, 1987). Halldordsottir & Larsen (1991) found a positive association between the risk of disease and the season of importation. Horses imported from Iceland during October to April (autumn–winter; Northern Hemisphere) had a significantly greater risk of developing allergic dermatitis than those imported during summer.

Exposure to biting flies of *Culicoides* spp. is considered central to the interpretation of these findings. These insects are not present in Iceland (Illies, 1978) but are endemic in the UK and mainland Europe. Intermittent exposure of horses imported during the autumn and winter may predispose to hypersensitivity (Halldordsottir & Larsen, 1991). This emphasizes the importance of recognizing environmental factors in AD. However, Icelandic horses with allergic dermatitis, irrespective of their country of birth, have an increased risk of respiratory disease (chronic rhinitis, chronic obstructive pulmonary disease), suggesting that there is a breed predisposition to the development of hypersensitivity to multiple allergens.

Pets and people

Most studies of human AD have not shown an association between the presence of household pets and exacerbation of disease. However, there is a significant association between dogs with AD and humans in the same household with AD, asthma and/or hay fever (Shaw, unpublished data) when compared with households with nonAD dogs. House dust mites are recognized as major allergens in dogs with AD and the association between allergic dogs and humans may reflect a common household exposure to house dust mite allergen.

In several studies (Table 18.3) there is a significant intradermal reactivity of dogs with AD to human and animal epithelia. Between 35 and 70% of dogs with AD reacted to human dander (Carlotti & Costargent, 1992; Sture et al., 1995). Although it is difficult to interpret these findings because the prevalence of such responses in normal dogs is not known, a high exposure to epithelia may play a direct role in the pathogenesis of canine AD. Alternatively, proliferation of house dust mite may be encouraged by an elevated environmental concentration of epidermal scale in a household shared by atopic dogs and humans.

Summary of key points

- Atopic dermatitis (AD) is recognized in several animal species but is best characterized in the dog.
- Canine AD mimics human AD clinically and immunologically.
- Major and minor diagnostic criteria developed for canine AD have close similarities to those described for human AD (Hanifin & Rajka, 1980).
- The most significant allergens associated with canine and feline AD are the house dust mites *D. farinae* and *D. pteronyssinus*.
- Allergen-specific IgE and IgG subclass antibodies are found in dogs with AD.
- There is a strong breed and familial predisposition for canine AD.
- Around 75% of dogs with AD are symptomatic by the age of three years, and 34% by the age of nine months.
- Dogs and horses with AD are more predisposed to ectoparasite hypersensitivity, but there have been no studies which document an association between AD and endoparasite infection.
- There is a significant association between dogs with AD and humans in the same household with AD, asthma and/or hay fever.

References

Bettany, S. (1998). Response to hyposensitisation in 29 atopic cats. In: Kwochka, K.W., Willemse, T. & von Tscharner, C. (eds.) *Advances in Veterinary Dermatology*, Vol. 3, pp. 517–18. Oxford: Butterworth-Heinemann.

Bond, R., Thorogood, S.C. & Lloyd, D.H. (1994). Evaluation of two enzyme-linked immunosorbent assays for the diagnosis of canine atopy. *Vet Rec*, **135**, 130–3.

Brostrom, H. & Larsson, A. (1987). Allergic dermatitis (sweet itch) of Icelandic horses in Sweden: an epidemiological study. *Equine Vet J*, **19**, 229–36.

Butler, J.M. (1983). Pruritic dermatitis in asthmatic Basenji–Greyhounds: a model for human atopic dermatitis. *J Am Acad Dermatol*, **8**, 33–8.

Carlotti, D.N. (1992). Feline atopy. In: Kirk, R.W. (ed.) *Current Veterinary Therapy, No. XI*, pp. 509–12. Philadelphia: Saunders.

Carlotti, D.N. & Prost, C. (1988). L'atopic feline. *Point Veterinaire*, **20**, 777–80.

Carlotti, D.N. & Costargent, F. (1992). Analysis of positive skin tests in 449 dogs with allergic dermatitis. *Pract Med Chirurg Animal Compagnie*, **27**, 53–69.

Chalmers, S. & Medleau, L. (1994). Feline allergic dermatosis, diagnosis and prognosis. *Vet Med*, **84**, 342–6.

Chamberlain, K.W. (1974). Inhalant allergic dermatitis. *Vet Clin N Am*, **4**, 29–36.

Codner, E.C. & Lessard, P. (1993). Comparison of intradermal allergy test and enzyme-linked immunosorbent assay in dogs with allergic skin disease. *J Am Vet Med Ass*, **202**, 739–43.

Corcoran, B.M., Foster, D.J. & Luis Fuentes, V. (1995). Feline asthma syndrome: a retrospective study of the clinical presentation in 29 cats. *J Small Anim Pract*, **36**, 481–8.

Day, M.J. (1996). Expression of major histocompatibility complex class II molecules by dermal inflammatory cells, epidermal Langerhans cells and keratinocytes in canine dermatological disease. *J Comp Pathol*, **115**, 317–26.

Day, M.J. & Penhale, W.J. (1988). Humoral immunity in disseminated *Aspergillus terreus* infection in the dog. *Vet Microbiol*, **16**, 283–94.

Day, M.J. & Mazza, G. (1995). Tissue immunoglobulin G subclasses observed in immune-mediated dermatopathy, deep pyoderma and hypersensitivity dermatitis in dogs. *Res Vet Sci*, **58**, 82–9.

Day, M.J., Corato, A. & Shaw, S.E. (1996). Subclass profile of allergen-specific IgG antibodies in atopic dogs. *Res Vet Sci*, **61**, 136–42.

DeBoer, D.J., Saban, R., Schultz, K.T. & Bjorling, D.E. (1992). Feline IgE: preliminary evidence of its existence and cross-reactivity with canine IgE. In: Ihrke, P.J., Mason, I.S. & White, S.D. (eds.) *Advances in Veterinary Dermatology*, Vol. 2, pp. 51–62. Oxford: Pergamon Press.

DeBoer, D.J., Ewing, K.M. & Schultz, K.T. (1993). Production and characterization of mouse monoclonal antibodies directed against canine IgE and IgG. *Vet Immunol Immunopathol*, **37**, 183–99.

Fadok, V.A. & Greiner, E.C. (1990). Equine insect hypersensitivity – skin test and biopsy results correlated with clinical data. *Equine Vet J*, **22**, 236–40.

Ferguson, E. & Scheidt, V.J. (1993). Hypoallergenic diets and skin disease. In: Ihrke, P.J., Mason, I.S. & White, S.D. (eds.) *Advances in Veterinary Dermatology*, Vol. 2, pp. 451–61. Oxford: Pergamon Press.

Foster, A.P. & O'Dair, H. (1993). Allergy testing for skin disease in the cat. In vivo and in vitro testing. *Vet Dermatol*, **4**, 111–5.

Foster, A.P., Duffus, W.P.H., Shaw, S.E. & Gruffydd-Jones, T.J. (1995). Studies on the isolation and characterisation of a cat reaginic antibody. *Res Vet Sci*, **58**, 70–4.

Frick, O.L. & Brooks, D.L. (1983). Immunoglobulin E antibodies to pollens augmented in dogs by virus vaccines. *Am J Vet Res*, **44**, 440–5.

Gilbert, S. & Halliwell, R.E.W. (1998). Assessment of an ELISA for the detection of allergen specific IgE in cats experimentally sensitised against house dust mites. In: Kwochka, K.W., Willemse, T. & von Tscharner, C. (eds.) *Advances in Veterinary Dermatology*, Vol. 3, pp. 520–1. Oxford: Butterworth-Heinemann.

Griffin, C.E. (1993). Canine atopic disease. In: Griffin, C.E., Kwochka, K.W. & MacDonald, J.M. (eds.) *Current Veterinary Dermatology: The Science and Art of Therapy*, pp. 99–105. St Louis: Mosby Year Book.

Gross, T.L., Ihrke, P.J. & Walder, E.J. (1992). *Veterinary Dermatopathology: A Macroscopic and Microscopic Evaluation of Canine and Feline Skin Disease*, pp. 114–16, St Louis: Mosby Year Book.

Halldordsottir, S. & Larsen, H.J. (1991). An epidemiological study of summer eczema in Icelandic horses in Norway. *Equine Vet J*, **23**, 296–9.

Halliwell, R.E.W. (1990). Clinical and immunological aspects of allergic skin diseases in domestic animals. In: von Tscharner, C. & Halliwell, R.E.W. (eds.) *Advances in Veterinary Dermatology*, Vol. 1, p. 91. Philadelphia: Bailliere Tindall.

Halliwell, R.E.W. & Schwartzman, R.M. (1971). Atopic disease in the dog. *Vet Rec*, **89**, 209–14.

Halliwell, R.E.W. & Gorman, N.T. (1989a). Atopic diseases. In: Halliwell, R.E.W. & Gorman, N.T. (eds.) *Veterinary Immunology*, pp. 232–52. Philadelphia: Saunders.

Halliwell, R.E.W. & Gorman, N.T. (1989b). Non-atopic allergic skin diseases. In: Halliwell, R.E.W. & Gorman, N.T. (eds.) *Veterinary Immunology*, pp. 265–84. Philadelphia: Saunders.

Hanifin, J.M. & Rajka, G. (1980). Diagnostic features of atopic dermatitis. *Acta Dermatol Venereol (Scand.)*, **92**, 44–7.

Hill, P.B., Moriello, K.A. & DeBoer, D.J. (1995). Concentrations of total serum IgE, IgA, and IgG in atopic and parasitized dogs. *Vet Immunol Immunopathol*, **44**, 105–13.

Hites, M.J., Kleinbeck, M.L., Loker, J.L. & Lee, K.W. (1989). Effect of immunotherapy on the serum concentrations of allergen-specific IgG antibodies in dog sera. *Vet Immunol Immunopathol*, **22**, 39–51.

Illies, J. (1978). Ceratopogonidae. In: Illies, J. (ed.) *Limno fauna Europea*, Stuttgart: Fisher Verlag.

Jackson, H.A., Miller, H.R.P. & Halliwell, R.E.W. (1996). Canine leucocyte histamine release: response to antigen and to anti-IgE. *Vet Immunol Immunopathol*, **53**, 195–206.

Jeffers, J.G., Shanley, K.J. & Meyer, E.K. (1991). Diagnostic testing of dogs for food hypersensitivity. *J Am Vet Med Assoc*, **198**, 245–50.

Katz, D.H. (1978). The allergic phenotype: manifestation of 'allergic breakthrough' and inbalance in normal 'dampening' of IgE antibody production. *Immunol Rev*, **41**, 177–80.

Kunkle, G. & Horner, S. (1992). Validity of skin testing for diagnosis of food allergy in dogs. *J Am Vet Med Assoc*, **200**, 677–80.

Kurotaki, T., Narayama, K., Oyamada, T., Yoshikawa, H. & Yoshikawa, T. (1994). Immunopathological study on equine insect hypersensitivity ('Kasen') in Japan. *J Comp Pathol*, **110**, 145–52.

Littlewood, J.D., Paterson, S. & Shaw, S.C. (1998). Atopy-like skin disease in the horse. In: Kwochka, K.W., Willemse, T. & von Tscharner, C. (eds.) *Advances in Veterinary Dermatology*, Vol. 3, pp. 563–4. Oxford: Butterworth-Heinemann.

Mason, I.S. & Lloyd, D.H. (1993). Scanning electron microscopical studies of the living epidermis and stratum coreum in dogs. In: Ihrke, P.J., Mason, I.S. & White, S.D. (eds.) *Advances in Veterinary Dermatology*, Vol. 2, pp. 131–9. Oxford: Pergamon Press.

Mason, K.V. (1993). Cutaneous malassezia. In: Griffin, C.E., Kwochka, K.W. & MacDonald, J.M. (eds.) *Current Veterinary Dermatology: The Science and Art of Therapy*, p. 44. St Louis: Mosby Year Book.

Mazza, G., Whiting, A.H., Day, M.J., & Duffus, W.P.H. (1994). Development of an enzyme-linked immunosorbent assay for the detection of IgG subclasses in the serum of normal and diseased dogs. *Res Vet Sci*, **57**, 133–9.

McEwan, N.A. (1990). Bacterial adherence to canine corneocytes. In: von Tscharner, C. & Halliwell, R.E.W. (eds.). *Advances in Veterinary Dermatology*, Vol. 1, p. 454. London: Balliere Tindall.

Miller, W.H., Scott, D.W., Wellington, J.R., Scarlett, J.M. & Panic, R. (1993). Evaluation of the performance of a serologic allergy system in atopic dogs. *J Am Anim Hosp Assoc*, **29**, 545–50.

Nimmo Wilkie, J.S., Yager, J.A., Wilkie, B.N. & Parker, W.M. (1991). Abnormal cutaneous response to mitogens and a contact allergen in dogs with atopic dermatitis. *Vet Immunol Immunopathol*, **28**, 97–106.

Ohlen, B.M. (1992). Projekt allergitester i Sverige. *Svensk Veterinar tidning*, **44**, 365–71.

Olivry, T., Moore, P.F., Affolter, V.K. & Naydan, D.K. (1996). Langerhans cell hyperplasia and surface IgE expression in canine atopic dermatitis. *Arch Dermatol Res*, **288**, 579–88.

Paradis, M. & Lecuyer, M. (1993). Evaluation of an in-office allergy screening test in nonatopic dogs having various intestinal parasites. *Canad Vet J*, **34**, 293–5.

Peng, Z., Simons, F.E.R. & Becker, A.B. (1993). Measurement of ragweed-specific IgE in canine serum by use of enzyme-linked immunosorbent assays, containing polyclonal and monoclonal antibodies. *Am J Vet Res*, **54**, 239–43.

Peters, J.E., Hirshman, C.A. & Malley, A. (1982). The basenji-greyhound dog model of asthma: leukocyte histamine release, serum IgE, and airway response to inhaled antigen. *J Immunol*, **129**, 1245–9.

Plant, J.D., Rosenkrantz, W.S. & Griffin, C.E. (1992). Factors associated with and prevalence of high Malassezia pachydermatis numbers on dog skin. *J Am Vet Med Assoc*, **201**, 879–82.

Prelaud, P. (1990). Basophil degranulation test in the diagnosis of canine allergic skin disease. In: Tscharner, C. von & Halliwell, R.E.W. (eds.) *Advances in Veterinary Dermatology*, Vol. 1, pp. 117–25. London: Bailliere Tindale.

Prost, C. (1998). Diagnosis of feline allergic skin diseases: a study of 90 cats. In: Kwochka, K.W., Willemse, T. & von Tscharner, C. (eds.) *Advances in Veterinary Dermatology*, Vol. 3, pp. 516–17. Oxford: Butterworth–Heinemann

Pucheu-Haston, C.M., Grier, T.J., Esch, R.E. & Bevier, D.E. (1996). Allergenic cross-reactivities in flea-reactive canine serum samples. *Am J Vet Res*, **57**, 1000–5.

Rhodes, K.H., Kendel, F., Soter, N.A. & Chinnici, R. (1987). Investigations into the immunopathogenesis of canine atopy. *Semin Vet Med Surg (Small Anim)*, **2**, 199–201.

Schick, R.O. & Fadok, V.A. (1986). Responses of atopic dogs to regional allergens: 268 cases 1981–1984. *J Am Vet Med Assoc*, **189**, 1493–6.

Schwartzman, R.M., Rockey, J.H. & Halliwell, R.E. (1971). Canine reaginic antibody. Characterisation of the spontaneous anti-ragweed and induced anti-dinitrophenyl reaginic antibodies of the atopic dog. *Clin Exp Immunol*, **9**, 549–69.

Schwartzman, R.M., Massicot, J.G. & Sogn, D.D. (1983). The atopic dog model: report of an attempt to establish a colony. *Int Arch Allergy Appl Immunol*, **72**, 97.

Scott, D.W. (1981). Observations on canine atopy. *J Am Anim Hosp Assoc*, **17**, 91–100.

Scott, D.W. & Miller, W.H. (1989). Epidermal dysplasia and Malassezia pachydermatis infection in West Highland white terriers. *Vet Dermatol*, **1**, 25–30.

Scott, D.W., Miller, W. & Griffin, C. (1995). Immunologic skin diseases. In: Scott, D.W., Miller, W. & Griffin, C., (eds.) *Small Animal Dermatology*, 5th edn, pp. 500–4. Philadelphia: Saunders.

Shearer, D.H. & Day, M.J. (1997). Aspects of the humoral immune response to *Staphylococcus intermedius* in dogs with superficial pyodermia, deep pyoderma and anal furunculosis. *Vet Immunol Immunopathol*, **58**, 107–20.

Sinke, J.D., Thepen, T., Bihari, I.C., Rutten, V.P.M.G. & Willemse, T. (1998). Immunophenotyping of skin-infiltrating T cell subsets in dogs with atopic dermatitis. In: Kwachka, K.W., Willemse, T. & von Tscharner, C. (eds.) *Advances in Veterinary Dermatology*, Vol. 3, pp. 503–4. Oxford: Butterworth-Heinemann.

Sture, G.H., Halliwell, R.E.W., Thoday, K.L., van den Broek, A.H.M., Henfrey, J.I., Lloyd, D.H., Mason, I.S. & Ferguson, E. (1995). Canine atopic disease: the prevalance of positive intradermal skin tests at two sites in the north and south of Great Britain. *Vet Immunol Immunopathol*, **44**, 293–308.

Van Stee, E.W. (1983). Risk factors in canine atopy. *Calif Vet*, **4**, 8–13.

Vollsett, I. (1985). Atopic dermatitis in Norwegian dogs. *Nordisk Vet Dermatol*, **37**, 97–106.

Vriesendorp, H.M., Smid-Mercx, B.M., Visser, T.P., Halliwell, R.E.W. & Schwartzman, R.M. (1975). Serological DL-A typing of normal and atopic dogs. *Transplant Proc*, **7**, 375–7.

Willemse, A. (1984a). Investigation on canine atopic dermatitis. PhD Thesis, University of Utrecht.

Willemse, A. (1984b). Canine atopic disease: investigations of eosinophils and the nasal mucosa. *Am J Vet Res*, **45**, 1867–9.

Willemse, A. (1986). Atopic skin disease: a review and a recon-sideration of diagnostic criteria. *J Small Anim Pract*, **27**, 771–8.

Willemse, A. & Van den Brom, W.E. (1983). Investigations of the symptomatology and the significance of immediate skin test reactivity in canine atopic dermatitis. *Res Vet Sci*, **34**, 261–5.

Willemse, A., Van den Brom, W.E & Rijnberk, A. (1984). Effect of hyposensitisation on atopic dermatitis in dogs. *J Am Vet Med Assoc*, **184**, 1277–80.

Willemse, A., Noordzij, A., Rutten, V.P.M.G. & Bernadina, W.E. (1985a). Induction of non-IgE anaphylactic antibodies in dogs. *Clin Exp Immunol*, **59**, 351–8.

Willemse, A., Noordzij, A., van den Brom, W.E. & Rutten, V.P.M.G. (1985b). Allergen specific IgGd antibodies in dogs with atopic dermatitis as determined by the enzyme linked immunosorbent assay. *Clin Exp Immunol*, **59**, 359–63.

Williams, H., Burney, P.G.J., Hay, R.J., Archer, C.B., Shipley, M.J., Hunter, J.J.A., Bingham, E.A., Finlay, A.Y., Pembroke, A.C., Graham-Brown, R.A.C., Atherton, D.A., Lewis-Jones, M.S., Holden, C.A., Harper, J.I., Champion, R.H., Poyner, T.P., Launer, J. & David, T.J. (1994a). The UK working party's diagnostic criteria for atopic dermatitis. I. Derivation of a minimum set of discriminators for atopic dermatitis. *Br J Dermatol*, **131**, 383–96.

Williams, H., Burney, P.G.J., Strachan, D. & Hay, R.J. (1994b). The UK working party's diagnostic criteria for atopic dermatitis. II. Observer variation of clinical diagnosis and signs of atopic dermatitis. *Br J Dermatol*, **131**, 397–405.

Williams, H., Burney, P.G.J., Pembroke, A.C. & Hay, R.J. (1994c). The UK working party's diagnostic criteria for atopic dermatitis. III. Independent hospital validation. *Br J Dermatol*, **131**, 406–16.

PART VI

Conclusions

19

The future research agenda

Hywel C. Williams

Where are we now?

This book has summarized something about the burden and causes of atopic dermatitis (AD) throughout the world. Because the subject is so vast, there will be some gaps in coverage of the material, even in a text dedicated to the epidemiology of AD. Like any printed material, some of the data in this book will be out of date within a few years, and important breakthroughs will occur. Despite these limitations, it is worth pausing for a moment to look back and see where research into the epidemiology of AD has taken us so far, in order to identify the major gaps for the future research agenda. The author has resisted the temptation to draw figures depicting his own personal theory on the causes of AD as (*a*) it is likely to be wrong, and (*b*) it will certainly be incomplete. Instead, it is considered more useful to summarize some areas of notable progress to be followed by a section on areas of notable ignorance, and then to highlight what needs to be done to address those gaps. It is hoped that this will inspire future researchers to study this interesting yet enigmatic disease.

Ten areas of notable progress

Disease definition

Even as recently as the late 1970s, at least 12 synonyms for atopic dermatitis were in use in Europe alone, and it is unclear whether these names referred to the same clinical concept. The Hanifin,

Lobitz and Rajka consensus criteria marked an important milestone in listing the main clinical features of AD (Hanifin & Lobitz, 1977; Hanifin & Rajka, 1980), but they were unsuitable for epidemiological studies. As Chapter 1 highlighted, these criteria have formed the building blocks for more refined sets of criteria of known validity and repeatability which are easy to use in epidemiological studies. Disease definition had been a major obstacle preventing any meaningful comparison between population-based studies. The recently developed diagnostic criteria require more validation, but should permit a more standardized approach towards defining AD in a way that any researcher can understand and replicate (Williams, 1997a).

A better understanding of disease burden

Studies such as the International Study of Asthma and Allergies in Childhood (ISAAC) have been instrumental in piecing together a picture of the burden of AD symptoms throughout the world (Williams et al., 1999). Even though the results of this questionnaire-based study need to be validated with more objective measures, the phenomenal task of gathering data on over half a million children in 56 countries in all five continents of the world using a strict standardized approach should not be underestimated. This feat is even more astonishing when one considers that participation of ISAAC collaborators was voluntary. The ISAAC study has suggested that AD is a major problem worldwide, and that it is not a problem confined to northern and western

Europe. Other studies of the burden of AD have looked more closely at its effects on sufferers and their carers. Thus, it has been shown that AD can have serious psychological effects on children and their families (Lawson et al., 1998; Absolon et al., 1997), and that such morbidity is comparable to other 'important' non-communicable diseases (Emerson et al., 1997; Su et al., 1997).

Studies which have documented the cost of atopic dermatitis

In addition to collecting information on 'how common' and 'how miserable' AD can be, it is also essential to document its cost, given that all health care systems have finite resources. Such information is of paramount importance for raising the public health profile of AD from one of neglect or indifference to its rightful place alongside asthma and other common childhood infections. Indeed, studies performed to date suggest that the direct costs of AD to the State in the UK (Herd et al., 1996a; Emerson, Williams & Allen, 1998a), Australia (Su et al., 1997) and USA (Lapidus, Schwarz & Honig, 1993) are very high indeed, and that additional personal financial costs for special clothing, bedding, laundry and visits to doctors can also be substantial (Herd et al., 1996a). Without such economic studies, there is little hope of the voices of AD sufferers being heard in rationed health care systems, both in terms of provision of care and investment into research and development.

Geographical associations

It is surprising that so few ecological studies have been performed with AD as a starting point for epidemiological research. Yet in the last five years, geographical studies have suggested strong possible links between the environment and AD prevalence. At a global level, the ISAAC study has suggested that there is a distinct pattern of AD symptoms which cannot be easily explained by current risk factors (Williams et al., 1999). At a national level, strong

regional variation of AD prevalence has been documented within the UK which cannot be explained by known confounders (Peters & Golding, 1987; McNally, 1998). At a smaller spatial scale, striking associations between water hardness have been noted in younger children (McNally et al., 1998). Although such preliminary ecological associations need to be replicated at an individual level, such studies have generated ideas about new constellations of potentially harmful exposures which might be amenable to public health manipulation.

Socioeconomic correlations

At first, the positive social class gradient of AD and its link with smaller family size may be perceived as interesting but useless information in that it does not identify specific exposures that can be acted upon through a public health approach (Williams, 1997b). Yet, these findings have been helpful in confirming that environmental factors account for a large part of the variation in prevalence of AD, and that time would be well spent in researching correlates of attributes such as socioeconomic advantage and smaller family size. History has also taught us that changes in factors such as hygiene and social class have resulted in a far greater impact on the health of populations than even the most specific medical interventions such as immunizations (McKeown, 1975). We should not eschew population interventions that aim to alter the structure of society, especially in view of the finding that changes in societal structure associated with a 'western' lifestyle may be responsible for much of the AD epidemic today (Williams, 1995a).

Migrant studies which point to a strong role of the environment

There is now strong evidence that there is a range of environmental factors which are crucial for determining the expression of AD. The rising prevalence of AD discussed by Diepgen in Chapter 7, along with its links with wealth and geography (Chapter 10) point strongly to environmental influences. The migrant studies described by Burrell-Morris and Williams in Chapter 13 suggest that people who are genetically similar can experience large rises in prevalence when they move to countries where there are high pre-existing levels of disease prevalence. Although migrant studies have their own drawbacks, they suggest that environmental factors might be critical in determining the expression of AD. This is welcome news to epidemiologists as it brings them one step nearer to their ultimate aim of disease prevention.

Progress in cell biology and understanding the skin immune system

Although the balance of AD research over the last 20 years has perhaps been skewed too much towards 'basic' science, this should not prevent us from acknowledging the major advances in understanding the role of the skin immune system in AD (Cooper, 1994; Boguniewicz & Leung, 1998). We have moved a long way from thinking about AD as a disease of mast cells and excessive IgE production, to one where an imbalance of helper T lymphocytes (Th1 and Th2 cells) and their cytokines play a key role (Leung, 1995). Some believe that, in AD, there is a switch from the normal T helper cell profile to one where there is increased Th2 activity, resulting in cytokines such as IL-4, IL-5 and IL-10 which stimulate B lymphocytes, eosinophils and mast cells, and decreased γ interferon, all of which may mediate the tissue damage seen in AD (Chapter 2). That such a switch might occur as a result of immunizations (Shaheen et al., 1996; Dalton et al., 1998) or decreased infections (Strachan, 1989), perhaps at a critical time of lymphocyte maturation opens up exciting new windows for possible prevention (Shaheen, 1997). The discovery that Langerhans cells play a key part in presenting specific IgE to lymphocytes has partly explained how an allergen might induce an allergic reaction (Fokkens et al., 1990), and further work with aeroallergen patch tests suggest that delayed-type immune reactions might be just as important as IgE-mediated disease (Buckley et al., 1992). Thestrup-Pedersen's theory (see Chapter 11) on aberrant clones of T lymphocytes which are determined in early life gains some support from the transferability of AD from affected individuals to previously unaffected bone-marrow recipients (Bellou et al., 1997). Other work, reviewed by Japanese scientists, has postulated a possible role for defective barrier function of the skin in AD (Ogawa & Yoshiike, 1993), and how such a defect may be central to the inflammatory responses which follow. It is important to incorporate the dimension of time when considering questions such as which cells and cytokines are involved in AD, as these may vary according to whether the lesions are acute or chronic (Leung, 1995).

Genetic epidemiology

Although some readers might have placed this in the section on notable ignorance, the author has chosen to place it in this section because of the real likelihood of major breakthroughs in this area over the next five to ten years. Schultz Larsen summarized the evidence for supposing that there is a strong genetic component to AD in Chapter 8, although some recent twin studies in the UK (published only in abstract form) have suggested that heritability may be as low as 0.36 and 0.11 in the monozygotic and dizygotic twins, respectively (Swale et al., 1998). Other groups are currently homing in on specific candidate genes which explain some, but not all, AD cases. It is likely that several genes will be discovered, some determining IgE reactivity, some determining defective barrier function, some predicting disease chronicity and susceptibility to secondary infections with *Staphylococcus aureus*, and others determining whether subjects will develop concomitant inhalant allergy (Cox et al., 1998). Genetic discoveries also open up the possibility of exploring the interaction that may occur between disease genotype and environmental factors (Diepgen & Blettner, 1997), rather than relying on family history of atopy as a surrogate measure of genotype, as is currently the case. This seems a very exciting area which could lead to better targeting of 'high risk groups' for screening or intervention studies.

Studies pointing to the role of the early environment

Since most cases of AD begin in the first five years of life, it seems plausible that risk factors acting early in life are important for determining disease incidence. In Chapter 9, Godfrey provides strong evidence that many noncommunicable modern diseases might be 'programmed' during intrauterine or perinatal life, and that AD itself might also be subject to such 'programming'. If, indeed, simple exposures during pregnancy such as iron supplementation or other dietary factors are risk factors for AD, then this opens up genuine possibilities for primary prevention, or even prevention of sensitization (Hide, 1995), since pregnant mothers are often highly motivated to do anything they can to prevent problems in their unborn child. Another study has suggested that asthma development may be reduced over an 18-month period in a subset of AD infants born to atopic mothers when given an antihistamine (ETAC Study Group, 1998).

Studies suggesting that disease prevention is possible

The pioneering work of the late David Hide has shown that prevention of atopic disease including AD may well be possible through interventions such as dietary manipulation in early life or measures aimed at reducing house dust mite allergen levels around the home (Arshad et al., 1992). Whether such interventions prevent AD for good, or whether they simply delay the onset of disease or reduce its severity, is too early to say at present (Hide et al., 1994). Other studies have also supported the notion that a proportion of AD can be prevented, and in Chapter 16, Mar and Marks suggest that this could be as large as 50%. Disease prevention is so much more desirable than treating sick individuals who present themselves to health care workers after a long chain

of pathological events and needing expensive and potentially toxic drugs which at best only diminish the disease process (Williams, 1998a).

Ten areas of notable ignorance

The lamentable volume of research into the epidemiology of atopic dermatitis

Considering the prevalence and morbidity of AD, few biologists would disagree that the quantity of research into the epidemiology of AD over the last 30 years has been pitiful. This 'inverse research law', i.e. the observation that the quality and quantity of research into a skin disease is inversely proportional to its prevalence, has been noted previously (Williams, 1995b). Past research has been dominated by a belief that the key to understanding AD lies in reducing it to a cellular or subcellular level (Figure 19.1). For example, in a Medline search of 680 articles published between January 1966 and May 1998 where atopic dermatitis was the main focus, 179 and 67 references were found for 'immunology' and 'pathology or physiopathology', respectively, compared with 21 and 11 references for 'epidemiology' and 'prevention and control', respectively. Whilst the enormous investment in research into the cellular and molecular biology of AD characterized by the last 30 years has produced some interesting findings, such studies of the disease *process* have resulted in very few discoveries that are of use to AD sufferers – either in terms of disease prevention or treatment. This is not the same as saying that molecular or cellular research is not important but, like the tree in Figure 19.1, simply that the *balance* of research has been too one-sided. Basic science and epidemiology will always need each other in order to make sense of each other's findings (Williams, 1997c).

Even within the study of allergic diseases, AD does not seem to figure with any prominence. Thus, in a recent textbook of allergy (Middleton et al., 1998), 12 pages were devoted to AD compared with 142 for asthma. This is a pity as the skin offers a unique

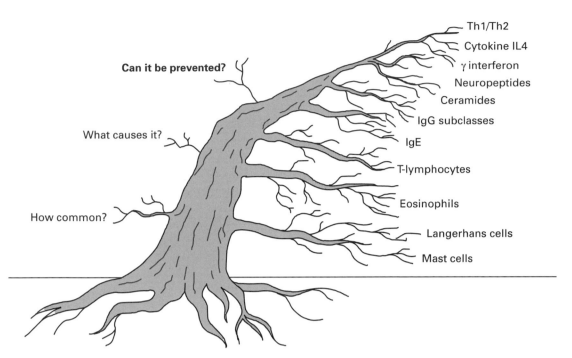

Fig. 19.1. The tree of research into atopic dermatitis over the last 20 years has been an unbalanced one

opportunity of directly visualizing the interaction between allergens and the body and for serving as a model for chronic inflammatory diseases (Leung, 1995).

Research of insufficient scientific rigour

A profusion of poor quality or misleading research is almost as undesirable as no research at all. Although poor quality studies are occasionally useful in generating debate and hypotheses, the general quality of studies which purport to be 'epidemiological' studies of AD has been variable. Many studies which the author is asked to peer review for journals still fail to specify how AD was defined, to provide an adequate description of the sampling strategy, or to discuss the possible roles of chance, bias and confounding as alternative explanations for study findings. Such disregard for basic epidemiological principles is likely to result in erroneous conclu-

sions, and it is essential that dermatologists and other clinicians work alongside professional epidemiologists in order to improve aspects of study design and report writing. Societies such as those mentioned at the end of this chapter have been instrumental in increasing the multiprofessional balance of researchers necessary for studying the epidemiology of AD.

Lack of measures of atopic dermatitis severity for use in epidemiological studies

Measuring the severity of AD may be just as important as recording the presence or absence of the disease. For example, an intervention might reduce the severity of the disease in a population to a level which is easy to cope with, yet the overall prevalence of the disease remains the same. Similarly, studies of the natural history of AD need to document the points at which the disease no longer becomes 'a problem', even though the person may still carry some of the stigmata of the condition. Yet, apart from one abstract published by Rajka and Langeland

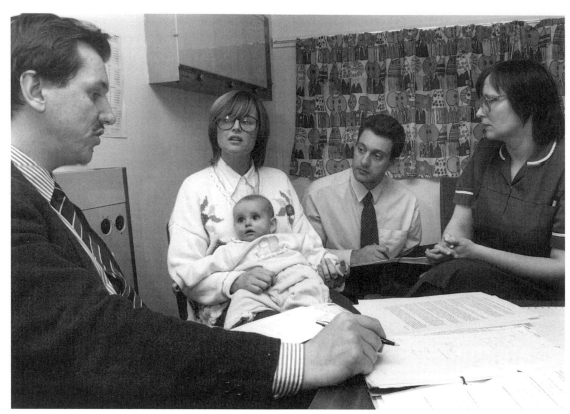

Fig. 19.2. 'Will my child's eczema get better doctor?' and 'will (s)he go on to develop asthma, doctor?' are questions frequently asked by parents, but ones which are difficult to answer given our current data

Preliminary work by our research group has taken the work of Rajka and Langeland further by testing the construct validity and practical usefulness of their original suggestion (Emerson et al., 1998).

in abstract form in 1989 (Rajka & Langeland, 1989), no severity criteria have been developed for specific use in epidemiological studies of AD that are easy to administer in questionnaire form, which measure something important to patients and which capture the chronicity of the disease. Severity measures for AD that have been developed for use in clinical trials such as SCORAD (European Task Force, 1993), are unsuitable for epidemiological studies as they require a detailed physical examination, and because many attempt to measure body surface area of disease involvement – a task which is probably impossible to record reliably given the ill-defined nature of AD (Charman, Venn & Williams, 1999).

A poor understanding of the natural history of atopic dermatitis

Chapter 3 summarized what is known about the natural history of AD, and concluded that no prospective population-based studies have specifically been set up to examine issues of natural history for AD. This is a shame as issues of natural history are so important to sufferers and their families (Figure 19.2). Such studies could easily produce useful results in a relatively short time given the early onset of AD. Little is known about which factors determine disease chronicity and even less is known about which factors predict that a child with AD will go on to develop asthma or hay fever. Such information could be very helpful in targeting interventions for those at high risk.

Failure to consider the aetiological fraction of the purported risk factors for atopic dermatitis

Most analytical studies on AD examine a similar spectrum of risk factors, with positive associations highlighted by means of measures of relative risk. However, the magnitude of these risk factors and their public health importance has seldom been considered in terms of the absolute risk reduction that could be achieved by reduction or eradication of the exposure. Even for the house dust mite, we still do not know if there is a critical threshold above which the risk of AD is considerably elevated, or what proportion of all cases of AD could be eradicated by decreasing house dust mite levels by different amounts and methods. The German Multicentre Allergy Study (MAS) should be in a position to answer this question in the very near future (Edenharter et al., 1998). It may well turn out that simple interventions on common exposures such as turning off a radiator in a child's bedroom could have a large public health impact even though the relative risk for such an exposure is quite small (McNally, 1998). In other words, a little bit of harm affecting a lot of people can add up to more than a lot of harm affecting a few people from a population perspective (Williams, 1996a).

The relative role of allergic and nonallergic factors in atopic dermatitis

In Chapter 1, we pointed out that it is still unclear whether 'atopy' is a prerequisite for development of AD, and whether nonallergic factors such as irritants, water, climate and microbial organisms are just as important as exposure to specific allergens in causing disease flare-ups. As Archer points out in Chapter 2, nonIgE mechanisms may be just as important in AD. Although atopy is clearly related to AD, perhaps too much emphasis has been placed on allergic factors at the expense of other modifiable risk factors. As a result of this skewed emphasis, a

large and profitable 'allergy testing' industry has flourished in many countries. Whilst tests such as skin prick tests, RAST tests, aeroallergen patch tests, and double-blind food challenges, have been useful in the field of research, their positive predictive value for disease improvement when such a test result is acted upon is still unclear (David, 1991).

The limited knowledge of adult atopic dermatitis

It is easy to understand why the study of childhood AD has dominated most of the epidemiological studies described in this book: the condition is more common in childhood, the effects of the disease may be critical for the child's development, and children attending nurseries and schools make an easily accessible population for researchers (Williams et al., 1995). However, as Herd pointed out in his study of an entire town population in Scotland (Herd et al., 1996b), adults over 16 years still constitute around one third of the total AD cases in a given community. Furthermore, such adults often suffer from more severe or chronic disease than their juvenile counterparts, and the effects of AD on their employment and social activities may be considerable. We must not, therefore, ignore the study of AD in adults. We know little about the validity of diagnostic criteria in this group (Williams et al., 1994), the natural history of the disease, or whether risk factors for disease occurrence or persistence are similar to those for childhood AD.

The relationship of atopic dermatitis to other types of dermatitis

Whilst it has been possible to define what constitutes a typical case of childhood AD, defining the relationship of typical AD to other types of dermatitis, has not been studied systematically. Thus, it is unclear whether seasonal occurrences of vesicles along the sides of the fingers represent a variant of AD, or whether the discoid eczema lesions occurring in a child with otherwise typical flexural AD is part of the same disease process. Studies which use approaches such as cluster analysis or numerical taxonomy offer one way forward to identifying groups of closely related disease reaction patterns (Burton, 1981).

Treatment of established disease (tertiary prevention)

Although new and possibly powerful treatment modalities such as tacrolimus (Nakagawa et al., 1994) or topical phosphodiesterase inhibitors (Hanifin et al., 1996) may be around the corner, the mainstay of treatment for the majority of AD sufferers is still topical corticosteroid preparations and emollients. Yet, despite being used for over 30 years, the evidential basis for using emollients and different corticosteroid strategies is quite weak. We still do not know how effective emollients are in AD, which ones are the best, and whether pouring expensive emollients into a bath offers any significant advantage over simple cheap emollients applied to the skin after bathing. Topical corticosteroids have also been around for 30 years, yet we still do not know if the benefit to risk ratio is better for potent preparations applied for a few days, as opposed to weaker preparations used for longer periods. It is also difficult for a clinician to make a rational choice when faced with the 30 or so preparations currently available for prescription (Williams, 1998b).

Nearly all clinical trials of AD have focused on short-term outcome measures such as reduction in itching, scaling and erythema after 4 to 6 weeks' treatment. Whilst it is nice to know that a drug will help to control the appearance and symptoms of AD during an acute exacerbation, what is needed for a chronic intermittent disease like AD is knowledge of whether these drugs alter the natural history of the disease. It is possible, for instance, that topical corticosteroids, whilst providing short-term benefit, might actually increase the number of exacerbations. Although long-term trials are likely to cost more, clinicians should insist on such data for AD, since it is a chronic intermittent disease in most people.

Nonpharmacological treatments have tended to be ignored in AD. Despite promising results in observational studies of psychological approaches such as habit reversal (Norén, 1995), these have not been tested in prospective randomized trials. In view of the recent strong link between water hardness and AD prevalence (McNally et al., 1998), it seems now essential to conduct a randomized controlled trial on the possible benefits of water softeners.

Similarly, different models of delivering care to the AD patient, such as educational support, liaison nurses, involvement of patients in the management of their own disease, pharmacists' advice and specialist eczema clinics (Lawton et al., 1997), have yet to be fully evaluated.

The relationship between the need, supply and demand for atopic dermatitis treatment

Knowing how many people could benefit from medical care, and what proportion of such people actually seek such care and why, is of vital importance to health care planners (Stevens & Gabbay, 1991). It is odd, therefore, that these questions seem to have been completely ignored to date for a common problem like AD. One study in Nottingham, UK, has suggested that disease severity is not the only determinant of referral to secondary care, and that most AD cases are managed in the community (Emerson, Williams & Allen, 1998b). Many milder cases of AD probably manage with advice from family members, friends and pharmacists, but it is not known whether this advice is truly helpful or whether it simply delays appropriate diagnosis and treatment (Williams, 1995c). It would be useful to know whether treatment of AD is perceived as a need in some developing countries, and how well local medical systems meet these needs and at what cost when compared with local traditional healers (Hay et al., 1994; Ryan, 1994).

What should we do in the future?

Where should we direct our future efforts?

The simple answer to the above question is 'to address the areas of notable ignorance'. Some further consideration needs to be given to some strategic points regarding study design and choice of study subjects.

Cohort studies are often disregarded in dermatology because of their large resource implications. Yet they should be considered more often for studies of atopic dermatitis, perhaps in collaboration with other groups who are prospectively recording asthma outcomes. Unlike skin cancer, where it takes decades for the disease to develop and the incidence of such events is low, Chapter 3 suggests that most cases of AD become manifest in the first two years of life. This, plus the fact that the disease is so common, makes consideration of the cohort study more attractive for funding organizations, providing of course that the study design is appropriate to the question posed (Safavi & Lawrence, 1997). Such prospective studies are suitable for common diseases like AD, and they are able to separate causes and effects according to their temporal sequence, and record more accurate data on potentially harmful or protective exposures.

Secondary analyses of existing cohort studies that have collected (but ignored) eczema data may also be a fruitful area for research (Williams, Pottier & Strachan, 1993; Williams, Strachan & Hay, 1994). Even simple ecological analyses of such studies may generate important hypotheses which may be relevant today (McNally, Phillips & Williams, 1998).

Given the early onset of AD and the evidence that factors occurring early in life may be critical in determining predisposition to disease, studies which measure exposures in early life seem a sensible area to concentrate efforts at present.

In addition to studying risk factors for increased disease occurrence, there should be more study of factors which appear to protect against AD, e.g. by studying communities which are 'healthy' from the AD perspective (Evans, 1993). Countries in the ISAAC study which appear to have very low prevalence of AD may be a useful starting point in this respect (Williams et al., 1999).

More randomized controlled trials aimed at disease prevention, which separate the effects of the various interventions such as diet or reduction in house dust mite, are needed in different communities in order to assess the potential for disease prevention on a wider scale.

Systematic reviews on the prevention and treatment of AD, of the type carried out by the Cochrane Skin Group (Williams et al., 1998), are needed in order to summarize what we already know in an explicit and unbiased way and to identify the major gaps in our present knowledge. Currently, there is an on-going project at our centre which seeks to summarize all of the randomized controlled clinical trial evidence for treatments of AD, but this will need to be constantly updated as new trials or previously unpublished trials become available.

Where does clinical and public health policy need to be modified?

The organization of health care services for AD sufferers is not based on any formal needs assessment anywhere in the world at present. It is no longer acceptable to rely on a demand-led service with implicit rationing by doctors, since such a system might favour the better educated, aggressive or wealthy. What is needed is to consider the problem of AD in the entire community in order to develop an appropriate service response. It is essential, therefore, that public health planners gather epidemiological data on disease incidence, prevalence and severity in order to begin to estimate their population's unmet needs, and then to view these data in the context of current service organization and evidence of cost effectiveness of interventions, including prevention (Williams & Wright, 1998).

Much can be done about the consistency and quality of information on AD provided to patients by various health professionals such as nurses, pharmacists, health visitors and local healers. In addition, health service managers have a role to play in regulating some aspects of the allergy testing industry on the basis of evidence of its usefulness.

There is a striking lack of training for primary care doctors in dermatology who paradoxically have most contact with AD sufferers. This needs to be addressed by central Government and the appropriate training colleges. Attitudes of nondermatologist doctors also need to change so that skin examination becomes a routine part of the assessment of any patient (Charman, Williams & Kinnear, 1998). Physicians and surgeons need to overcome their tendency to 'look through the skin' rather than 'at the skin' (Monk et al., 1983). These changes are probably best influenced by modifying medical undergraduate curricula and through role models. Dermatology textbooks also need to give more space for important epidemiological findings when discussing AD, rather than spending most of the text discussing theories of pathophysiology in great detail (Holden & Parish, 1998).

There is a need for patients and their representatives to campaign politically to ensure that their voice is heard amongst competing demands in the world of politics. The work of the Skin Care Campaign in the UK is an example of what can be achieved in a relatively short time (APPGS, 1997). These issues are not the sole concern of developed industrialized countries as indications are that AD is reaching epidemic levels in developing countries as well (Williams et al., 1999).

What is limiting progress?

Some methodological difficulties, such as lack of severity measures for AD that can be used in questionnaire-based surveys, are limiting progress in some studies, although these are likely to be overcome in the next few years. Disease definition should no longer impede progress, yet many researchers still cling to older consensus criteria of unknown validity for reasons which are unclear (Rothe & Grant-Kels, 1996; Williams, 1996b).

Conceptual difficulties, such as the issue of whether predisposition to AD is necessary for disease expression, will perhaps only be sorted out when the genetic basis of AD becomes clearer. It is unclear whether biological markers such as positive skin prick tests represent part of the disease (in the sense that they define atopy) or whether they indicate a specific exposure (i.e. a person is allergic to one type of grass pollen as opposed to another). Not all purported risk factors will prove to be true risk factors – some will be spurious because of con-

founding or bias, and some may exert their effect only in the presence of other factors, i.e. effect modifiers (Phillips & Davey-Smith, 1997). It also needs to be understood that risk factors for sensitization, disease incidence and disease chronicity are not necessarily the same. The tendency in the past to group AD with asthma unreservedly has not always been helpful, as the determinants of the two conditions may be quite different.

Another conceptual error is trying to look for just one hypothesis to explain AD occurrence across several countries. In some parts of the world, geographical variations may be due to an inverse relationship with helminthic parasites (Moqbel & Pritchard, 1990), whereas in other areas it may be cold winds or high house dust mite populations (Dowse et al., 1985).

When considering risk factors, it is important to consider the *timing* of exposure in addition to a simple exposure yes/no category. It is possible that exposure to some agents at a certain age of thymic development may result in lifelong tolerance (Hanson et al., 1977), whereas at another age it could result in sensitization. This has been studied only scantily to date (de Jong et al., 1997).

There will always be ethical obstacles to answering some epidemiological questions, e.g. it is unlikely that there will ever be a randomized study of breast feeding versus bottle feeding to see whether prolonged breast feeding protects against AD, and the uptake of participants in nonrandomized studies is likely to be strongly biased by parental perceptions (Saarinen & Kajosaari, 1995; Kramer, 1988).

Funding is always an issue for further research, but it is hard to see why a research body should turn down a good research proposal for an epidemiological study on AD simply on the grounds of low priority, given the wealth of data that we now have on disease prevalence, morbidity and costs. Hopefully, as more research becomes publicly accountable, the balance of research will shift away from studies of disease process at a cellular level, to studies of groups of patients and human populations.

Failure to consult with other disciplines is also a potential barrier to progress, i.e. dermatologists

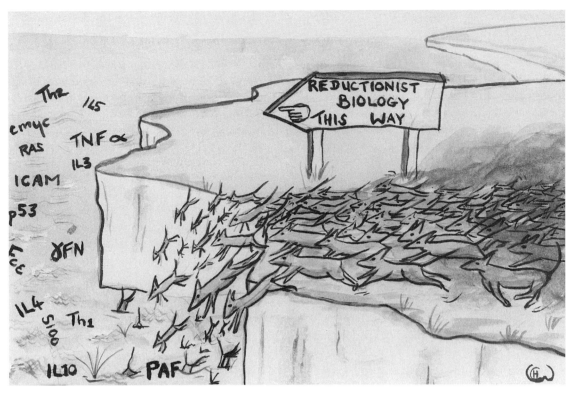

Fig. 19.3. It is odd that discovering the causes of AD by means of population research has attracted fewer young researchers than research fields such as molecular and cellular biology

'dabbling' in epidemiology without appropriate training. Some of the most interesting breakthroughs which the author has had the privilege to be involved with have come through collaborations with professional epidemiologists, asthma specialists, medical geographers and statisticians, and with researchers from more than one country. Better communication in the form of e-mail discussion lists and web sites is one way forward.

Conclusions

Despite the above list of possible reasons which might limit research into the epidemiology of AD, the author is still at a loss to explain why so little interest has been shown in this disease. Perhaps it is because chronic nonfatal skin diseases which

rarely invoke drama in the media do not attract young researchers, or that performing painstaking counts of cases in population studies is not as attractive as running western blots or conducting experiments on transgenic mice (Figure 19.3). Whatever the reason, the epidemic of AD will not go away, and it will not be long before we all have at least one member of our family affected by the condition.

This book has tried to capture some of the facts and concepts surrounding the epidemiology of atopic dermatitis as we approach the next millennium. Unlike cardiovascular epidemiology, where researchers have identified at least 246 possible risk factors (Hopkins & Williams, 1981) and are having to look harder and harder for smaller and smaller risk factors and interactions, the land of atopic dermatitis epidemiology is still relatively unchartered, with large and important risk factors and challenges out there for researchers to discover. That is, if they dare.

Summary of key points

- Areas of notable progress in the epidemiology of atopic dermatitis (AD) over recent years include better disease definitions, and the quantification of disability and costs.
- Migrant studies, geographical studies, and the finding that AD is linked with wealth and small families suggest that environmental factors are important for disease expression.
- Some evidence suggests that the early environment may be critical for programming of later disease.
- Advances in genetics and molecular biology over the next few years will permit a better understanding of the interaction between genes and environment.
- Disease prevention is already possible to some degree.
- Areas of notable ignorance include the lack of a severity measure for AD that can be used in epidemiological surveys, and a poor understanding of the natural history of the disease.
- Allergic factors in AD have sometimes been studied to the exclusion of important nonallergic factors.
- Little is known about the epidemiology of AD in adults.
- We do not have a clear understanding of how AD relates to other eczematous conditions such as dyshidrotic eczema.
- The relationship between the need, supply and demand for AD health services in different countries is currently a public health scotoma.
- The evidential basis for many commonly used treatments for established AD is weak.
- Systematic reviews produced by the Cochrane Skin Group will help to summarize what is known about prevention and treatment of AD, and to identify gaps for future research.
- Past AD research has leaned too heavily in favour of cellular biology.
- The cohort study design should be considered more often in AD research because AD is a common disease with early onset.
- Prevention studies should employ a randomized design which separates the effects of different interventions.
- Although lack of severity measures and inadequate funding are genuine obstacles which limit progress in some areas of AD research, conceptual obstacles such as the failure to think in population terms may be more common.
- Dermatologists need to work closely with epidemiologists and asthma specialists in order to make sense of their findings.
- The epidemiology of AD is a rich research resource for important aetiological and methodological discoveries and for preventing human suffering on a global scale.

References

Absolon, C.M., Cottrell, D., Eldridge, S.M. & Glover, M.T. (1997). Psychological disturbance in atopic eczema: the extent of the problem in school-aged children. *Br J Dermatol*, **137**, 241–5.

APPGS. All Party Parliamentary Group on Skin (1997). An investigation into the adequacy of service provision and treatments for patients with skin diseases in the UK. London: House of Commons.

Arshad, S.H., Matthews, S., Gant, C. & Hide, D. (1992). Effect of allergen avoidance on development of allergic disorders in infancy. *Lancet*, **339**, 1493–7.

Bellou, A., Kanny, G., Gremont, S. & Moneret-Vautrin, D.A. (1997). Transfer of atopy following bone marrow transplantation. *Ann Allergy, Asthma Immunol*, **78**, 513–6.

Boguniewicz, M. & Leung, D.Y.M. (1998). Atopic dermatitis. In: Middleton, E., Reed, C.E. & Ellis, E.F. (eds.) *Allergy; Principles and Practice*, 5th edn., pp. 1123–4. New York: Mosby.

Buckley, C.C., Ivison, C., Poulter, L.W. & Rustin, H.A. (1992). FcεR11/CD23 receptor. Distribution in patch test reactions to aeroallergens in atopic dermatitis. *J Invest Dermatol*, **99**, 184–8.

Burton, J.L. (1981). The logic of dermatological diagnosis. *Clin Exp Dermatol*, **6**, 1–21.

Charman, C., Venn, A.J. & Williams, H.C. (1999). Measurement of body surface area involvement in atopic eczema: an impossible task? *Br J Dermatol*, **140**, 109–11.

Charman, C., Williams, H.C. & Kinnear, W. (1998). Recognition of dermatological conditions by junior doctors on general medical wards. *J R Coll Phys*, **32**, 146–8.

Cooper, K.D. (1994). Atopic dermatitis: recent trends in pathogenesis and therapy. *J Invest Dermatol*, **102**, 128–37.

Cox, H.E., Moffatt, M.M., Faux, J. et al. (1998). Association of atopic dermatitis to the beta subunit of the high affinity immunoglobulin E receptor. *Br J Dermatol*, **138**, 182–7.

Dalton, S.J., Haeney, M.R., Patel, L. & David, T.J. (1998). Exacerbation of atopic dermatitis after bacillus Calmete-Guérin vaccination. *J R Soc Med*, **91**, 133–4.

David, T.J. (1991). Conventional allergy tests. *Arch Dis Childh*, **66**, 281.

de Jong, M.H., Scharp, V.T.M., de Groot, C.J. et al. (1997). Brief neonatal exposure to cow milk protein does not influence expression of atopy in the first two years of life (results of the 'BOKAAL-study'). *Proc Europ Soc Paediat Res*, **42**, 385 (abstract).

Diepgen, T.L. & Blettner, M. (1997). Genetic epidemiology of atopy. In: Grob, J.J. (ed.) *Epidemiology and Prevention of Skin Diseases*, pp. 231–6. Oxford: Blackwell Scientific.

Dowse, G.K., Turner, K.J., Stewart, G.A. et al. (1985). The association between *Dermatophagoides* mites and the increasing prevalence of asthma in village communities within Papua New Guinea highlands. *J Allergy Clin Immunol*, **75**, 75–83.

Edenharter, G., Bergmann, R.L., Bergmann, K.E., Wahn, V., Forster, J., Zepp, F. & Wahn, U. (1998). Cord blood-IgE as risk factor and predictor for atopic diseases. *Clin Exp Allergy*, **28**, 671–8.

Emerson, R.M., Williams, H.C., Allen, B.R., Mehta, R. & Finlay, A.Y. (1997). How much disability does atopic eczema cause compared with other common childhood health problems? *Br J Dermatol*, **137** (Suppl. 50), 19.

Emerson, R.M., Williams, H.C. & Allen, B.R. (1998a). What are the prescribing costs for atopic dermatitis in young children? *Br J Dermatol*, **139** (Suppl. 51), 21–2.

Emerson, R.M., Williams, H.C. & Allen, B.R. (1998b). Severity distribution of atopic dermatitis in the community and its relationship to secondary referral. *Br J Dermatol*, **139**, 73–6.

Emerson, R.M., Charman, C.R., Williams, H.C. & Allen, B.R. (1998). Modified Rajka and Langeland severity assessment (MRSA) for atopic dermatitis: a useful tool for epidemiological studies? *Br J Dermatol*, **139** (Suppl. 51), 65.

ETAC Study Group (1998). Allergic factors associated with the development of asthma and the influence of cetirizine in a double-blind, randomised, placebo-controlled trial: first results of ETAC®. *Pediat Allergy Immunol* **9**, 116–24.

European Task Force on Atopic Dermatitis (1993). Severity scoring of atopic dermatitis: the SCORAD Index. *Dermatology*, **186**, 23–31.

Evans, A. (ed.) (1993). Epilogue. In: *Causation and Disease*, pp. 229–30. London: Plenum Medical Book Company.

Fokkens, W.J., Bruijnzeel-Koomen, C.A.F.M., Vroom, Th. M. et al. (1990). The Langerhans cell: an underestimated cell in atopic disease. *Clin Exp Allergy*, **20**, 627–38.

Hanifin, J.M. & Lobitz, W.C. Jr. (1977). Newer concepts in atopic dermatitis. *Arch Dermatol*, **113**, 663–70.

Hanifin, J.M. & Rajka, G. (1980). Diagnostic features of atopic dermatitis. *Acta Dermatol Venereol (Stockh.)*, Suppl. 92, 44–7.

Hanifin, J.M., Chan, S.C., Cheng, J.B. et al. (1996). Type 4 phosphodiesterase inhibitors have clinical and *in vitro* anti-inflammatory effects in atopic dermatitis. *J Invest Dermatol*, **107**, 51–6.

Hanson, D.G., Vaz, N., Maia, L. et al. (1977). Inhibition of specific immune responses by feeding protein antigen. *Int Arch Allergy Immunol*, **55**, 1518–24.

Hay, R.J., Castanon, R.E., Hernandez, H.A. et al. (1994). Wastage of family income on skin disease in Mexico. *Br Med J*, **309**, 848.

Herd, R.M., Tidman, M.J., Prescott, R.J. & Hunter, J.A.A. (1996a). The cost of atopic eczema. *Br J Dermatol*, **135**, 20–3.

Herd, R.M., Tidman, M.J., Prescott, R.J. & Hunter, J.A.A. (1996b). Prevalence of atopic eczema in the community: the Lothian atopic dermatitis study. *Br J Dermatol*, **135**, 18–19.

Hide, D.W. (1995). Allergy prevention – an attainable objective? *Europ J Clin Nutr*, **49** (Suppl. 1), S71–76.

Hide, D.W., Matthews, S., Matthews, L. et al. (1994). Effect of allergen avoidance in infancy on allergic manifestations at age two years. *J Allergy Clin Immunol*, **93**, 842–6.

Holden, C.E. & Parish, W.E. (1998). Atopic dermatitis. In: Champion, R.H., Burton, J.L., Burns, D.A. & Breathnach, S.M. (eds.) *Textbook of Dermatology*, 6th edn., pp. 681–708. Oxford: Blackwell Scientific.

Hopkins, P.N. & Williams, R.R. (1981). A survey of 246 suggested coronary risk factors. *Atherosclerosis*, **40**, 1–52.

Kramer, M.S. (1988). Does breast feeding help protect against atopic disease? Biology, methodology, and a golden jubilee of controversy. *J Pediat*, **112**, 181–90.

Lapidus, C.S., Schwarz, D.F. & Honig, P.J. (1993). Atopic dermatitis in children: who cares? who pays? *J Am Acad Dermatol*, **28**, 699–703.

Lawson, V., Lewis-Jones, S., Finlay, A., Reid, P. & Owens, R.G. (1998). The family impact of childhood atopic dermatitis: the Dermatitis Family Impact questionnaire. *Br J Dermatol*, **138**, 107–13.

Lawton, S., Newham, S., Cox, M. et al. (1997). Managing atopic eczema; running a specialist clinic. *Professional Nurse*, **12**, 706–11.

Leung, D.Y.M. (1995). Atopic dermatitis: the skin as a window into the pathogenesis of chronic allergic diseases. *J Allergy Clin Immunol*, **96**, 302–18.

McKeown, T. (1975). The medical contribution. In: Black, N., Boswell, D., Gray, A., Murphy, S. & Popay, J. (eds.) *Health and Disease*, pp. 107–14. Milton Keynes: Open University Press.

McNally, N. (1998). The spatial epidemiology of atopic eczema. PhD Thesis. University of Nottingham.

McNally, N., Williams, H.C., Phillips, D.R. et al. (1998). Atopic eczema and water hardness. *Lancet*, **352**, 527–31.

McNally, N.J., Phillips, D.R. & Williams, H.C. (1998). The problem of atopic eczema: aetiological clues from the environment and lifestyles. *Soc Sci Med*, **46**, 729–41.

Middleton, C.E., Reed, E.F., Ellis, J. et al. (1998). *Allergy: Principles and Practice*, 5th edn. New York: Mosby.

Monk, B.E., Clement, M.I., Pembroke, A.C. & du Vivier, A. (1983). Lesson of the week: the incidental melanoma. *Br Med J*, **287**, 485–6.

Moqbel, R. & Pritchard, D.I. (1990). Parasites and allergy; evidence for a 'cause and effect' relationship. *Clin Exp Allergy*, **20**, 611–18.

Nakagawa, H., Etoh, T., Ishibashi, Y. et al. (1994). Tracolimus ointment for atopic dermatitis. *Lancet*, **344**, 883.

Norén, P. (1995). Habit reversal: a turning point in the treatment of atopic dermatitis. *Clin Exp Dermatol*, **20**, 2–5.

Norén, P. & Melin, L. (1989). The effect of combined topical steroids and habit reversal treatment in patients with atopic dermatitis. *Br J Dermatol*, **121**, 359–66.

Ogawa, H. & Yoshiike, T. (1993). A speculative view of atopic dermatitis: barrier dysfunction in pathogenesis. *J Dermatol Sci*, **5**, 197–204.

Peters, T.J. & Golding, J. (1987). The epidemiology of childhood eczema: II. Statistical analyses to identify independent early predictors. *Paediat Perinatal Epidemiol*, **1**, 80–94.

Phillips, A. & Davey-Smith, G. (1997). Confounding. In: Williams, H.C. & Strachan, D.P. (eds.) *The Challenge of Dermato-epidemiology*, pp. 75–85. Boca Raton: CRC Press.

Rajka, G. & Langeland, T. (1989). Grading the severity of atopic dermatitis. *Acta Dermatol Venereol (Stockh.)*, Suppl. 144, 13–14.

Rothe, M.J. & Grant-Kels, J.M. (1996). Diagnostic criteria for atopic dermatitis. *Lancet*, **348**, 769–70.

Ryan, T.J. (1994). Healthy skin for all. *Int J Dermatol*, **33**, 829–35.

Saarinen, U.M. & Kajosaari, M. (1995). Breastfeeding as prophylaxis against atopic disease: prospective follow-up study until 17 years old. *Lancet*, **346**, 1065–9.

Safavi, K. & Lawrence, R.C. (1997). Making comparisons: moving from rates to inference. In: Williams, H.C. & Strachan, D.P. (eds.) *The Challenge of Dermato-epidemiology*, pp. 37–47. Boca Raton: CRC Press.

Shaheen, S. (1997). Discovering the causes of atopy. *Br Med J*, **314**, 987–8.

Shaheen, S.O., Aaby, P., Hall, A.J. et al. (1996). Cell-mediated immunity after measles infection in Guinea-Bissau: historical cohort study. *Br Med J*, **313**, 969–74.

Stevens, A. & Gabbay, J. (1991). Needs assessment, needs assessment. *Hlth Trends*, **23**, 20–3.

Strachan, D.P. (1989). Hay fever, hygiene, and household size. *Br Med J*, **299**, 1259–60.

Su, J.C., Kemp, A.S., Varigos, G.A. & Nolan, T.M. (1997). Atopic eczema: its impact on the family and financial cost. *Arch Dis Childh*, **76**, 159–62.

Swale, V., Sasieni, P., MacGregor, A. et al. (1998). Heritability of common skin diseases using the twin model. A UK twin study. *Br J Dermatol*, **139** (Suppl. 51), 15–16.

Williams, H.C. (1995a). Atopic eczema – why we should look to the environment. *Br Med J*, **311**, 1241–2.

Williams, H.C. (1995b). Introduction to atopic dermatitis session. *Nouv Dermatol*, **14** (Suppl. 1), 50.

Williams, H.C. (1995c). Extended role for pharmacists in caring for skin conditions: a welcome development which needs further evaluation. *J Clin Pharm Therap*, **20**, 307–12.

Williams, H.C. (1996a). Relative and attributable risk and its relevance to prevention of contact dermatitis. In: Elsner, P., Lachapelle, J.M., Wahlberg, J. & Maibach, H.I. (eds.) *Prevention of Contact Dermatitis*, pp. 1–17. Basel: Karger.

Williams, H.C. (1996b). Diagnostic criteria for atopic dermatitis. *Lancet*, **348**, 1391–2.

Williams, H.C. (1997a). Atopic dermatitis. In: Williams, H.C. & Strachan, D.P. (eds.) *The Challenge of Dermato-epidemiology*, pp. 125–44. Boca Raton: CRC Press.

Williams, H.C. (1997b). Socioeconomic aspects of atopic dermatitis. In: Grob, J.J. (ed.) *Epidemiology and Prevention of Skin Diseases*, pp. 236–40. Oxford: Blackwell Scientic.

Williams, H.C. (1997c). Introduction: the need for epidemiology in dermatology. In: Williams, H.C. & Strachan, D.P. (eds.) *The Challenge of Dermato-epidemiology*, pp. 37–48. Boca Raton: CRC Press.

Williams, H.C. (1998a). Epidemiology of skin disease. In: Champion, R.H., Burton, J.L., Burns, D.A. & Breathnach, S. (eds.) *Textbook of Dermatology*, 6th edn., pp. 139–57. Oxford: Blackwell Scientific.

Williams, H.C. (1998b). Too soon to market: problem is acute in dermatology. *Br Med J*, **316**, 299.

Williams, H.C., Pottier, A. & Strachan, D. (1993). Are viral warts seen more commonly in children with eczema? *Arch Dermatol*, **129**, 717–21.

Williams, H.C., Burney, P.G.J., Pembroke, A.C. & Hay, R.J. (1994). The UK working party's diagnostic criteria for atopic dermatitis. III: Independent hospital validation. *Br J Dermatol*, **131**, 406–16.

Williams, H.C., Strachan, D.P. & Hay, R.J. (1994). Childhood eczema: disease of the advantaged? *Br Med J*, **308**, 1132–5.

Williams, H.C., Pembroke, A.C., Forsdyke, H. et al. (1995). London-born black Caribbean children are at increased risk of atopic dermatitis. *J Am Acad Dermatol*, **32**, 212–17.

Williams, H.C., Adetugbo, K., Po, A.L.P. et al. (1998). The Cochrane Skin Group. *Arch Dermatol*, **134**, 1620–26.

Williams, R. & Wright, J. (1998). Health needs assessment. *Br Med J*, **316**, 1379–82.

Williams, H.C., Robertson, C.F., Stewart, A.W. et al. (1999). Worldwide variations in the prevalence of symptoms of atopic eczema in the International Study of Asthma and Allergies in Childhood. *J Allergy Clin Immunol*, **103**, 125–38.

Additional information

Useful further reading

Rajka, G. (1989). *Essentials of Atopic Dermatitis*. Berlin: Springer-Verlag.

Ruzicka, T., Ring, J. & Przybilla, B. (1991). *Handbook of Atopic Eczema*. Berlin: Springer-Verlag.

Burr, M.L. (1993). *Epidemiology of Clinical Allergy*. Basel: Karger.

Williams, H.C. & Strachan, D.P. (1997). *The Challenge of Dermato-epidemiology*. Boca Raton: CRC Press.

Grob, J.J., Stern, R.S., MacKie, R.M. & Weinstock, W.A. (1997). *Epidemiology and Prevention of Skin Diseases*. Oxford: Blackwell Scientific.

The Cochrane Library (CD-ROM updated each quarter). Oxford: Update Software Ltd.

Useful addresses and web sites

Dermato-epidemiology organizations

IDEA – the International Dermato-Epidemiology Association.
Contact: Dr. Carolyn Charman, Honorary Secretary, Dermato-Epidemiology Research Unit, Queen's Medical Centre, Nottingham NG7 2UH.
Fax: +44 (0)115 970 9003,
e-mail: carolyn.charman@nottingham.ac.uk

EDEN – the European Dermato-epidemiology Network
Contact: Professor Luigi Naldi, Clinica Dermatologica, Ospedali Riuniti di Bergamo, Largo Barozzi 1, 24100 Bergamo. Fax: +39 35 253070

BEES – the British Epidermo-epidemiology Society
Contact: Professor Hywel Williams, Dermato-Epidemiology Research Unit, Queen's Medical Centre, Nottingham NG7 2UH. Fax: +44 (0)115 970 9003

The Cochrane Skin Group
Contact: Dr Tina Leonard, Co-ordinator, Dermato-Epidemiology Research Unit, Queen's Medical Centre, Nottingham NG7 2UH.
Fax: +44 (0)115 970 9003,
e-mail: tina.leonard@nottingham.ac.uk
Web site: http://www.nottingham.ac.uk/~muzd/

The International Study of Asthma and Allergies in Childhood.
Web site: http://isaac.auckland.ac.nz

SCORAD.
Web site: http://scorad. sante.univ-nantes.fr/

Patient organizations

The National Eczema Society,
163 Eversholt Street,
London NW1 1BU
Fax: +44 (0)171–388 5882

Index